Y.-W. Bahk   E. E. Kim   T. Isawa

Nuclear Imaging of the Chest

Springer-Verlag Berlin Heidelberg GmbH

Y.-W. Bahk   E.E. Kim   T. Isawa

Nuclear Imaging of the Chest

With Contributions by

Y.-W. Bahk, H.-S. Bom, K. Chiyotani, S.-K. Chung,
K. Honma, T. Imai, T. Isawa, C. K. Kim, E. E. Kim,
D.-S. Lee, J. Lee, M.-C. Lee, A. M. Mahmud,
N. Narita, H. Shida, T. Teshima, D. F. Worsley

With 217 Figures, 36 in Color, and 25 Tables

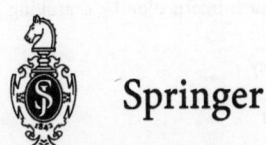

Springer

Yong-Whee Bahk, M.D., Ph.D., F.K.A.S.T.
Professor Emeritus (CUMC)
Senior Consultant, Department of Radiology
Samsung Cheil General Hospital
1–23, Mukjong-dong, Jung-gu
Seoul 100-380, Korea

E. Edmund Kim, M.D.
Professor of Radiology and Medicine
Chief, Experimental Nuclear Medicine
University of Texas, MD Anderson Cancer Center
1515 Holcombe Boulevard
77030 Houston, TX 77030, USA

Toyoharu Isawa, M.D., Ph.D.
Director of Yokohama Higashi National Hospital
215 Iwai-cho, Hodogaya-ku
Yokohama 240, Japan

ISBN 978-3-642-80389-5   ISBN 978-3-642-80387-1 (eBook)
DOI 10.1007/978-3-642-80387-1

Library of Congress Cataloging-in-Publication Data. Bahk, Yong-Whee, Nuclear imaging of the chest / Y. W. Bahk, E. E. Kim, T. Isawa. p. cm.
(alk. paper). 1. Chest – Radionuclide imaging. I. Kim, E. Edmund. II. Isawa, Toyoharu. III. Title. [DNLM: 1. Thoracic Radiography. 2. Thoracic Diseases – diagnosis. 3. Heart Diseases – radionuclide imaging. 4. Lung Diseases – radionuclide imaging.]
RC941.P25 1998 617.5′407575–dc21 DNLM/DLC for Library of Congress 97-29699

Production: ProEdit GmbH, 69126 Heidelberg, Germany
Cover design: Anna Deus, Heidelberg, Germany
Typesetting: K+V Fotosatz, 64743 Beerfelden, Germany

*This book is dedicated
to our wives Yeun-Soo (Cho) Bahk,
Bo Kim, and Masako Isawa,
and children*

Foreword

The book is the collaborative effort of Korean and Japanese authors with international contributors, who describe how nuclear medicine imaging in patients with heart, lung, mediastinal and chest wall disease can help to decrease the amount of unnecessary or inappropriate care, help prevent future complications of disease by making early diagnosis possible, help in the effective selection of procedures, and help to assure that all studies are of high quality and interpreted with maximum accuracy. Used properly by physicians who understand the basic principles covered by these authors, nuclear imaging not only improves patient care, but saves money. Knowledge of the information covered in this book can help insure that patients get the right procedure and the right care in the right setting and in the right amount.

Differential diagnosis of diseases of the chest, necessary for the effective care of patients with disease of the heart, lungs, mediastinum or chest wall, remains a difficult task, even when the responsible physician has available the fruits of the enormous scientific and technical advances that have been made since the first lung perfusion scan was introduced in 1963. Measurement and imaging of regional lung perfusion and then shortly thereafter regional ventilation by means of radioactive tracers moved nuclear medicine from its principal concern with thyroid and hematological diseases into the main stream of medical practice.

Since 1963, nuclear imaging of the chest has been jointed by the invention of exquisite, anatomically oriented procedures, computed tomography, and magnetic resonance imaging. The integration of these three diagnostic modalities is the focus and strength of this book, written primarily from a radiologist's viewpoint. For example, the effective use of nuclear imaging in the diagnosis of common diseases such as pulmonary embolism and chronic obstructive pulmonary disease requires skill, knowledge, and experience, all of which are reflected by the authors of this book.

Anatomy and histopathology remain the principal basis for making a diagnosis, but these two approaches suffer from being descriptive, subjective, not quantifiable, and, in the case of biopsies, based on the study of dead tissue. The era of histopathology as the dominant concept in medical practice is coming to an end, being supplemented by a molecular as well as a cellular approach to disease, the approach taken by nuclear imaging.

The authors of this unique multimodality book headed by Professor Yong-Whee Bahk, well known radiology-oriented nuclear physician, describe how the present approach to chest disease goes beyond anatomy into the domains of physiology and in vivo biochemistry. For example, in patients with lung nodules a single biopsy will at times not reveal the true nature of the disease, such as the presence and extent of malignancy. Far greater accuracy in staging of disease and in the planning of treatment is possible through nuclear medicine procedures. Similarly, Tc-99m aerosol lung imaging can delineate subtle functional and morphologic alterations in airways and airspaces in many bronchopulmonary diseases such as smoker's lung, chronic bronchitis, and bronchial asthma the detection of which has not been satisfactory so far by other imaging modalities.

Nuclear medicine does not just provide new tests for old diseases, but new ways of defining and detecting disease. Chemical changes can almost always be detected before clinical signs of disease making it possible to be more specific in characterization of the disease.

The cyclotron has more recently returned to the development of radiotracers for nuclear imaging based on the production of carbon-11 and fluorine-18, the workhorses of positron emission tomography (PET). The use of PET is included in this book, together with the use of more readily available tracers such as gallium-67 citrate.

The increasing role of primary physicians and the expected decrease in the number of specialists make a textbook, such as this, that covers one third of the body, more important than ever. Primary physicians have to become increasingly familiar with the broad spectrum of advances that have been made in scientific medicine, including the safe and effective use of radioactive tracers, the basis of nuclear imaging. Specialists and students will be able to learn the basic principles upon which the clinical applications are based. In the chapters of clinical applications, the authors describe how nuclear imaging can be used to answer the four questions that characterize the practice of medicine: What is wrong? What is going to happen? How did it happen? What can be done about it?

This book will serve as a textbook for those physicians who specialize in diseases of the chest, as well as for medical students and others who wish to learn how nuclear imaging can be integrated with radiographic imaging to provide better care of patients. The book will be useful to clinicians, radiologists, nuclear medicine specialists and medical students.

Henry N. Wagner
Baltimore, August 1997

Preface

The chest, or thorax, is a portion of the body that contains several seemingly different but in fact closely interrelated organ systems, carrying out in particular such complex vital functions as respiration and blood circulation. In addition to the cardiovascular and respiratory systems, the thorax is comprised anatomically of the mediastinum with the esophagus, thymus, lymphatics, and nerves, the bony thoracic cage and spine with various bones and articulations, and the chest wall with the breasts and lymphatics.

Many new and highly refined modalities are now at our disposal for the diagnosis of thoracic diseases. These include plain and contrast radiography, angiocardiography, coronary angiography, conventional X-ray tomography, computed X-ray tomography, magnetic resonance imaging, ultrasonography, and nuclear imaging. Each of these modalities has its own merits and drawbacks. For example, radiography has the highest spatial resolution of all – 50–80 line pair/mm resolution. This is a virtually ideal means for demonstrating the microstructures of airways and interstitia of the lung and the large and small vessels of the heart and lung. On the other hand, however, it is less useful than the ventilation-perfusion scan, ^{99m}Tc-DTPA and -phytate aerosol pulmonary imaging, and cine-scintigraphy for dynamic functional assessment of pulmonary gas exchange, bronchial epithelial permeability, and bronchial ciliary motion. It is less suited for both biochemical and metabolic profile studies of the myocardium than nuclear cardiac single-photon emission computed tomography. As is well known, nuclear blood-pool scan and myocardial imaging provide unique information obtainable by no other means about the cardiac ejection and myocardial viability. Tumor scans using ^{67}Ga, ^{201}Tl, and ^{99m}Tc-sestamibi are an important development in thoracic oncology, raising the specificity and sensitivity of the diagnosis of lung and breast cancers to a level that is unattainable by other imaging modalities. ^{99m}Tc-labeled methylene disphosphonate or oxidronate bone imaging with the aid of pinhole magnification has greatly enhanced the diagnosis of many specific thoracic bone diseases and improved the diagnosis of obscure, occult, and subtle bone diseases in the thorax.

Since the early 1960s nuclear imaging sciences have grown steadily, and made great strides particularly during the past decade. Using refined gamma-camera systems with positron emission tomography and single-photon emission computed tomography, new nuclear-medicine techniques, and specific radiopharmaceuticals, it is now possible to image and assess a number of hitherto undiagnosable diseases of the brain, heart, lung, liver, kidney, skeleton, digestive system, endocrine glands, and other systems.

However, with the unavoidable subspecialization of medicine nuclear imaging diagnosis has also become diverse for some specific organs and diseases, without integrating closely interrelated organs, functions, or diseases into an unity. The thorax is no exception to this, being a typical model of complex yet well-concerted body parts. In fact, the individual nuclear imagings of the heart, lung, blood vessels, breast, bony cage, and other thoracic organs and tissues as well as tumor and inflammation are dealt with as if they were independent and unrelated one another. Naturally, very little has been written in book form about the diagnosis and monitoring of a large variety of thoracic diseases. We have long felt that such a book is very needed for the promotion of holistic grasping, understanding, and studying the seemingly heterogeneous yet closely interrelated organs and systems in the chest.

In accordance with this need, therefore, the principal aims of this book are the objective selection, collective formulation, and systematic presentation of information regarding various nuclear scan diagnoses of as many thoracic diseases of both general and specific types as possible. Where necessary and feasible, nuclear images, aerosol ventilation scans, and bone scintigraphy in particular are correlated with and validated against other imaging modalities such as radiography, computed tomography, and magnetic resonance imaging.

Part I of this volume deals with the physical bases of imaging in the thorax: on the one hand the anatomy and physiology of the lung and, on the other, scintigraphic techniques and radiopharmaceuticals. Part II, on clinical applications of these techniques, considers the diagnosis of diseases of the heart and vessels, the lungs, the mediastinum with the esophagus and lymphatics, and the bony thorax as well as the breast and axilla.

It has indeed been a pleasant surprise that all of the contributors invited so gladly agreed to participate in this publication and so faithfully observed the general guidelines and time constraints, enabling us to complete the project in a relatively short time span of just over one year. Each is known for research in particular facets of the topics presented here. They all deserve our heartiest respect and warm salute. We extend many thanks to our technical, photographic, and secretarial colleagues for their superb work. We also gratefully acknowledge the excellent cooperation and support of our friends at Springer-Verlag in Heidelberg, Dr. Ute Heilmann in particular. Without their expertise, knowledge, and skill the publication of this textbook would not have been possible. Finally, we are all very thankful to our wives and children for their affectionate encouragement and untiring assistance.

It is humbly hoped that this textbook will meet the perceived needs of general practitioners and thoracic physicians and surgeons as well as nuclear physicians and radiologists in the diagnosis, management, and research of a variety of thoracic diseases in an integrated and interrelated manner.

August 1997   Y.-W. Bahk, Seoul
                                               E. E. Kim, Houston
                                               T. Isawa, Yokohama

Contents

Clinical Applications

7 Pneumoconiosis

H. Shida, K. Chiyotani, and K. Honma

8 Lung Cancer

E.E. Kim

H.S. Bom and J. Lee

List of Contributors

Yong-Whee Bahk, M.D., Ph.D., F.K.A.S.T.
Professor Emeritus (CUMC)
Senior Consultant, Department of Radiology
Samsung Cheil Hospital
Seoul, Korea

Hee-Seung Bom, M.D.
Associate Professor of Medicine
Director, Department of Nuclear Medicine
Chonnam University Hospital
Kwangju, Korea

Keizo Chiyotani, M.D.
Director
Rosai Hospital for Silicosis
Tochigi, Japan

Soo-Kyo Chung, M.D.
Professor of Radiology
Director, Department of Nuclear Medicine
Catholic University Medical College
Seoul, Korea

Koichi Honma, M.D.
Associate Professor
Department of Pathology
Dokkyo University Faculty of Medicine
Tochigi, Japan

TERUHIKO IMAI, M.D.
Assistant Professor of Radiology
Department of Oncoradiology
Nara Medical University
Kashihara, Japan

TOYOHARU ISAWA, M.D., Ph.D.
Director, Yokohama Higashi National Hospital
Yokohama, Japan

CHUN KI KIM, M.D.
Associate Professor of Radiology
Associate Director, Department of Nuclear Medicine
Mount Sinai School of Medicine, Mount Sinai Hospital
New York, N.Y., USA

E. EDMUND KIM, M.D.
Professor of Radiology and Medicine
Chief, Experimental Nuclear Medicine
University of Texas, MD Anderson Cancer Center
Houston, Texas, USA

DONG-SOO LEE, M.D.
Associate Professor of Nuclear Medicine
Seoul National University Hospital
Seoul, Korea

JAETAE LEE, M.D.
Associate Professor of Nuclear Medicine
Kyungbuk University Hospital
Taegu, Korea

MYONG-CHUL LEE, M.D.
Professor of Nuclear Medicine
Seoul National University Hospital
Seoul, Korea

A. M. MAHMUD, M.B.B.S., Ph.D.
Research Fellow in Respiratory Medicine
Institute for Development, Aging and Cancer
Tohoku University
Sendai, Japan

NOBUHIRO NARITA, M.D.
Professor and Chairman
Second Department of Medicine
Nara Medical University
Kashihara, Japan

HISAO SHIDA, M.D.
Senior Consultant in Diagnostic Radiology
Rosai Hospital for Silicosis
Professor of Radiological Sciences
International University of Health and Welfare
Tochigi, Japan

TAKEO TESHIMA, M.D.
Chief, Department of Medicine
Sendai Kohsei Hospital
Sendai, Japan

D. F. WORSLEY, M.D.
Assistant Professor of Radiology
University of British Columbia
Division of Nuclear Medicine, Department of Radiology
Vancouver Hospital and Health Sciences Center
Vancouver, BC, Canada

Basics

1 Introduction

Y.-W. BAHK

A number of nuclear imaging techniques have been developed over the past four decades to detect and assess diseases of the chest or thorax, the region controlling the vital functions of respiration, circulation, and body temperature. These techniques use various radiopharmaceuticals and highly refined gamma camera systems, including multihead cameras, single photon emission computed tomography (SPECT) and positron emission tomography (PET). The thorax is very complex both anatomically and functionally; in addition to the heart, great vessels, and lungs, it includes the mediastinum with the lymphatics, thymus, nervous tissue, esophagus, bony cage with the sternum and thoracic vertebrae, and external chest wall, and lymphatics. Each of these organs and structures represents an important object of nuclear thoracic imaging, and the range of techniques available for them varies widely and some are specific and unique.

Of the various thoracic diseases, pulmonary embolism (PE) has received most attention in thoracic nuclear imaging, for three reasons: it manifests in many different clinical contexts, it is a leading cause of morbidity and mortality, and it can be assessed efficiently and noninvasively by perfusion and inhalation scans. To be accurate, PE is not a disease per se but a clinical condition that can reflect a complication of venous thrombosis, right cardiac clots, bone fractures with fat emboli, pregnancy, or malignant tumors. In about 95% of PE cases emboli arise from deep venous thrombosis in the lower extremities [25].

The means presently available for clinical diagnosis of PE are generally not reliable. However, a normal pulmonary perfusion scan does rule out the presence of PE with reasonable certainty, although abnormal findings on perfusion scan require specificity [11]. Retrospective and prospective correlation studies of PE with contrast pulmonary angiography confirm the diagnostic efficacy of ventilation-perfusion (V-Q), which shows increasing specificity and a high probability of approximately 90% predictive value; the predictive value of even a low-probability scan approaches 90% [25]. For this reason probably the most frequent indication for contrast pulmonary angiography is a ventilation-perfusion scan of intermediate probability.

Because emphasis on thromboembolism as a systemic disease is again becoming a part of clinical routine, the integrated long-leg nuclear venogram is considered a reasonable approach. Importantly, lung perfusion SPECT enables the detection of a mismatch zone in the middle of a lung abnormality which a planar scan portrays as a "uniformly matched lesion." Properly performed and interpreted, contrast pulmonary angiography remains the most reliable test of PE; however, spiral computed tomography (CT) and magnetic resonance imaging (MRI) are gradually emerging as a potent noninvasive adjuncts in the diagnosis of PE in the segmental branches [9]. The direct imaging of thrombi using radiolabeled thrombolytic agents or antibodies to the components of blood clotting process now seems more promising than ever.

Unlike the perfusion scan, the ventilation scan has not yet become uniformly established, which accounts for the variability in interpretative criteria [24]. Ventilation scan using radioaerosols has not been fully explored, resulting in inadequate recognition of many valuable signs, including particularly central airways deposition, which has been regarded as undesirable. Research on this subject seldom pays sufficient attention to the diagnostic significance of various airway deposition phenomena, although these are indeed valuable and often unique signs of bronchial diseases, as discussed in this textbook. Normal airways do not of course accumulate visible microaerosols, and any visible airway deposition therefore indicates that the airways are abnormal [3]. For instance, arboriform airway deposition represents either chronic bronchitis or smoker's lung, the broomstick sign suggests chronic bronchitis [3], and segmental bronchial deposition is the pathognomonic sign of bronchial obstruction [5]. Occupational diseases of the lung such as pneumoconiosis are other interesting objects of ventilation and perfusion scans and of ^{67}Ga scans. A comprehensive multimodality correlation study has recently been carried out using pulmonary nuclear imaging, radiography, CT, and autopsy specimens in mixed dust pneumoconiosis, silicosis, and its related diseases [21].

Ventilation and perfusion scans are valuable tools for quantitative assessment of regional pulmonary gas exchange. In addition to gas exchange, the lung has other important functions including mucociliary clearance, pulmonary epithelial permeability, and metabolic function. Mucociliary clearance is the first-line defense in the respiratory system. It is well known that mucus overlying the airway surface is propelled orad by the coordinated beating of the cilia in the bronchial epithelium. Aerosol imaging is the only tool for noninvasively assessing the mucociliary clearance in vivo with reasonable accuracy [14], and cine-scintigraphy using aerosol has shown mucus transport to occur in the retrograde and contralateral directions in chronic obstructive pulmonary disease [15]. Most recently, the ^{99m}Tc-labeled human serum albumin aerosol cine-scintigraphy has been used in the quantitative evaluation of bolus movement in diffuse panbronchiolitis before and after erythromycin treatment [12].

^{99m}Tc-labeled diethylene triamine pentaacetic acid (DTPA) aerosols are known to deposit within the lung periphery and to be cleared across the alveolar-capillary membranes [20], and a test could conceivably be developed using a gamma camera system or a simple probe to assess regional changes in alveolar-capillary membrane permeability. In other words, the ^{99m}Tc-DTPA aerosol scan may be used to evaluate diseases associated with disruption of the pulmonary epithelium, such as exposure to toxic inhalants, adult respiratory distress syndrome, and hyaline membrane disease. An association has been suggested between epithelial damage in such disorders and increased DTPA clearance, although the exact mechanism is yet unknown. Quantitative evaluation of clearance patterns would permit early diagnosis of epithelial damages or diseases, and help to distinguish between the alveolar and cardiogenic types of edema. In normal subjects, ^{99m}Tc-DTPA is cleared from the lung with a half-life of approximately 80 min, using submicronic ^{99m}Tc-DTPA aerosols. A possible limitation to this test is that DPTA clearance increases as the alveolar surface area for gas exchange increases. Other likely limiting factors include cigarette smoking, which may induce increased DTPA clearance, and the instability of DTPA during nebulization process and in vivo. Therefore a strict quality control scheme such as chromatography of ^{99m}Tc-DTPA before and after nebulization is a prerequisite for assured results.

Nuclear cardiac imaging is another important development in nuclear medicine and cardiology, and its unique value is widely recognized [4]. Myocardial perfusion SPECT has become a useful noninvasive reference test for coronary arterial disease, replacing angiography. Indeed, normal results on myocardial SPECT assure a long and trouble-free life, while a persistent perfusion defect indicates coronary stenosis. Myocardial SPECT is an excellent means for evaluating myocardial function following any invasive or noninvasive treatment. On the other hand, questions regarding myocardial viability from its definition to the endpoints of treatment must still be answered [16]. Cellular metabolism, membrane integrity, inotropic reserve, and cellular integrity of the myocardium are four major concerns of cardiology. Dobutamine-gated myocardial SPECT with ^{99m}Tc-labeled methoxyisobutylisonitrile or ^{201}Tl can be used to assess membrane integrity and inotropic reserve, and gated PET to assess cellular metabolism and inotropic reserve. It is thought that these tests will eventually lead to understanding the pathophysiological implications of the stunning and hibernation of the myocardium. The ejection fraction, a reliable predictor of long-term outcome of cardiac patients, can readily be calculated using myocardial-gated SPECT, with an excellent reproducibility [10]. [^{18}F]Fluoro-2-deoxyglucose (FDG), PET, and SPECT are well suited for evaluating myocardial glucose metabolism. A mismatched uptake of [^{18}F]FDG in hypoperfused segments entails a poor prognosis, and both PET and SPECT have been used to screen potential recipients of heart transplants to estimate benefit of bypass surgery.

The continued refinement of gamma camera systems and the advent of tumor-specific radiopharmaceuticals have led to a reorientation in the direction of scan techniques for the viability study of thoracic tumors. SPECT using ^{67}Ga-citrate has recently been used to assess the therapeutic effect of lymphoma and lung cancers [8]. Performed along with CT or MRI, ^{67}Ga imaging can provide valuable information about hilar and mediastinal cancer. ^{99m}Tc-methoxyisobutylisonitrile and ^{201}Tl have emerged as useful viability test agents in thoracic tumors, showing relatively high sensitivity and specificity in detecting, for example, breast cancer. PET and SPECT with [^{18}F]FDG have been shown to be useful in differentiating residual or recurrent tumor from posttreatment changes [13].

The lung, traditionally viewed as the body's respiratory organ, is receiving increasing attention as a metabolic organ. For example, the lung is known to modulate arterial blood composition by several mechanisms: removing active substances from or releasing substances into the plasma, temporarily withholding substances from circulation, and activating or inactivating substances that pass through the lungs. Most procedures thus far proposed for noninvasively assessing pulmonary metabolic functions estimate the plasma clearance that is transported by pulmonary endothelial cells.

The mediastinum contains, among other things, the lymphatics and esophagus, which are known, respectively, as the seat of primary and metastatic cancers and achalasia with gastric regurgitation and Barrett's ulceration, which causes distressing symptoms. As discussed above, ^{67}Ga imaging provides valuable information about mediastinal and hilar malignancies, ^{99m}Tc-MIBI and ^{201}Tl are useful agents in testing tumor viability, and [^{18}F]FDG PET and SPECT have been shown effective in discriminating residual and recurrent tumor. Nuclear imaging is a potent diagnostic tool in achalasia, which is characterized by abolished esophageal peristalsis and the failure of the lower esophageal sphincter to relax after swallowing. The radionuclide test for esophageal emptying provides reliable information concerning the severity of disease and can thus be used for objective monitoring of the disease course. ^{99m}Tc-pertechnetate esophageal scintigraphy, especially with an acidified transport medium, is a simple yet sensitive test of gastroesophageal reflux and ectopic gastric epithelium in patients with Barrett's esophagus [17].

Skeletal nuclear imaging is an important diagnostic test for diseases of the bony thoracic cage. Until recently, most bone scans were performed for the clinical staging of lung or breast cancer by detecting metastasis either at an initial or follow-up visit [7]. However, this is being used increasingly in clinical studies of many bony thoracic cage diseases, as this textbook describes. Bone scan is extremely sensitive, but relatively low in specificity; this is due to the fact that scan agents are nonspecific, and the spatial and contrast resolution of planar scans and SPECT are not high enough. Fortunately, the pinhole magnification technique [1] and pinhole SPECT [2] have been shown to remarkably enhance both the sensitivity and specificity of bone scan. Pinhole bone scintigraphy with ^{99m}Tc-methylene disphosphonate or oxidronate help in reaching a specific diagnosis in many thoracic bone diseases such as condensing osteitis and Friedrich's disease of the clavicle, Paget's disease [1] and Tietze's disease [26]. On the other hand, Piccolo [19] has noted an interesting extraskeletal ^{99m}Tc-MDP uptake to occur in lung and breast cancers. He ascribed the phenomenon to the increased vascularization in these tumors.

Breast cancer continues to be the most aggressive and diagnostically challenging disease in women and thus one of the major areas of recent advances in nuclear imaging diagnosis. The two popular radiopharmaceuticals currently used for nuclear imaging of the breast are ^{99m}Tc-sestamibi and ^{201}Tl chloride. Of these, ^{99m}Tc-sestamibi scintimammography has a high accuracy of 94.4% and 84.2% in detecting, respectively, primary breast cancer and the axillary lymphnode metastasis [22]. Nuclear mammography has also been shown to significantly improve the specificity of conventional mammography for detecting breast cancer [18]. It is thus more likely than ever that ^{99m}Tc-sestamibi scintimammography will become an essential element in the repertoire of thoracic nuclear imaging. Intramammary lymphoscintigraphy with ^{99m}Tc-antimony sulfide colloid (^{99m}Tc-Sb$_2$S$_3$) has been used successfully to determine lymphatic drainage patterns in breast cancers [23], and ^{201}Tl breast scan has also been reported to be highly accurate in detecting primary breast cancer [6].

References

1. Bahk YW (1994) Combined scintigraphic and radiographic diagnosis of bone and joint diseases. Springer, Berlin Heidelberg New York
2. Bahk YW (1996) Pinhole scan versus SPECT in the diagnosis of bone and joint diseases: an improved scan delineation of structure and physiochemical profile. In: Torizuka K (ed) The syllabus of educational lecture of the 6th Asia and Oceania congress of nuclear medicine and biology. Kyoto, pp 1–8
3. Bahk YW, Chung SK (1994) Radioaerosol lung scanning in chronic obstructive pulmonary disease (COPD) and related disorders. In: Bahk YW, Isawa T (eds) Radioaerosol imaging of the lung. International Atomic Energy Agency, Vienna, pp 88–135
4. Berman DS, Kiat H, Friedman ID et al (1995) Clinical applications of exercise muscular cardiology studies in the era of healthcare reform. Am J Cardiol 75:3D–13D
5. Chung SK, Kim HH, Bahk YW (1997) Prestenotic bronchial radioaerosol deposition: a new lung scan sign of bronchial obstruction. J Nucl Med 38:23–26
6. Cimitan M, Volpe R, Candiani E et al (1995) The use of thallium-201 in the preoperative detection of breast cancer: an adjunct to mammography and ultrasonography. Eur J Nucl Med 22:1110–1117
7. Coleman RE, Rubens RD, Fogelman I (1988) Reappraisal of the baseline bone scan in breast cancer. J Nucl Med 29:1045–1049
8. Front D, Israel O (1995) The role of Ga-67 scintigraphy in evaluating the results of therapy of lymphoma patients. Semin Nucl Med 25:60–71
9. Gefter WB, Hatabu H, Holland GA et al (1995) Pulmonary thromboembolism: recent development in diagnosis with CT and MR imaging. Radiology 197:561–574
10. Germano G, Kiat H, Karvanogh PB et al (1995) Automatic quantification of ejection fraction from gated myocardial perfusion SPECT. J Nucl Med 36:2138–2147
11. Hull RD, Feldstein W, Stein PD, Pineo GF (1996) Cost-effectiveness of pulmonary embolism diagnosis. Arch Intern Med 156:68–72
12. Imai T, Sasaki Y, Ohishi H et al (1995) Clinical aerosol inhalation of cine-scintigraphy to evaluate mucociliary transport system in diffuse panbronchiolitis. J Nucl Med 36:1355–1362
13. Inoue T, Kim EE, Komaki K et al (1995) Detecting recurrent or residual lung cancer with FDG-PET. J Nucl Med 36:788–793
14. Isawa T, Teshima T, Hirano T et al (1984) Mucociliary clearance mechanism in smoking and nonsmoking normal subjects. J Nucl Med 25:352–359
15. Isawa T, Teshima T, Hirano T et al (1984) Lung clearance mechanisms of obstructive airways disease. J Nucl Med 25:447–454
16. Iskandrian AS (1996) Myocardial viability: unresolved issues. J Nucl Med 37:794–797
17. Kaul B, Petersen H, Grette K et al (1985) Scintigraphy, pH measurement and radiography in the evaluation of gastroesophageal reflux. Scan J Gastroenterol 20:289–294

18. Khalkhali I, Cutrone J, Mena I et al (1995) Technetium-99m-sestamibi scintimam-mography of breast lesions: clinical and pathological follow-up. J Nucl Med 36:1784–1789
19. Piccolo S, Lastoria S, Mainolfi C et al (1995) Tc-99m methylene diphosphonate scintimammography to image primary breast cancer. J Nucl Med 36:718–724
20. Rinderknecht J, Shapiro L, Krauthammer M et al (1980) Accelerated clearance of small solutes from the lungs in interstitial lung disease. Am Rev Respir Dis 121:105–117
21. Shida H, Chiyotani K, Honma K et al (1996) Radiologic and pathologic character-istics of mixed dust pneumoconiosis. Radiographics 16:483–498
22. Taillefer R, Robidoux A, Lambert R et al (1995) Technetium-99m-sestamibi prone scintimammography to detect primary breast cancer and axillary lymph node in-volvement. J Nucl Med 36:1758–1765
23. Uren RF, Howman-Giles RB, Thompson JF et al (1995) Mammary lymphoscinti-graphy in breast cancer. J Nucl Med 36:1775–1780
24. Worsley DF, Alavi A (1995) Comprehensive analysis of the results of the PIOPED diagnosis. J Nucl Med 36:2380–2387
25. Worsley DF, Palevsky HI, Alavi A (1994) Clinical characteristics of patients with pulmonary embolism and low or very low probability lung scan interpretations. Arch Intern Med 154:2737–2741
26. Yang WJ, Bahk YW, Chung SK et al (1994) Pinhole skeletal scintigraphic manifes-tations of Tietze's disease. Eur J Nucl Med 21:947–952

2 Anatomy and Physiology

T. Isawa

The lung is responsible for both respiratory and nonrespiratory functions. The former consists of gas exchange and includes ventilation, perfusion, and diffusion (Fig. 2.1), while the latter involves mucociliary clearance, pulmonary epithelial permeability, lung uptake of various substances, metabolism, etc. (Fig. 2.2). This chapter describes respiratory lung function briefly from the standpoints of ventilation, blood flow or perfusion, and ventilation-perfusion relationships, and nonrespiratory lung function from the standpoints of pulmonary epithelial permeability, and lung uptake of various substances. Mucociliary clearance, another very important nonrespiratory lung function is described in Chap. 10.

Respiratory Lung Function

Ventilation

Airways

Function

The airways are passages for air ventilation for gas exchange, which takes place in the terminal respiratory units. The major function of ventilation is arterialization of the mixed venous blood. A volume of oxygen equal to that used by the body must be supplied each minute to the alveoli and pulmonary capillary beds by ventilation, and a volume of carbon dioxide nearly equal to that of the entire lung must be removed by ventilation.

Anatomic Dead Space

The extrapulmonary airways in the thorax are the trachea, carina, and proximal part of the main bronchi. Following the dichotomous (less frequently, trichotomous) branching of the intrapulmonary airways, the airways become narrower, shorter, and numerous as they penetrate more deeply into the lung until they become terminal bronchioles. Characteristically, the airways above

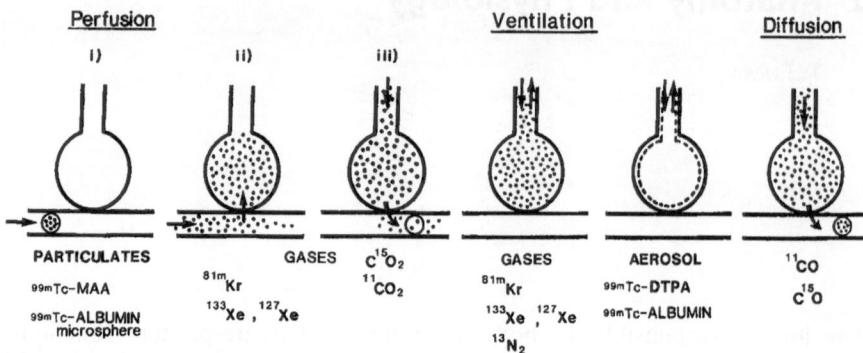

Fig. 2.1. Respiratory lung function. Perfusion can be studied with particulates such as ^{99m}Tc-MAA or with radioactive gases such as dissolved ^{133}Xe, or positron emitters. Ventilation with radioactive gases or radioaerosols such as ^{99m}Tc-labeled human serum albumin aerosol. Diffusion by carbon monoxide labeled with positron emitters

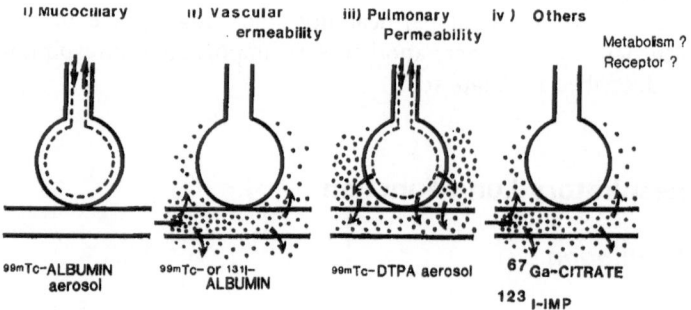

Fig. 2.2. Nonrespiratory lung function. Mucociliary clearance by inhaled radioaerosol such as ^{99m}Tc-labeled human serum albumin aerosol, vascular endothelial permeability by injecting ^{99m}Tc-labeled albumin, pulmonary epithelial permeability by ^{99m}Tc-DTPA aerosol, and other nonrespiratory lung functions by taking up injected or inhaled substances such as [^{123}I]IMP

the terminal bronchioles are ciliated and reinforced by the cartilage. According to Weibel, branching is repeated an average of 16 times before the airway reaches the terminal bronchiole [1]. The airways lead the inspired gas to the gas-exchanging units of the lung. Because there are no alveoli for gas exchange, the conducting airways themselves represent anatomic dead space.

Acinus or Respiratory Zone

The terminal bronchioles divide into respiratory bronchioles that also have alveoli on the walls. After branching several times the alveolar ducts are reached, which are completely surrounded by the alveoli. The conglomerate of alveoli subtended by an alveolar duct is called the alveolar sac, the wall of which consists of alveoli. The acinus is the region distal to the terminal bronchiole, or all of the lung structure subtended from the terminal bronchiole, comprising the respiratory bronchioles, alveolar ducts, alveolar sacs, and the alveoli [2]; this is also referred to as the transitional and respiratory zone because the nonalveolated regions of the respiratory bronchioles do not, strictly, participate in gas exchange [1].

The acinus can be as large as 8.5 mm; the distance from the terminal bronchiole to the distal acinar edge is approximately 5–10 mm [2]. Roentgenologically the acinus is considered as a functional or respiratory unit, in contrast to the conductive airways proximal to the terminal bronchiole.

Although the distance from the terminal bronchiole to the most distal alveolus is very short, the respiratory zone makes up most of the lung volume (lung volume minus the anatomical dead space). When the cross-sectional area of the airways of each generation is calculated, there is relatively little change in the cross-sectional area until the 16th or terminal bronchioles [1]. However, near this level the cross-sectional area increases very rapidly. West compares the shape of the combined airways to that of a trumpet, or even a thumbtack [3]. Because of this rapid change in cross-sectional area at the terminal bronchiole level the convective or bulk flow in the conductive zone of the airways gradually becomes diffusive in the neighborhood of the terminal bronchiole.

This means that inhaled aerosols reaching the terminal bronchioles in convective flow tend to sediment at or near the terminal bronchioles. Nondiffusible suspended or particulate matter remains away from the alveolar walls and is expelled in the subsequent expiration [4]. This is why it is difficult to deposit particulates or aerosols on the alveolar walls, and why large inspired volumes and breath holding are important for obtaining efficient alveolar deposition of inhaled aerosols, especially of aerosols smaller than 1 μm.

Cilia

Ciliated epithelial cells occur at all levels in the trachea, bronchi, and bronchioles, all the way to the respiratory bronchioles, but are not found in the alveoli themselves. In the smaller bronchioles, however, the ciliated cells are less frequent and their cilia shorter [5]. Mucus-secreting goblet cells are abundant in epithelia of the trachea and larger bronchial airways but become less frequent in the smaller airways, disappearing at the level of or distal to the terminal bronchioles in normal subjects. The respiratory bronchioles lack mucus-secreting cells but have other secretory cells that are believed to produce a serous secretion; this watery fluid was shown by Gil and Weibel in electron microscope studies, to be coated at the liquid-air interface by osmophilic film that they believe to be of the same nature as the surfactant film covering the alveolar surface, but is thicker in the bronchioles than in the alveoli [6].

Lung Volumes

Subdivisions

The following aspects of lung capacity and volume can be differentiated:
- Total lung capacity (TLC) is the volume of gas contained in the lungs at maximal inspiration.
- Vital capacity (VC) is the volume of gas that can be exhaled from TLC.
- Residual volume (RV) is the volume of gas remaining in the lung after maximal expiration.
- Tidal volume (V_T) is the volume of gas inspired or expired during each respiratory excursion.
- Functional residual capacity (FRC) is the volume of gas remaining in the lungs at the end of a normal expiration.
- Inspiratory reserve volume (IRV) is the maximal amount of gas that can be inspired from the end-inspiratory position of resting tidal ventilation.
- Expiratory reserve volume (ERV) is the maximal volume of gas that can be expired from the end-expiratory level of tidal ventilation.

Total or minute ventilation is the total volume of gas exhaled per minute. This is equivalent to $V_T \times$respiratory frequency.

Here we must understand the fundamental concept of dead space. This is a portion of lung ventilation that is wasted or does not participate in gas exchange. The most important types of dead space are anatomic and physiological. Anatomic dead space is simply the volume of the conducting airways, as described above; this increases with the size of the lung or the FRC. The portion of inspired air that traverses the conductive airways and enters alveoli in volume per minute is called alveolar ventilation. Not all of the alveolar ventilation is equally effective in arterializing the mixed venous blood.

Physiological Dead Space

Inspired air that enters alveoli lacking pulmonary capillary blood supply is wasted. This area is called "alveolar dead space." When the inspired air enters alveoli with blood supply but supply which is reduced, such that a portion of the inspired air is wasted, there is also "alveolar dead space." While anatomical dead space is determined by the anatomy of the lung, determining physiological dead space requires a functional measurement of the lung's efficiency in eliminating carbon dioxide. This can be calculated by the following equation (rewritten Bohr's equation):

$$V_D/V_T = (Pa_{CO_2} - P_{ECO_2})/Pa_{CO_2}$$

assuming that Pa_{CO_2} is equal to the P_{CO_2} of alveolar gas; E refers mixed expired gas [7].

When the lung is normal, physiological dead space is virtually the equivalent of anatomic dead space. Physiological dead space is increased in the presence of ventilation-perfusion inequality. The concept of physiological dead space is important in understanding mismatching of ventilation and blood flow (perfusion) in the lung.

Inequality of Ventilation

Measurements of ventilation distribution in the upright position show more ventilation near the lung bases, while those in the supine position show less difference between the lung apex and the base. In the lateral decubitus position the under lung has more ventilation than the upper counterpart [8].

Why does this inequality of ventilation occur? Because of the lung's own weight the intrapleural pressure becomes more negative toward the lung apex in the upright position, and the transpulmonary pressure, or the pressure to expand the lung, increases larger toward the lung apex and decreases near the lung base. An analogy can be found in a coiling spring. When the spring is hung from the ceiling, the distance between the coils becomes greater in the upper part of the spring than the lower part due to the weight of the spring itself. When an additional weight is applied at the lower end of the spring, the distance between the coils in the lower part of the spring also becomes larger. This type of inequality of ventilation is thus due to a gravitational effect [9].

Further reasons for inequality in lung ventilation include uneven time constants [10], asymmetry of the structure of the small lung units [11], series inequality [12], and closing volume [13].

Blood Flow

Gas is exchanged between ventilation and blood flow or perfusion. The perfusion distribution in the lung can easily be assessed using radioactive particulates such as ^{99m}Tc-labeled macroaggregated albumin (MAA) or dissolved radioactive gases such as ^{133}Xe or ^{81m}Kr.

Gravitational Effect

Because the pulmonary circulation is a low-pressure system, with systolic pressure normally being about 25 mmHg, diastolic pressure 8 mmHg, and mean pressure 15 mmHg [14], the distribution of the pulmonary arterial blood flow is affected by body posture. The adult lung is approximately 30 cm long, and a hydrostatic pressure between the lung apex and the base is 30 cm blood, or 23 mmHg.

Because the lung resembles a manometer, when a tracer is injected with the subject in the upright position, the distribution of radioactivity represents the perfusion distribution in the lung in the same upright position.

When the tracer is injected in the supine position, the distribution of radio-activity represents the perfusion distribution in the supine position. As described above, the lower lung shows greater perfusion per unit lung volume than does the upper lung, due to the hydrostatic pressure difference, but in the supine position there is only little difference in the perfusion distribution between the upper and lower lungs. This is the "gravitational effect" on perfusion in the lung.

Zone Theory

West has proposed a model to explain the relationships between alveolar pressure (P_A), pulmonary arterial pressure (Pa), and pulmonary venous pressure (Pv) [15]. The lung is divided into three zones, according to the relative magnitudes of the P_A, Pa, and Pv, as shown in Fig. 2.3. Zone 1 is the lung region in which P_A exceeds Pa. The collapsible capillaries close because the pressure outside exceeds the pressure inside. Zone 2 is that part of the lung where Pa exceeds P_A, but P_A exceeds Pv. Perfusion is determined by the pressure difference between Pa and P_A instead of the arterial-venous pressure difference. Thus the linear increase in perfusion in zone 2 is explained by the hydrostatic pressure increase in Pa in the zone where P_A remains constant. Zone 3 is the part of the lung in which Pv exceeds P_A. The pressure difference responsible for the blood flow is Pa minus Pv, and the rate of increase in zone 3 is less than that in zone 2.

At the lowermost lung region below zone 3, however, blood flow decreases and is not regulated by the above mechanisms. As indicated, the alveoli are

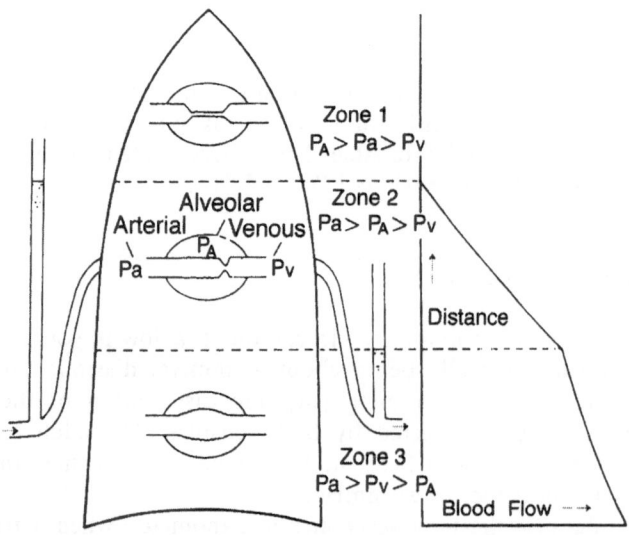

Fig. 2.3. Relationships between pulmonary arterial pressure (*Pa*), pulmonary venous pressure (*Pv*) and alveolar pressure (*P_A*) in zones 1–3. (From [3])

less well expanded at the base than at the apex because of distortion of the elastic lung caused by its weight. As a result the extra-alveolar vessels are relatively narrow, resulting in increased resistance and decreased blood flow. In other words, Pa is less than interstitial pressure (P_I). This lung zone is named zone 4 [16]. In mitral valvular diseases, for example, the extra-alveolar vessels are narrowed by the interstitial edema inducing the high P_I. The reversal of perfusion in mitral valvular diseases is considered to be due to the increase in this zone 4.

Factors Affecting Perfusion Distribution

Pathological factors that affect perfusion distribution in the lungs include:

- Vascular obstruction such as pulmonary embolism where perfusion distal to the vascular obstruction is either absent or extremely diminished
- Parenchymal lung diseases such as pneumonia, pulmonary tuberculosis, lung abscess, pulmonary interstitial fibrosis, and cyst and bulla formation where local perfusion is decreased
- Vascular compression and/or invasion such as bronchogenic carcinoma, especially a hilar lesion which can reduce the blood flow to the entire ipsilateral lung by compressing the pulmonary artery
- Vascular stenosis or agenesis where perfusion distal to the stenosis is diminished or absent, and there is no vascular channel for blood flow in the case of pulmonary artery agenesis.

Hypoxic Pulmonary Vasoconstriction

In addition to the above factors, alveolar hypoxia (low oxygen tension in the alveoli; Fig. 2.4) associated with ventilatory disturbance plays a crucial role in:

- Obstructive airways disease such as pulmonary emphysema, bronchitis, bronchial asthma, panbronchiolitis, and bronchiectasis where regional perfusion is decreased
- Bronchial obstruction due to intraluminal tumors or foreign substances such as a swallowed foreign body where distal to the obstruction perfusion is diminished or absent

In pulmonary emphysema the pulmonary vascular destruction associated with alveolar wall destruction and stretching of the vascular beds also contribute to the decrease in regional perfusion. Uneven ventilation distribution inducing regional alveolar hypoxia causes decreased perfusion in the corresponding lung regions and results in uneven perfusion distribution in the lung [17].

Fig. 2.4. Comparison of perfusion partition to the right and left lungs. When the left lung was given hypoxic gases and the right lung inhaled 100% oxygen, the lungs (*left*) that breathed air showed perfusion partition to the right and left lungs (*right*). The lung that was given hypoxic gas for inhalation showed decreased perfusion partition, indicating hypoxic pulmonary vasoconstriction depending on the degree of alveolar hypoxia

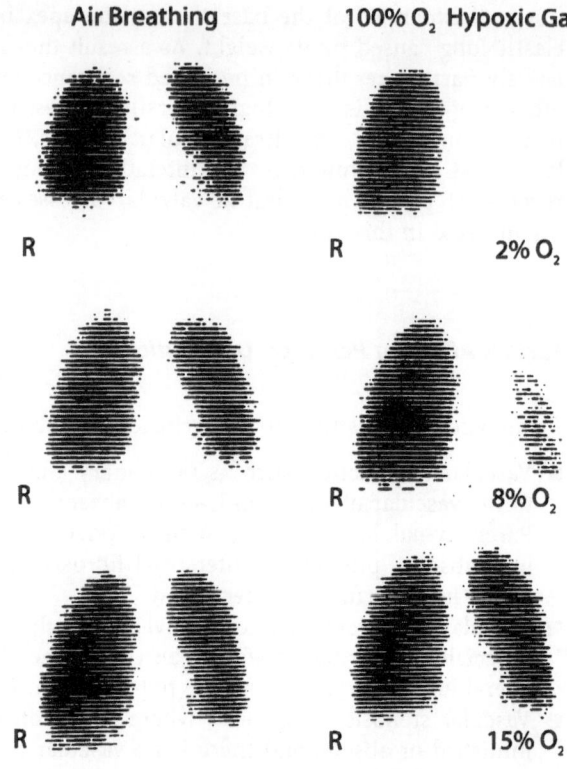

Diffusion

It is believed that the exchange of oxygen and carbon dioxide takes place by diffusion between the blood in the pulmonary capillaries and the air inhaled into the alveoli. The lung functions most efficiently when ventilation and blood flow match one another well. Mismatching of ventilation and perfusion is the most common cause of hypoxemia.

Ventilation-Perfusion Relationship

The introduction by West et al. [15] of radioisotopes to elucidate the topographical distribution of ventilation and perfusion marked a substantial innovation.

Normal

It has been found that both ventilation and blood flow per unit lung volume decrease from the lung base to the apex of the upright lung (Fig. 2.5a) although the gravity effect is less for ventilation than for blood flow (Fig. 2.5b). The upper lung (zone 1) is overventilated but underperfused, and the lung base (zone 3) is overperfused but underventilated [15].

Fig. 2.5 a. Perfusion distribution. ^{133}Xe dissolved in saline was injected into a healthy 53-year-old man at TLC level with breath held in the sitting position. The distribution of radioactivity indicates perfusion distribution at TLC. Note more perfusion distribution at the lung base than the apex. **b** Ventilation distribution. ^{133}Xe gas was inhaled from residual volume to TLC, and breath was held. The distribution of radioactivity indicates ventilation distribution at TLC. The distribution of radioactivity is more uniform than in **a,** but still indicates more radioactivity in the lung base than at the apex

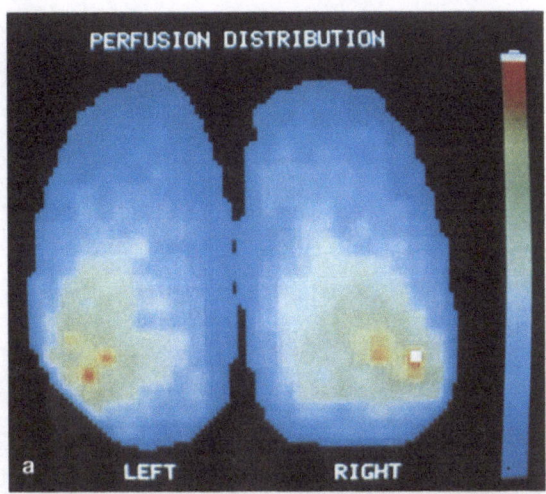

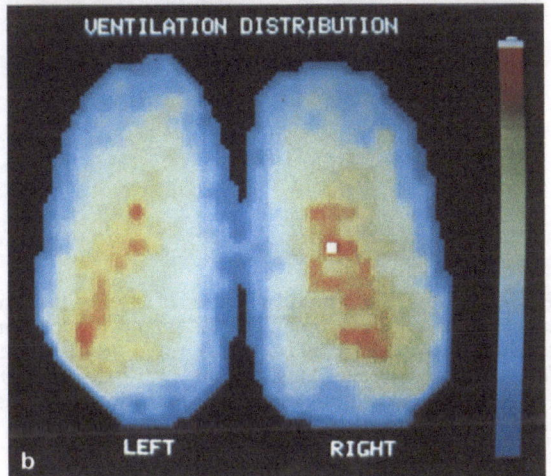

The use of ^{133}Xe gas following the procedures illustrated in Fig. 2.6 can clarify the ventilation distribution per lung volume, perfusion distribution per lung volume, and ventilation and perfusion relationships (Fig. 2.5c). Perfusion distribution can be studied by injecting ^{99m}Tc-MAA instead of using dissolved ^{133}Xe gas. Ventilation distribution can be studied by inhaling ^{99m}Kr gas or Technegas [18].

Pulmonary Embolism

In cases of pulmonary embolism, for example, radioaerosols can be used as inhalation agent, with perfusion images then compared to radioaerosol inhalation images. Mismatch between the distribution of injected MAA and

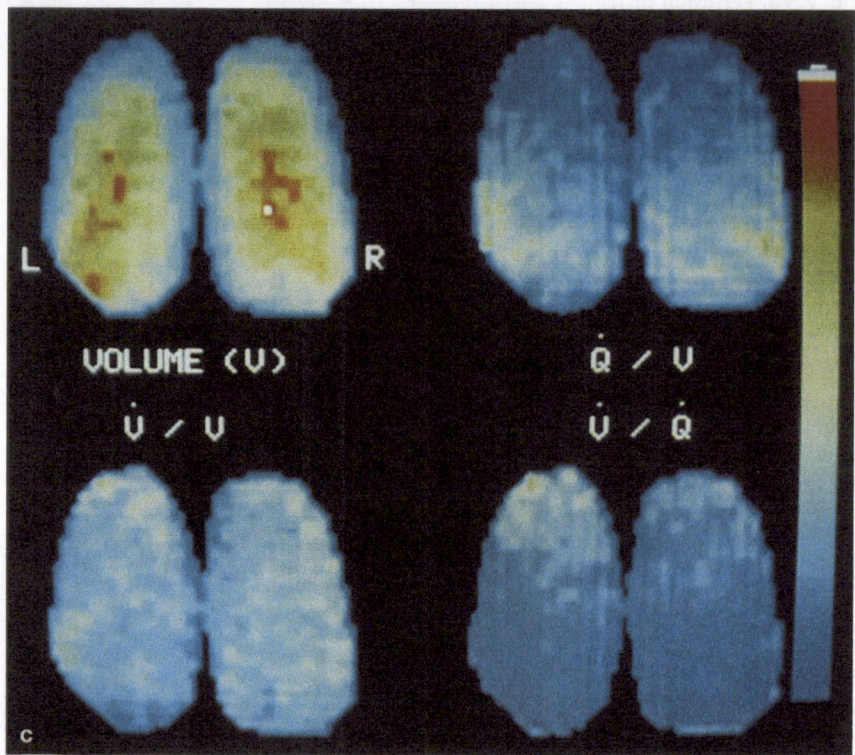

Fig. 2.5c. *Upper left*, the distribution of ^{133}Xe in the lungs after equilibrium is reached between the radioactivity in the lungs and the ^{133}Xe in the closed circuit, indicating the lung volume (*V*) at TLC; *upper right*, perfusion versus lung volume ($\dot{Q}/V$); *lower left*, ventilation versus lung volume ($\dot{V}/V$); *lower right*, ventilation versus perfusion ($\dot{V}/\dot{Q}$) or topographical ventilation-perfusion relationships in the lungs, indicating larger $\dot{V}/\dot{Q}$ ration at the lung apex than the lung base

inhaled radioaerosol in the same position or absent perfusion distribution in the normally ventilated lung regions (Fig. 2.7) yields the diagnosis of pulmonary vascular disease or pulmonary embolism when clinical situations are compatible with the diagnosis.

Airways Disease

In the case of airways disease the matching of ventilation and perfusion can be seen between the inhalation and perfusion images, and the diagnosis of airways disease can be made (Fig. 2.8). In parenchymal disease there is a matching of inhalation and perfusion images in addition to abnormal densities on chest X-rays.

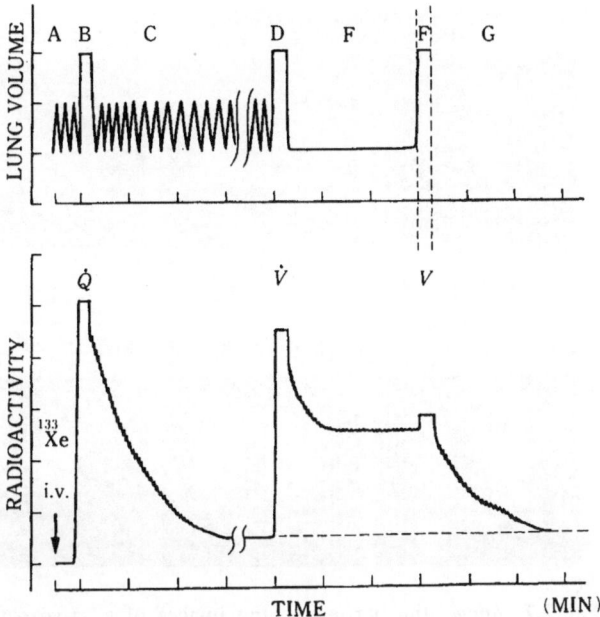

Fig. 2.6. Respiratory maneuver to obtain the perfusion ($\dot{Q}$) image, ventilation ($\dot{V}$) image, and lung volume image (V) at the same lung volume, here at TLC. The inhalation of ^{133}Xe was provided via a closed-circuit container. Dissolved ^{133}Xe was injected intravenously while the subject holds his breath at TLC (B, $\dot{Q}$). Injected ^{133}Xe is washed out by breathing air. The subject inhaled ^{133}Xe from a closed-circuit from residual volume to TLC and held his breath (D, $\dot{V}$). He continued breathing from the closed circuit, and when radioactivity in the lungs and the closed circuit reached equilibrium, he breathed from the closed circuit to TLC level and held his breath (F, V)

Nonrespiratory Lung Function

Nonrespiratory lung functions are those not directly related to gas exchange (Fig. 2.2). Mucociliary clearance is one of these functions and is discussed in detail in Chap. 10. Here we briefly consider pulmonary epithelial permeability and lung uptake of various substances.

Pulmonary Epithelial Permeability

The use of ^{99m}Tc-labeled diethylene triamine pentaacetic acid (DTPA) aerosol was first introduced in 1968 as an inhalation agent for studying regional lung diffusing capacity in patients with pulmonary sarcoidosis and alveolar proteinosis. It was expected that clearance of the inhaled ^{99m}Tc-DTPA aerosol from the lung would be slower; however, the result was the opposite, and the trial proved unsuccessful because quantification was impossible without computers which were not available at the time. Clearance from the lung seemed very rapid [19].

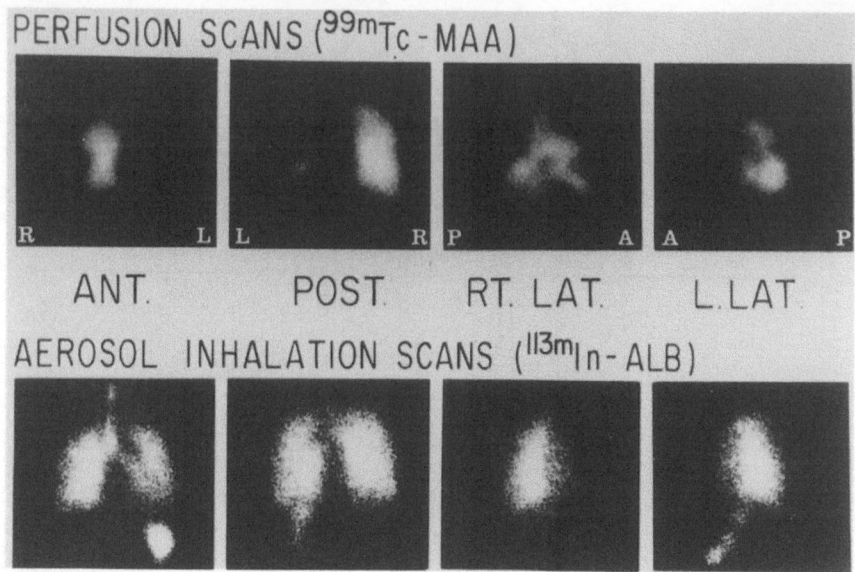

PERFUSION SCANS (^{99m}Tc - MAA)

R   L L   R P   A A   P

ANT.   POST.   RT. LAT.   L.LAT.

AEROSOL INHALATION SCANS (^{113m}In - ALB)

Fig. 2.7. *Above,* the perfusion lung images of a 23-year-old woman complaining of chest pain and dyspnea whose chest X-rays were within normal limits. Perfusion in the left lung was virtually absent while that in the right showed multiple perfusion defects. *Below,* immediately after perfusion study with ^{99m}Tc-MAA, radioaerosol inhalation lung imaging was carried out using ^{113m}In-labeled albumin aerosol. The right and left lungs showed normal inhalation lung images, indicating ventilation and perfusion mismatch or perfusion defects in normally ventilated lung region

Using computers for analysis, Taplin et al. later found the clearance of inhaled ^{99m}Tc-DTPA aerosol from the lung to be accelerated in patients with interstitial lung diseases [20]. Minty et al. found that the pulmonary clearance of inhaled ^{99m}Tc-DTPA aerosol from the lung is also accelerated in smokers [21, 22], but that it rapidly normalizes after the cessation of smoking [23]. The ^{99m}Tc-DTPA aerosol inhalation method is now widely accepted as a useful test for evaluating pulmonary epithelial permeability.

Fig. 2.8 a. Perfusion (*left*) and radioaerosol inhalation (*right*) lung images from an 18-year-old woman complaining of chest pain, dyspnea, and wheezing who had been treated for pulmonary embolism at another hospital. Note the matched perfusion and ventilation images indicating the airways disease. *Above,* posterior views; *below,* left lateral view. **b** Perfusion (*left*) and radioaerosol inhalation (*right*) lung images of the same patient after 2 weeks' treatment using a bronchodilator and antibiotics under the diagnosis of asthmatic bronchitis. Perfusion and inhalation lung images returned normal. *Above,* posterior views; *below,* left lateral view

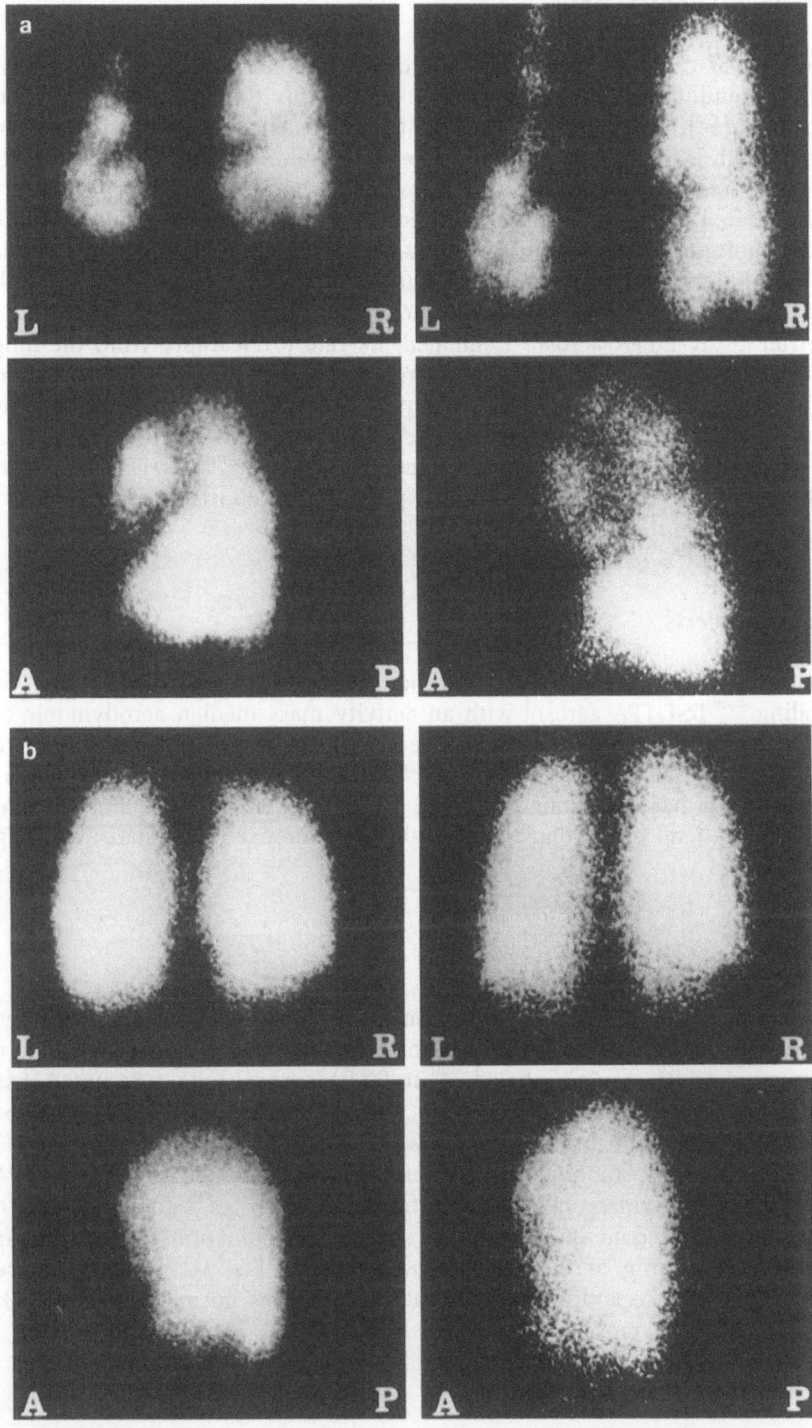

Pathophysiological Basis

The alveolar-capillary barrier consists of the alveolar airway barrier in series with an endothelial barrier and in parallel with the interstitial lymphatic pathways [24]. Pulmonary epithelium forms an extremely tight barrier that is one-tenth as permeable as capillary endothelium for hydrophylic molecules and prevents the alveolar lumen from being flooded [25]. Permeability is likely related to the intercellular junctions which are the main site of hydrophilic molecules crossing the membranes. The pore radius of the alveolar epithelial tight junctions is reported to be 0.8–1.0 nm whereas that of the capillary endothelium is 0.4–8.0 nm [26].

After ^{99m}Tc-DTPA aerosol is inhaled, its rate of clearance from the lungs depends upon condition of the lung. When the alveolar epithelium is intact, it produces resistance to ^{99m}Tc-DTPA particles passing through the intercellular epithelial junctions; however, when the intercellular epithelial junctions are widened due to some pathological condition, ^{99m}Tc-DTPA is cleared more rapidly. Positive end-expiratory pressure is reported to clear inhaled ^{99m}Tc-DTPA more rapidly [27–30].

Normal Subjects

In normal nonsmokers (n=23) clearance half-life ($t_{\frac{1}{2}}$) is 78.7±18.5 min when inhaling ^{99m}Tc-DTPA aerosol with an activity mass median aerodynamic diameter (AMAD) of 0.86 μm and a geometric standard deviation (GSD) of 1.75. The corresponding figure with ^{99m}Tc-DTPA aerosol of 1.00 μm AMAD and 1.78 GSD has been found to be 58.5±23.0 min (n=10) [31]. Smaller aerosol particles tend to prolong $t_{\frac{1}{2}}$, although the difference is not statistically significant.

Smoking

Clearance of ^{99m}Tc-DTPA has been found faster in smokers [21, 22]. Our own study showed that when seven smokers (average cigarette consumption 16 pack-years or BI of 160) inhaled ^{99m}Tc-DTPA aerosol with 0.86 μm AMAD and 1.75 GSD, the $t_{\frac{1}{2}}$ was 25.7±15.8 min. The difference between the $t_{\frac{1}{2}}$ of normal nonsmokers and that of smokers was statistically significant (Fig. 2.9). It is not known why smoking induces faster clearance of inhaled ^{99m}Tc-DTPA. Horseradish peroxidase labeled with tranferrin instilled into the alveoli of dogs was observed to increase in the intercellular junctions after smoking, indicating widening of the intercellular junctions [32, 33]. It has been reported that the acceleration of permeability becomes normalized in 3 weeks after cessation of smoking [23].

Fig. 2.9. Clearance half-life of ^{99m}Tc-DTPA aerosol (BARC) is accelerated in smokers ($n=7$, mean BI 160) than in nonsmokers ($n=23$)

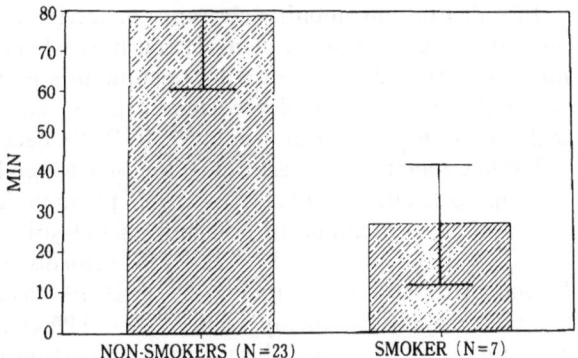

Interstitial Lung Diseases

Patients with biopsy-confirmed idiopathic interstitial pneumonia show significantly faster clearance of inhaled ^{99m}Tc-DTPA aerosol than do nonsmoking normal subjects, but there is no correlation between abnormal clearance of ^{99m}Tc-DTPA aerosol and abnormal diffusing capacity measured by carbon monoxide [31]. Clearance is accelerated not only in idiopathic interstitial pneumonia but also in interstitial pneumonia due to sarcoidosis [20], systemic sclerosis [27], radiation pneumonitis, or radiation fibrosis [34].

It has been speculated that the intercellular junctions are widened by increased retractive forces due to fibrosis [27], and that the increase precedes alveolitis or a residue of subsiding active disease in sarcoidosis [35]. According to our experimental fibrosis induced in rat by bleomycin, clearance of ^{99m}Tc-DTPA aerosol definitely increased 2 weeks after instillation of bleomycin, but no definite tendency was discernible thereafter because of partial recovery and partial fibrosis developing in the same lung. Microscopic examination indicated that there was thinning, detachment, or denudation of the alveolar epithelium, and that the basement membrane was directly exposed to the alveolar surface. Electron microscopy did not confirm the widening of the intercellular junctions. We believe that the epithelial damage and loss of epithelial covering of the basement membrane contribute to some extent to the faster clearance of inhaled ^{99m}Tc-DTPA aerosol [36].

Other Pathological Conditions

Increase in pulmonary clearance of inhaled ^{99m}Tc-DTPA is consistently reported with noncardiogenic pulmonary edema such as in adult respiratory distress syndrome (ARDS) and infantile respiratory distress syndrome [37–41], but the increase is not a uniform finding in cardiogenic pulmonary edema. Depletion of surfactant seems responsible for increased permeability in ARDS [42]. The respiratory bronchioli are suggested as being the sites where permeability is accelerated [40].

In radiation pneumonitis clearance is accelerated not only in the pneumonic lesions but also in the contralateral lung where no radiological abnormalities are observed [34]. Radiation pneumonitis is thought to be caused by alveolar damage and alveolar edema [43]. As radiation pneumonitis recovers with steroid therapy, clearance of ^{99m}Tc-DTPA becomes prolonged.

Hyaline membrane disease [44], long-term free base cocaine use [45], glue sniffing [46], and *Pneumocystis carinii* pneumonia complicated by AIDS or HIV-positive hemophilia in nonsmokers [47–50] are reported to show accelerated clearance of inhaled ^{99m}Tc-DTPA aerosols from the lung. Especially in *Pneumocystis carinii* pneumonia ^{99m}Tc-DTPA clearance returns toward normal with response to therapy, and ^{99m}Tc-DTPA clearance study is reported to be more useful than ^{67}Ga chest scans in detecting *Pneumocystis carinii* pneumonia when chest X-rays and/or PaO$_2$ are within normal limits [51].

Urban Pollution and Pulmonary Epithelial Permeability

The $t_{\frac{1}{2}}$ following ^{99m}Tc-DTPA aerosol inhalation also differs in nonsmoking normal subjects living in different places. An international cooperative study has shown that $t_{\frac{1}{2}}$ in healthy nonsmokers depends on the severity of air pollution, especially the amount of suspended particulates in the air. The study was carried out under the auspices of the International Atomic Energy Agency in ten cities in eastern, southern, and southeastern countries of Asia using the same aerosol generator (Bhabha Atomic Research Centre, Bombay; BARC) [52] and the same agent ^{99m}Tc-DTPA for aerosol generation [53]. There were highly significant correlations between $t_{\frac{1}{2}}$ and total suspended particulates (Fig. 2.10) and between $t_{\frac{1}{2}}$ and total pollutants (Fig. 2.11).

Lung Uptake of Various Substances

[^{123}I]IMP

The use of N-isopropyl-[^{123}I]p-iodoamphetamine (^{123}I-IMP) as a brain scan agent was first described in 1980 [54]. The agent accumulates in the lungs immediately after intravenous injection, and the possibility has been suggested of its depicting amine receptors in the lungs [55]. The incidental finding that the agent accumulates in the regions of bronchogenic carcinoma triggered wide interest [56]. Why it accumulates in the lung and precisely where are not known, but it is has been documented to accumulate in the inflammatory and atelectatic lesions surrounding bronchogenic carcinoma [57–59], diffuse interstitial lung diseases [60], and adenocarcinoma of the lung [61]; clearance of [^{123}I]IMP from the lung is delayed in smokers [62, 63] and in those suffering from bronchial asthma [64]. Inhaled [^{123}I]IMP passes through the pulmonary epithelium intracellularly whereas inhaled ^{99m}Tc-DTPA passes intercellularly because the former is lipophilic and the latter

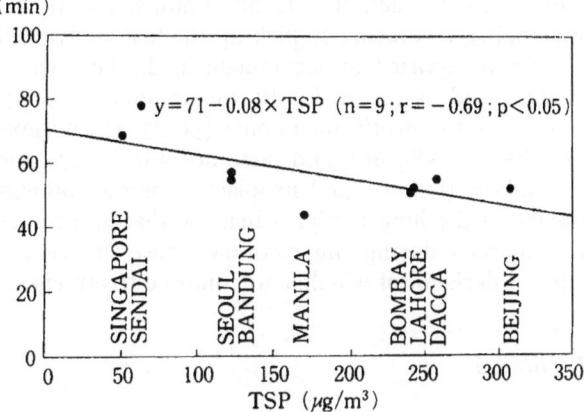

Fig. 2.10. Clearance half-life of ^{99m}Tc-DTPA aerosol in normal nonsmokers is accelerated as the level of total suspended particulates (*TSP*) increases

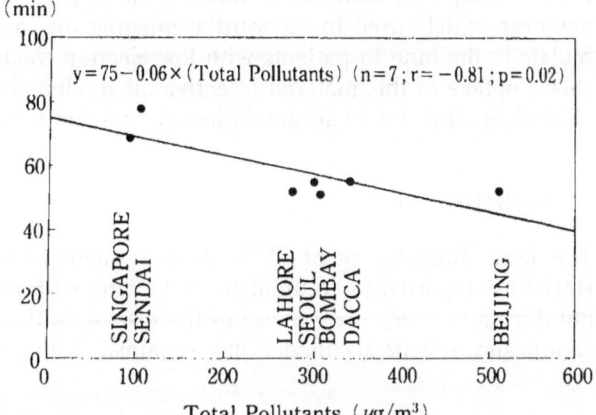

Fig. 2.11. Clearance half-life of ^{99m}Tc-DTPA aerosol in normal nonsmokers is accelerated as the level of total pollutants increases

hydrophilic. When there is a damage to the pulmonary epithelium, clearance of the former is delayed but that of the latter accelerated [65].

^{67}Ga Citrate

The use of ^{67}Ga-citrate as a tumor scanning agent was first reported in 1969 [66], and it subsequently became widely used for imaging epithelial and lymphoreticular neoplasms [67, 68]; however, investigators have also noted its concentration in inflammatory lesions [69, 70].

Injected ^{67}Ga binds to serum tranferrin and localizes in lysosomes or lysosomelike granules of the cell [71]. The information provided by ^{67}Ga for detecting the primary site of bronchogenic cancer has been so disappointing [72] that interest has gradually shifted to using this agent to determine the "activity" of interstitial lung diseases [73, 74]. The mechanism by which ^{67}Ga shows disease "activity" is not known, but it is speculated that activated macrophages voraciously pick up the isotope [74, 75].

[67]Ga is reported to accumulate in the lung with cryptogenic fibrosing alveolitis and hypersensitivity pneumonia [76, 77], rheumatoid lung [78], *Pneumocystis carinii* pneumonia [51, 79–83], occupational lung diseases such as asbestosis [84–86], and pneumoconiosis [87], radiation pneumonitis [88], sarcoidosis [89, 90], and neoplastic angioendotheliosis of the lung [91]. [67]Ga uptake in the lung is high when the disease process is in active stage but is less marked during the recovery phase or regression, thus facilitating the clinical decision of whether to continue treatment, especially in sarcoidosis.

[123I]MIBG

The structure of [123I]metaiodo-benzyl-guanidine (MIBG) has a structure similar to that of norepinephrine (NE) and behaves as NE at the sympathetic nerve endings. In addition to imaging the sympathetic function, [123I]MIBG has been widely used in myocardial imaging [92, 93]. It is reported to accumulate in the lung in patients with low ejection fraction [94]. Another report shows uptake of this material in active tuberculous lesion of the lung [95]. Its clinical significance or accumulation mechanism is not known.

^{99m}Tc-HMDP

The bone imaging agent ^{99m}Tc-hydroxy-methylene diphosphonate (^{99m}Tc-HMDP) is reported to accumulate in the lung with radiation pneumonitis but not during the very early phase of the disease [96]. Again, neither its clinical significance nor its accumulation mechanism is known.

References

1. Weibel ER (1963) Morphometry of the lung. Academic, New York, pp 1–151
2. Groskin SA (1993) Subsegmental anatomy of the lung. In: Heitzman ER (ed) The lung, 3rd edn. Mosby-Year Book, St Louis, pp 43–69
3. West JB, Dollery CT, Naimark A (1964) Distribution of blood flow in isolated lung; relation to vascular and alveolar pressure. J Appl Physiol 19:713–724
4. Altshuler B, Palmes ED, Yarmus L, Nelson N (1959) Intrapulmonary mixing of gases studied with aerosols. J Appl Physiol 14:321–327
5. Greenwood MF, Holland P (1972) The mammalian respiratory tract surface. A scanning electron microscopic study. Lab Invest 27:296–304
6. Gil J, Weibel ER (1971) Extracellular lining of bronchioles after perfusion-fixing of rat lungs for electron microscopy. Anat Rec 169:185–200
7. Forster RE, II, DuBois AB, Briscoe WA, Fisher AB (1986) Physiologic dead space. In: The lung. Physiologic basis of pulmonary function tests, 3rd edn. Year Book Medical, Chicago, pp 266–267
8. Isawa T, Okubo K, Oka S (1969) Postural effect on regional ventilation. Tohoku J Exp Med 97:101–112
9. Milic-Emili J, Henderson JAM, Dolovich MB, Trop D, Kaneko K (1966) Regional distribution of inspired gas in the lung. J Appl Physiol 21:749–759

10. Otis AB, McKerrow CB, Bartlett A, Mead J, McIlroy MB, Selverstone NJ, Radford EP Jr (1956) Mechanical factors in distribution of pulmonary ventilation. J Appl Physiol 8:427–443
11. Engel L (1978) Gas mixing within the acinus of the lung. J Appl Physiol 54:416–423
12. Cumming G, Crank J, Horsfield K, Parker I (1966) Gaseous diffusion in the human airways of the human lung. Respir Physiol 1:58–74
13. Sutherland PW, Katsura T, Milic-Emili J (1968) Previous volume history of the lung and regional distribution of gas. A Appl Physiol 25:566–574
14. Criley JM, Ross RS (1971) Introduction to methods. In: Cardiopulmonary physiology. Tampa Tracing, Oldsman, pp 1–34
15. West JB (1965) Inequality of blood flow and ventilation in the normal lung. In: Ventilation/blood flow and gas exchange. Blackwell Scientific, Oxford, pp 17–33
16. Hughes JMB, Glazier JB, Malorey JE, West JB (1967) Effect of interstitial pressure on pulmonary blood flow. Lancet 1:192–193
17. Isawa T (1995) Pulmonary nuclear medicine (in Japanese). Kinkodo, Sendai, pp 1–223
18. Isawa T, Teshima T, Anazawa Y, Miki M, Soni PS (1994) Technegas versus krypton-81m gas as an inhalation agent. Comparison of pulmonary distribution at total lung capacity. Nucl Med Commun 19:1085–1090
19. Taplin GV, Isawa T (1968) Regional alveolar liquid diffusibility by lung scintigraphy. California University, Los Angeles Report UCLA 12-686, UC-48, Biology and Medicine, pp 4–48
20. Rinderknecht J, Shapiro L, Krauthammer M. Taplin G, Wasserman K, Uszler JM, Effros RM (1980) Accelerated clearance of small solutes from the lungs in interstitial lung disease. Am Rev Respir Dis 121:105–117
21. Jones JG, Lawler P, Crawley JCW, Minty BD, Hulands G, Veall N (1980) Increased alveolar permeability in cigarette smokers. Lancet 1:66–68
22. Jones JG, Minty BD, Royston D, Royston JP (1983) Carboxyhaemoglobin and pulmonary epithelial permeability in man. Thorax 38:129–133
23. Minty BD, Jordan C, Jones JG (1981) Rapid improvement in abnormal pulmonary epithelial permeability after stopping cigarettes. BMJ 282:1183–1186
24. Staub NC (1983) Alveolar flooding and clearance. Am Rev Respir Dis 127:S44–S51
25. Gorin AB, Stewart PA (1979) Differential permeability of endothelial and epithelial barriers to albumin flux. J Appl Physiol 47:1315–1324
26. Taylor AE, Gaar K (1970) Estimation of equivalent pore radii of pulmonary capillary and alveolar membranes. Am J Physiol 218:1133–1140
27. Chopra KS, Taplin GV, Tashkin DP, Elam D (1979) Lung clearance of soluble aerosols of different molecular weights in systemic sclerosis. Thorax 34:63–67
28. Marks JD, Luce JM, Lazar NM, Wu JNS, Lipavsky A, Murray JF (1985) Effect of increases in lung volume on clearance of aerosolized solute from human lungs. J Appl Physiol 59:1242–1248
29. Nolop KB, Maxwell DL, Royston D, Hughes JMB (1986) The effect of raised thoracic pressure and volume of 99mTc-DTPA clearance in humans. J Appl Physiol 60:1493–1498
30. Peterson BT, James HL, McLarty JW (1988) Effects of lung volume on clearance of solutes from the air spaces of lungs. J Appl Physiol 64:1068–1075
31. Anazawa Y, Isawa T, Teshima T, Miki M, Motomiya M (1991) Pulmonary epithelial permeability in normal subjects and patients with idiopathic interstitial pneumonia. J Jpn Soc Chest Dis 29:1439–1443
32. Boucher RC, Johnson J, Inoue S, Hulbert W, Hogg JC (1980) The effect of cigarette smoke on the permeability of guinea pig airways. Lab Invest 43:94–100
33. Hogg JC (1983) The effect of smoking on airway permeability (editorial). Chest 83:1–2
34. Anazawa Y, Isawa T, Teshima T, Miki M, Motomiya M (1992) Changes in pulmonary epithelial permeability due to thoracic irradiation. J Jpn Soc Chest Dis 30:862–867

35. Jacob MP, Baughman RP, Hughes J, Fernandez-Ulloa M (1985) Radioaerosol lung clearance in patients with active pulmonary sarcoidosis. Am Rev Respir Dis 131:687–689
36. Anazawa Y, Isawa T, Teshima T, Miki M, Motomiya M (1992) Pulmonary epithelial permeability in rats with bleomycin-induced pneumonitis. J Jpn Soc Chest Dis 30:1222–1228
37. Braude S, Apperley J, Krausz T, Goldman JM, Royston D (1985) Adult respiratory distress syndrome after allogenic bone marrow transplantation: evidence for a neutrophil-independent mechanism. Lancet 1:1239–1242
38. Braude S, Nolop KB, Hughes JMB, Barnes PJ, Royston D (1983) Comparison of lung vascular and epithelial permeability indices in the adult respiratory syndrome. Am Rev Respir Dis 133:1002–1005
39. Royston D, Minty BD, Higenbottam TW, Wallwork J, Jones GJ (1985) The effect of surgery with cardiopulmonary bypass on alveolar-capillary barrier function in human beings. Ann Thorac Surg 40:139–142
40. Mason GR, Effros RM, Uszler JM, Mena I (1985) Small solute clearance from the lungs of patients with cardiogenic and noncardiogenic pulmonary edema. Chest 88:327–334
41. Coates G, O'Brodovich H (1986) Measurement of pulmonary epithelial permeability with 99mTc-DTPA aerosol. Semin Nucl Med 16:275–284
42. Wollmer P, Evander E, Jonson B, Lachmann B (1986) Pulmonary clearance of inhaled 99mTc-DTPA: effect of surfactant depletion in rabbits. Clin Physiol 6:85–89
43. Gross NJ (1977) Pulmonary effects of radiation therapy. Ann Intern Med 86:81–92
44. Jefferies AL, Coates G, O'Brodovich H (1984) Pulmonary epithelial permeability in hyaline-membrane disease. N Engl J Med 311:1075–1080
45. Susskind H, Weber DA, Volkow ND, Hitzemann R (1991) Increased lung permeability following long-term use of free-base cocaine (crack). Chest 100:903–909
46. Sundram F (1994) Clinical application of radioaerosol studies – pulmonary embolism, inhalation burns and glue-sniffers and COPD. In: Bahk YW, Isawa T (eds) Radioaerosol imaging of the lung – an IAEA (CRP) group study. Benedict, Waegwan, pp 136–149
47. Mason GR, Duane GB, Mena I, Effros RM (1987) Accelerated solute clearance in pneumocystis carinii pneumonia. Am Rev Respir Dis 135:864–868
48. Meignan M, Guillon JM, Denis M, Joly P, Rosso J, Carette MR, Baud L, Parquin F, Plata F, Debre P, Akoun G, Austran B, Maynaud C (1990) Increased lung permeability in HIV-infected patients with isolated cytotoxic T-lymphocytic alveolitis. Am Rev Respir Dis 141:1241–1248
49. Van der Wall H, Murray IPC Jones PD, Mackey DWJ, Walker BM, Monaghan P (1991) Optimising technetium 99m diethylene triamine pentaacetate lung clearance in patients with the acquired immunodeficiency syndrome. Eur J Nucl Med 18:235–240
50. O'Doherty MJ, Page CL, Harrington C, Nunan T, Savidge G (1990) Hemophilia, AIDS and lung epithelial permeability. Eur J Haematol 44:252–256
51. Rosso J, Guillon JM, Parrot A, Denis M, Akoun G, Maynaud CH, Scherrer M, Meignan M (1992) Technetium-99m-DTPA aerosol and gallium-67 scanning in pulmonary complications of human immunodeficiency virus infection. J Nucl Med 33:81–87
52. Kotrappa P, Raghunath B, Subramanyam PSS, Raikar UR, Sharma SH (1977) Scintigraphy of lungs with dry aerosol generation and delivery system: concise communication. J Nucl Med 18:1082–1085
53. Nair G, Samuel AM, Nambi KSV, Isawa T, Bahk YW, Sundram FX, Buachum V, Ahmed K, Torres JF, Chou C, Shahid MA, Masjhur J (1997) Urban air pollution and altered lung function. An east, south and south-eastern Asian regional co-ordinated study (in preparation)
54. Winchell HS, Baldwin RM, Lin TH (1980) Development of 123-labeled amines for brain studies: localization of I-123 iodophenylalkyl amines in rat brain. J Nucl Med 21:940–946

55. Touya JJ, Rahimian J, Grubbs DE, Corbus HF, Bennett LR (1985) A noninvasive procedure for in vivo assay of a lung amine endothelial receptor. J Nucl Med 26:1302–1307
56. Hill TC, Holman BL, Lovett R, O'Leary DH, Front D, Magistrette P, Zimmerman RE, Moore S, Clouse ME, Wu JL, Lin TH, Baldwin RM (1982) Initial experience with SPECT (single photon emission computerized tomography) of the brain using N-isopropyl I-123 P-iodoamphetamine: concise communications. J Nucl Med 23:191–195
57. Nakajo M, Uchiyama N, Hiraki Y, Miyata Y, Iriki A, Hirotsu Y, Wakimoto J, Norimatsu Y (1988) Increased accumulation of iodine-123-IMP in the pulmonary lesion surrounding a lung cancer. Ann Nucl Med 2:49–53
58. Nakajo M, Shimada J, Shimozono M, Uchiyama N, Hiraki Y, Shinohara S (1988) Serial lung imaging with 123I-IMP in localized pulmonary lesions (in Japanese). Jpn J Nucl Med 25:441–450
59. Suematsu T, Narabayashi I, Takada Y, Ohbayashi K, Hirata Y, Oshitani T, Kanoh K, Sakamoto T, Komiyama T, Yoshino A, Tsubota N, Hatta T, Kadoh T, Yamamoto H (1989) Delayed lung scintigraphy with N-Isopropyl-I-123-p-Iodoamphetamine in lung cancer and inflammatory disease (in Japanese). Jpn J Nucl Med 26:45–53
60. Takahashi T, Kato K, Yanagisawa T, Maiya N, Tamura M (1991) ^{123}I-IMP clearance of the lung with diffuse lung disease (in Japanese). Jpn J Nucl Med 28:191–195
61. Suematsu T, Yoshida S, Yamamoto H, Maruta T, Ogawa K, Komoto E, Horio M, Narabayashi I (1991) A case of increased ^{123}I-IMP uptake in adenocarcinoma of the lung (in Japanese). Jpn J Nucl Med 28:293–296
62. Itasaka M, Ikeda H, Yakuwa N, Kato S, Takahashi K, Yasui S (1989) The study of the lung accumulation of I-123 IMP by the bronchoalveolar lavage (in Japanese). Jpn J Nucl Med 26:189–194
63. Katoh K, Takahashi T (1990) Effects of cigarette smoking on I-123 IMP clearance from the lung (in Japanese). Jpn J Nucl Med 27:1093–1098
64. Ikeda H, Komatsu M, Seino S, Takahashi K, Yasui S, Mariko M (1990) ^{123}I-IMP accumulation in the lung with bronchial asthma – early uptake and delayed washout (in Japanese). Jpn J Nucl Med 27:719–724
65. Kosuda S, Kawahara S, Ishibashi A, Tamura K, Kubo A, Hashimoto S (1991) Pulmonary inhalation scintigraphy using N-isopropyl-[I^{123}]iodoamphetamine (^{123}I-IMP) aerosol (in Japanese). Jpn J Nucl Med 28:577–583
66. Edwards CL, Hayes RL (1969) Tumor scanning with ^{67}gallium citrate. J Nucl Med 10:103–105
67. Freeman LM, Blaufax MD (1978) Gallium-67 citrate. Semin Nucl Med 8:181–270
68. Hoffer PB (1980) Status of gallium-67 in tumor detection. J Nucl Med 21:394–398
69. Lavender JP, Lowe J, Barker JR, Burn JI, Chaudhri MA (1971) Gallium 67 citrate scanning in neoplastic and inflammatory lesion. Br J Radiol 44:361–366
70. Littenberg RL, Taketa RM, Alazraki NP, Halpern SE, Ashburn WL (1973) Gallium-67 for localization of septic lesions. Ann Intern Med 79:403–406
71. Swartzendruber DC, Nelson B, Hayes RL (1971) Gallium-67 localization in lysosomal-like granules of leukemic and nonleukemic murine tissues. J Natl Cancer Inst 46:941–952
72. Siemsen JK, Grebe SF, Waxman AD (1978) The use of gallium-67 in pulmonary disorders. Semin Nucl Med 8:235–249
73. Niden AH, Mishkin FS, Khurana MML (1976) 67 Gallium citrate lung scans in interstitial lung disease. Chest 69:266–268
74. Crystal RG, Gadek JE, Ferrans VJ, Fulmer JD, Line BR, Hunninghake GW (1981) Interstitial lung disease: current concepts of pathogenesis, staging and therapy. Am J Med 70:542–568
75. Abe S (1990) Clinical usefulness of 67Ga scintigraphy in pulmonary sarcoidosis. J Jpn Soc Chest Dis 28:65–66
76. Vanderstappen M, Mornex JF, Lahneche B, Chauvot P, Bouvier JF, Wiesendanger T, Pages J, Webert P, Cordier JF, Brune J (1988) Gallium-67 scanning in the staging of cryptogenic fibrosing alveolitis and hypersensitivity pneumonia. Eur Respir J 1:517–522

77. Nimkin K, Oates E (1989) Gallium-67 lung uptake in extrinsic hypersensitivity pneumonia. Clin Nucl Med 14:451–452
78. Specht HD, Bakke AC, Braziel R, Miley A, Rashidi-Nezami S, Germain L (1991) Cellular basis for the elevated gallium-67 computed lung index in a rheumatoid lung patient. J Nucl Med 32:2288–2290
79. Charron M, Ackerman ES, Kolodny GM, Rosenthall L (1988) Focal lung uptake of gallium-67 in patients with acquired immunodeficiency syndrome secondary to pneumocystis carinii pneumonia. Eur J Nucl Med 14:424–426
80. Kramer EL, Sanger JH, Garay SM, Grossman RJ, Tiu S, Banner H (1989) Diagnostic implications of Ga-67 chest-scan patterns in human immunodeficiency virus-seropositive patients. Radiology 170:671–676
81. Reiss TF, Golden J (1990) Abnormal lung gallium-67 uptake preceding pulmonary physiologic impairment in an asymptomatic patients with pneumocystis carinii pneumonia. Chest 97:1261–1263
82. Kosuda S, Shioyama Y, Kutsukake Y, Tanaka J, Asumi M, Ito K, Kamata N, Suzuki K (1991) 67Ga citrate imaging in AIDS-related pneumocystis carinii pneumonia in Japan (in Japanese). Nippon Acta Radiol 51:59–65
83. Smith RL, Berkowitz KA, Lewis ML (1992) Pulmonary disposition analysis using bronchoalveolar lavage. J Nucl Med 33:512–515
84. Hayes AA, Thickbroom GW, Geulfi GR, Musk AS, Van der Schaaf AA (1990) Computer quantitation of gallium 67 lung uptake in crocidolite (blue asbestos) workers in Western Australia. Eur J Nucl Med 16: 855–858
85. Cordasco EM, O'Donnell J, MacIntyre W, Demeter S, Gonzalez L, Eren M, McMahon W, Burns D, Feiglin DHI (1990) Multiplane gallium tomography of occupational chest diseases. Am J Indust Med 17:285–297
86. Delclos GL, Flitcraft DG, Brousseau KP, Windsor NT, Nelson DL, Wilson RK, Lawrence EC (1989) Bronchoalveolar lavage analysis, gallium-67 lung scanning and soluble interleukin-2 receptor levels in asbestos exposure. Environ Res 48:164–178
87. Siemsen JK, Sargent EN, Grebe SF, Windsor DW, Wentz D, Jacobson G (1974) Pulmonary concentration of Ga^{67} in pneumoconiosis. Am J Roentgenol 120:815–820
88. Kataoka M, Kawamura M, Itoh H, Hamamoto K (1992) Ga-67 citrate scintigraphy for the early detection of radiation pneumonitis. Clin Nucl Med 17:27–31
89. Line BR, Hunninghake GW, Keogh BA, Jones AE, Johnston GS, Crystal RG (1981) Gallium-67 scanning to stage the alveolitis of sarcoidosis: correlation with clinical studies, pulmonary function studies, and bronchoalveolar lavage. Am Rev Respir Dis 123:440–446
90. Israel HL, Albertine KH, Park CH, Patrick H (1991) Whole-body gallium-67 scans. Role in diagnosis of sarcoidosis. Am Rev Respir Dis 144:1182–1186
91. Honda N, Machida K, Kamano T, Mamiya T, Takahashi T, Tamaki S, Itoyama S (1991) Gallium scintigraphy in neoplastic angioendotheliosis of the lung. Clin Nucl Med 16:43–46
92. Kleine RC, Swanson DP, Wieland DM, Thrall JH, Gross MD, Pitt B, Beierwaltes WH (1981) Myocardial imaging in man with I-123 metaiodobenzyl guanidine. J Nucl Med 22:129–132
93. Schofer JR, Spielmann R, Schuchert A, Weber K, Schluter M (1988) Iodine-123 meta-iodobenzyl-guanidine to demonstrate myocardial adrenergic nervous system disintegrity in patients with idiopathic dilated cardiomyopathy. JACC 12:1252–1258
94. Ohtsu I, Inoue M, Hasegawa S, Takeda T, Ishikawa E (1995) Lung uptake of ^{123}I-MIBG at myocardial scintigraphy (in Japanese). Jpn J Med Imaging 13:397 (abstract)
95. Onsel C, Sonmezoglu K, Camsari G, Atay S, Cetin S, Erdil YT, Uslu I, Uzun A, Kanmaz B, Sayman HB (1996) Technetium-99m MIBI scintigraphy in pulmonary tuberculosis. J Nucl Med 37:233–238
96. Suga K, Chouji T, Ariyoshi I, Nomura S, Nishikawa E, Nakanishi T (1990) Accumulation of ^{99m}Tc-HMDP to radiation pulmonary fibrosis of six cases. Jpn J Nucl Med 27:1343–1348

3 Radiopharmaceuticals and Imaging Techniques

Ventilation Scan

T. Isawa

Both radioactive gases such as ^{133}Xe and ^{81m}Kr and radioaerosols are used in daily practice for studying ventilation distribution in the lungs. Cyclotron-produced isotopes with ultrashort half-lives such as ^{19}Ne and ^{13}N are also used when a cyclotron is available nearby [1–4]. ^{19}Ne has physical half-life ($t_{\frac{1}{2}}$) of 17.4 s and ^{13}N one of 10 min. Positron emission tomography (PET) is used for positron emitters. We do not go into detail here about the use of positron emitters for ventilation study.

Radioactive gases are naturally more suitable than radioaerosols for studying the dynamic aspects of ventilation, whereas aerosols are convenient in clinical practice for taking multiple views of the lung images for comparison with perfusion counterpart.

Radioactive Gases

Single-Breath Method

In practice the single-breath method for inhalation of radioactive gases is used most frequently because it is very simple in technique and yields information regarding respirable space and air trapping in the lungs.

Radioactive gases are inhaled from the residual volume (RV) to the total lung capacity (TLC) levels by a single breath with the nose clipped, and then the breath is held for 10 s or so followed by breathing air. While the breath is held, the distribution of radioactive gases in the lungs is measured and imaged, that is, in the respirable space or the lung space connected to the airways. The lungs are then imaged during the washout period. Retention of radioactivity in the lung during the washout phase indicates that the lung space is a so-called slow space where the turn-over rate of ventilation is slow.

With a $t_{\frac{1}{2}}$ of 13 s, ^{81m}Kr is too short half-lived for the study of wash-out phase.

Tidal-Breathing Method

Repeated tidal breathing of a radioactive gas is made from a container of the radioactive gas, again, with the nose clipped. The container could be a shielded balloon or a spirometer. At a certain lung volume, for example, at the functional residual capacity (FRC), the breath is held. The lung image indicates the distribution of radioactivity at the lung volume during tidal breathing, in this instance at the FRC. The circuit is then switched to breathing air. The radioactivity in the lung during washout period is recorded and imaged. Delayed washout in any region indicates a lung space there of slow turn-over during the tidal breathing. This procedure provides more precise information about ventilation during the tidal resting breathing of air.

Equilibration Method

Radioactive gases are inhaled from a container in a closed circuit from a given respiratory level such as from the RV or the FRC to the TLC levels, and the breath is held to determine the distribution of ventilation in the lungs. The distribution of radioactivity in the lungs indicates the distribution of ventilation in the lung at TLC. The subject continues breathing the radioactive gas until an equilibration state of radioactivity is reached between the whole circuit and the subjects's lung, and then the breath is held at the TLC level. The distribution of radioactivity in the lungs represents the distribution of the lung volume at TLC. The circuit is then switched open to permit the breathing of air. The radioactivity in the lung during the washout phase is recorded and imaged. ^{81m}Kr gas is not suitable for washout study because of its short $t_{\frac{1}{2}}$.

In all the above procedures the exhaled gas must be collected in a container shielded by lead and reabsorbed in the lead-shielded activated charcoal for cooling before disposal.

Radioaerosols

Usual Radioaerosols

Aerosol Generators

Radioaerosols here are those generated either by jet nebulizers or by ultrasonic nebulizers. A recent addition is Technegas [5].

Aerosol Size

Radioaerosols for clinical use have an activity median aerodynamic diameter (AMAD) of less than 3 μm and are generated by commercially available jet

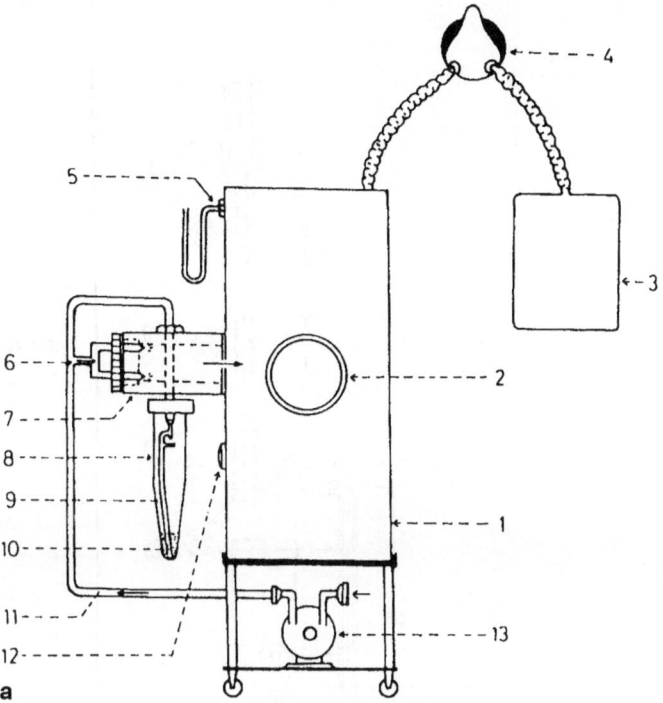

Fig. 3.1 a. Diagram of BARC nebulizer. *1*, Reservoir; *2*, viewing window; *3*, plastic bag; *4*, inhalation-exhalation nose cup; *5*, manometer; *6*, drying air; *7*, perspex block; *8*, test tube; *9*, nebulizer; *10*, activity; *11*, compressed air; *12*, safety valve; *13*, pressure vacuum pump (from [7])

or ultrasonic nebulizers. Table 3.1 in the section "Mucociliary Scan" shows the size of radioaerosol particles produced by various aerosol generators [6]. Particularly convenient for the purpose of ventilation study is the Indian-made jet nebulizer from the Bhabha Atomic Research Centre (BARC) in Bombay, made by assembling needles, test tubes, and an air compressor [7]. The BARC nebulizer produces aerosols with an AMAD of 0.84 μm and geometric standard deviation (GSD) of 1.73 when a reservoir is placed between the nebulizer and a mouthpiece (Fig. 3.1).

Inhalation Method

Aerosol is inhaled with resting tidal breathing either in the sitting position or in the supine position through a mouthpiece with the nose clipped. Aerosol tends to deposit more on the central large airways when inhaled with rapid, shallow breathing or hyperventilation maneuver. The same body position as in the perfusion study is preferred for inhalation of aerosol; this facilitates comparison of aerosol inhalation lung images with perfusion counter-

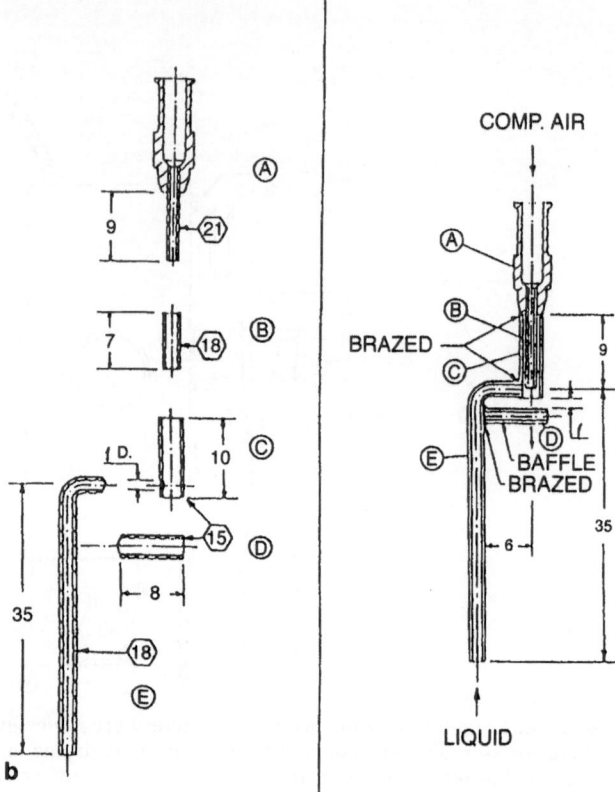

Fig. 3.1 b. Detailed description of the needle assembly inside the test tube. *15, 18, 21,* needle gauges (from [7])

parts. When ^{99m}Tc-labeled human serum albumin (^{99m}Tc-HSA) aerosol with AMAD of 1.93 μm and GSD of 1.52 is inhaled with resting tidal breathing, the alveolar deposition ratio is about 40% (or about 40% of initially inhaled aerosol in the lung remains there after 24 h) [8].

Technegas

Aerosol Generator

Technegas, an aerosol generator recently devised in Australia, produces aerosol particulates with characteristics of both an aerosol and a gas [5, 9].

Aerosol Size

Most Technegas particles measure almost 5 nm and are less than 10 nm in diameter. High-resolution electron microscopy has revealed that technetium crystals are coated with carbon layers [10].

Inhalation Method

Because Technegas particulates are so small, it is recommended that inhalation from RV to TLC level be followed by a period of breath holding [9]. Intrapulmonary distribution of inhaled Technegas is not exactly the same as that of a radioactive gas. Although visually the distribution of inhaled Technegas generally resembles that of [81m]Kr, qualitatively there is a little statistical difference in the distribution patterns between Technegas and [81m]Kr gas when compared at the TLC level of the lung volume following inhalation from RV levels [11]. The alveolar deposition ratio of Technegas is as high as 85% [9].

References

1. Valind SO, Rhodes CG, Clark J (1983) Quantitative measurements of regional ventilation using positron computed tomography and a short-lived inert gas-neon-19. Nucl Med Commun 4:149
2. Valind SO, Rhodes CG, Jonson B (1987) Quantification of regional ventilation in man using a short lived radiotracer - theoretical evaluation of the steady state model. J Nucl Med 28:1144–1154
3. Murata K, Itoh H, Senda M, Todo G, Yonekura Y, Torizuka K (1986) Ventilation imaging with positron emission tomography and nitrogen 13. Radiology 158:303–307
4. Senda M, Murata K, Itoh H, Yonekura Y, Torizuka K (1986) Quantitative evaluation of regional pulmonary ventilation using PET and nitrogen-13. J Nucl Med 27:268–273
5. Burch WM, Sullivan PJ, McLaren CJ (1986) Technegas - a new ventilation agent for lung scanning. Nucl Med Commun 7:865–871
6. Anazawa Y, Isawa T, Teshima T, Hirano T, Miki M, Konno K (1988) Measurement of size of aerosols produced by different generators and effect of physical factors on aerosol size. J Jpn Soc Chest Dis 26:867–963
7. Kotrappa P, Raghunath B, Subramanyam PSS, Soni PS, Raikar UR (1979) Constructional details of dry aerosol delivery system for scintigraphy of lungs. J Nucl Med 20:1000–1001
8. Isawa T, Teshima T, Hirano T, Anazawa M, Konno K, Motomiya M (1989) Normal values for quantitative parameters for evaluation of mucociliary clearance in the lungs. Tohoku J Exp Med 148:119–131
9. Isawa T, Teshima T, Anazawa Y, Miki M, Motomiya M (1991) Technegas for inhalation lung imaging. Nucl Med Commun 12:47–55
10. Isawa T, Lee B-T, Hiraga K (1996) High-resolution electron microscopy of technegas and pertechnegas. Nucl Med Commun 17:147–152
11. Isawa T, Teshima T, Anazawa Y, Miki M, Soni PS (1994) Technegas versus krypton-81m gas as an inhalation agent. Comparison of pulmonary distribution at total lung capacity. Clin Nucl Med 19:1085–1090

Mucociliary Scan

T. Isawa

Airway Mucus and Cilia

Mucociliary clearance is the first line of defense in the respiratory system. The mucus overlying the epithelial surface of the respiratory tract is propelled upward toward the larynx by coordinated beating of the cilia of the airway epithelium. The cilia line the epithelium of the respiratory mucosa from the nasal passages to the terminal bronchioles. In and distal to the terminal bronchiole the cilia are either poorly developed or absent [1].

The bronchial or ciliary surface is covered with mucus layer. Actually the cilia are dipped in the periciliary fluid, above which there is a mucus layer. A coordinated ciliary motion at the rate of about 1000/min normally transports the mucus layer toward the oropharynx. Mucociliary clearance or transport is orchestrated by interaction between the mucus layer and ciliary beats [2, 3].

Principle of Mucociliary Imaging

Bronchoscopic and radiographic methods have been used to study mucociliary clearance mechanisms, but these are generally invasive and require anesthesia of the airways and insertion of a bronchoscope [4–7]. For external measurement of mucociliary clearance radioactive materials are placed on the mucosal surface of the airways and sequential imaging is performed [8–10]. Transport of the radioactivity placed on the mucus layer is equivalent to the study of mucociliary clearance. Acute toxicity of cigarette smoke to mucociliary clearance has been easily evaluated in dogs by this method. The migration or transport of the droplet with mucus on the trachea is disturbed by forced smoking in a dose-response manner in the dog [10] (Chap. 10, Fig. 2). A large field-of-view gamma-camera is used for imaging.

Radioactivity is introduced onto the mucosal surface either as a radioactive droplet or as inhaled radioaerosols. The former method is generally invasive because it requires anesthesia of the airways and bronchoscopic procedures, whereas the latter is noninvasive and readily applicable in clinical practice.

Static Sequential or Follow-Up Lung Imaging

In addition to the lung imaging immediately following radioaerosol inhalation, sequential or follow-up lung images are taken at 30 min, 1, 2, 3 h and perhaps beyond to evaluate mucociliary transport in the lung, especially on the large airways such as the trachea. When excessive deposition of radioactivity or a hot spot is present on the airways, such as in bronchogenic carcinoma invading the main bronchus, repeated sequential lung imaging demonstrates whether the hot spot is cleared over time. If it is, mucociliary clearance function can be judged to be maintained, but if it is not, it is damaged (see Figs. 10.3, 10.4).

An inevitable disadvantage of this follow-up imaging, however, is that it is not always known how the radioactivity is cleared over time from the airways because there is no guarantee that the radioactivity under consideration is the same as that on the previous images, and whether a hot spot on the subsequent images is the same as that on the previous images is difficult to ascertain. In this sense sequential static images are not adequate means to study mucociliary clearance mechanisms in vivo in humans.

Transport direction or velocity can be determined by this method only with an adequately discrete hot spot.

Radioaerosol Inhalation Lung Cine-Scintigraphy

To avoid the above drawback radioactivity of the entire thorax including the trachea is measured continuously from immediately following radioaerosol inhalation for 90–120 min in sequential 10 s frame mode in 64×64 matrix. Each sequential 10 s data is recorded and stored in a computer. The raw data are either compiled for cinematographic display called "radioaerosol inhalation lung cine-scintigraphy" or used for quantitative analysis [11–13].

"Radioaerosol inhalation lung cine-scintigraphy" is displayed in cine mode on a cathode ray tube screen at the rate of 18 frames/s, and the cinematographic display is recorded by a movie camera or on video-tape.

This cinematographic display enables visualization of the features of actual mucous transport on the airways in vivo [11].

Mechanisms of Aerosol Deposition

Inhaled aerosol deposits on the airways by impaction, sedimentation, and diffusion. When turbulence occurs in the airways at the sites of stenosis or narrowing caused by mucous deposition, cancerous protrusion of the airway mucosa, excessive narrowing of the airways in obstructive airways disease, etc, excessive deposition of inhaled aerosol or "hot spots" appear regionally, corresponding to the stenotic lesions [14].

Agents Used for Mucociliary Clearance

Radioactive Droplet

Any agent that stays on the airway mucous layer following placement through bronchoscopy can be used, including $^{99m}TcO_4^-$ (technetium pertech-

Table 3.1. Activity median aerodynamic diameter (AMAD) and GSD under standard conditions (temperature 37°C, relative humidity 100%, test agent ^{99m}Tc-albumin) measured by cascade impactor (Andersen sampler)

Nebulizer	AMAD (μm)	GSD
Jet nebulizers		
OEM-1 (USA)	1.96	1.65
OEM-2 (USA)	1.19	1.86
Ultravent (USA)	1.04	1.71
Penicillin nebulizer glass (Japan)	1.76	1.70
BARC with reservoir (India)	0.84	1.73
BARC without reservoir (India)	1.57	1.80
Ultasonic nebulizers		
Mistogen EN-142 (USA)	1.93	1.52
Omuron NE-U11 (Japan)	1.62	1.50
Devilbiss (USA)	1.78	1.60

netate), ^{99m}Tc-HSA, ^{99m}Tc-millimicrosphere, ^{99m}Tc-albumin microsphere, ^{99m}Tc-labeled macroaggregated albumin (^{99m}Tc-MAA) [15]. A ^{99m}Tc-MAA droplet size in the order of 0.025–0.05 ml placed through a tube inserted into the bronchoscope is practical and convenient.

Anesthesia of the airway mucosa and oropharynx is required for placing a radioactive droplet on the tracheal or bronchial mucosa. This is tedious and cumbersome and causes the patient such discomfort that the actual clinical application of this method is limited.

Radioaerosol

Radioaerosol generated by either a jet nebulizer, ultrasonic nebulizer, spinning-disc atomizer under special circumstances, or other inhalers is inhaled through a mouthpiece with the nose clipped. An agent that is not absorbed or dispersed through the airway mucosa is ideal. Either ^{99m}Tc-sulfur colloid, ^{99m}Tc-phytate or ^{99m}Tc-HSA can be used to study mucociliary clearance mechanisms. We generally use ^{99m}Tc-HSA aerosol generated by a jet nebulizer or an ultrasonic nebulizer. Aerosols with a GSD (or σ_g) of 1.1 or less are termed monodisperse aerosols, while those with GSD greater than 1.1 are called polydisperse aerosols. The size of inhaled radioaerosol, hygroscopy and breathing pattern determine the sites of deposition in the lungs [14, 16]. The size of various aerosols is shown in Table 3.1.

We adopt normal tidal breathing for inhaling radioaerosol. In studying mucociliary clearance an AMAD of less than 5–6 μm but greater than 1 μm is most suitable, as has been shown by Morrow and Yu [17]. The author personally uses ^{99m}Tc-HSA aerosol with AMAD of 1.93 μm with GSD of 1.52 inhaled by the normal tidal breathing for studying mucociliary clearance in the lungs.

References

1. Sleigh MA (1977) The nature and action of respiratory tract cilia. In: Brain JD, Proctor DF, Reid LM (eds) Respiratory defense mechanisms, I. Marcel Dekker, New York, pp 247-288
2. Lucas AM, Douglas LC (1934) Principles of underlying ciliary activity in the respiratory tract. II. A comparison of nasal clearance in man, monkey and other mammals. Arch Otolaryngol 20:518-541
3. Wanner A (1977) Clinical aspects of mucociliary transport. Am Rev Respir Dis 116:73-125
4. Hilding AC (1957) Ciliary streaming in the bronchial tree and the time element in carcinogenesis. N Engl J Med 256:634-640
5. Berke HL, Roslinski LM (1971) The roentgenographic determination of tracheal mucociliary transport rate in the rat. Am Ind Hyg Assoc J 32:174
6. Sackner MA, Rosen MJ, Wanner A (1973) Estimation of tracheal mucous velocity by bronchofiberscopy. J Appl Physiol 34:495-499
7. Friedman M, Scott FD, Poole DO, Dougherty R, Chapman GA, Watson H, Sackner MA (1977) A new roentgenographic method for estimating mucous velocity in airways. Am Rev Respir Dis 115:67-72
8. Sakakura Y, Proctor DF (1972) The effect of various conditions on tracheal mucociliary transport in dogs. Proc Soc Exp Biol Med 140:870-879
9. Baetjer AM (1967) Effect of ambient temperature and vapor pressure on cilia-mucus clearance rate. J Appl Physiol 23:498-504
10. Isawa T, Hirano T, Teshima T, Konno K (1980) Effect of nonfiltered and filtered cigarette smoke on mucociliary clearance mechanism. Tohoku J Exp Med 130:189-197
11. Isawa T, Teshima T, Hirano T, Ebina A, Konno K (1981) Radioaerosol inhalation lung cine-scintigraphy: a preliminary report. Tohoku J Exp Med 134:245-255
12. Isawa T, Teshima T, Hirano T, Ebina A, Konno K (1984) Mucociliary clearance mechanisms in smoking and nonsmoking normal subjects. J Nucl Med 25:352-359
13. Isawa T, Teshima T, Hirano T, Ebina A, Motomiya M, Konno K (1984) Lung clearance mechanisms in obstructive airways disease. J Nucl Med 25:447-454
14. Isawa T, Wasserman K, Taplin GV (1970) Lung scintigraphy and pulmonary function studies in obstructive airways disease. Am Rev Respir Dis 102:161-172
15. Hirano T (1988) Mucociliary clearance mechanisms. I. Canine tracheal mucous velocity and different particles sizes (in Japanese). Kohkenshi 40:107-113
16. Miki M, Isawa T, Teshima T, Anazawa Y, Motomiya M (1992) Difference in inhaled aerosol deposition patterns in the lungs due to three different sized aerosols. Nucl Med Commun 13:553-562
17. Morrow PE, Yu CP (1993) Models of aerosol behavior in airways and alveoli. In: Moren F, Dolovich MB, Newhouse MT, Newman SP (eds) Aerosols in Medicine. Principles, diagnosis and therapy. Elsevier Science, Amsterdam, pp 157-193

Perfusion Lung Scanning

C.K. Kim

The clinical use of perfusion lung scanning for the diagnosis of pulmonary embolism was first described by several investigators using ^{131}I-labeled macroaggregates of albumin in the early and middle 1960s [7, 10, 11]. Currently the radiopharmaceutical of choice for perfusion lung scanning is ^{99m}Tc macroaggregated albumin (MAA), which can easily be prepared with kits provided by several manufacturers. ^{99m}Tc-MAA is in the range of 10–150 μm, with over 90% of particles measuring 10–90 μm. After preparation this agent can be used for 6–8 h. However, the vial should be resuspended before drawing each dose as the particles may settle. Following the intravenous administration of these radiotracers particles pass through the right atrium and ventricle, then lodge in precapillary arterioles in the lungs since the particle size is larger than the capillary diameter. The distribution of particles within the lungs is proportional to regional pulmonary blood flow at the time of injection. The particles break down into smaller particles which leave the pulmonary capillary bed with a biological half-life in the lung of approximately 2–6 h.

^{99m}Tc-labeled human albumin microspheres (^{99m}Tc-HAM) is an alternative pulmonary perfusion imaging agent which has physical characteristics superior to ^{99m}Tc-MAA. ^{99m}Tc-HAM particles are more homogeneous in size (25–60 μm) and more stable in the lungs, with a slower breakdown than that of ^{99m}Tc-MAA. However, there is no practical difference between the two tracers for imaging. The incidence of adverse reactions to ^{99m}Tc-HAM has been reported to be much higher than that to ^{99m}Tc-MAA [4, 9].

The administered activity of ^{99m}Tc-MAA is generally 74–148 MBq (2–4 mCi) and contains 200 000–500 000 particles. The normal adult human lung contains approximately 300×10^6 precapillary arterioles and 300×10^9 capillaries, and in routine clinical use therefore only about 0.1% of precapillary arterioles are transiently blocked. The number of particles injected should be reduced in patients with pulmonary hypertension, right to left intracardiac or intrapulmonary shunts, children, and those who have undergone pneumonectomy or single lung transplantation. For an adult patient a minimum of 60 000 particles are required to obtain an even distribution of activity within the pulmonary arterial circulation to and avoid potential false-positive interpretations [8]. Injection of too few particles may result in an inhomogenous distribution of activity, with focal hot spots within both lungs (see Chap. 4, Fig. 7). Alternatively, drawing of a significant amount of blood into the syringe before injection may cause clot formation, with further aggregation of the particles, which can yield focal hot spots within the lungs when injected. Although no significant side effects to the patient have been reported, focal hot spots, when large, may overlap with perfusion defects. If any doubt exists, the study should be repeated.

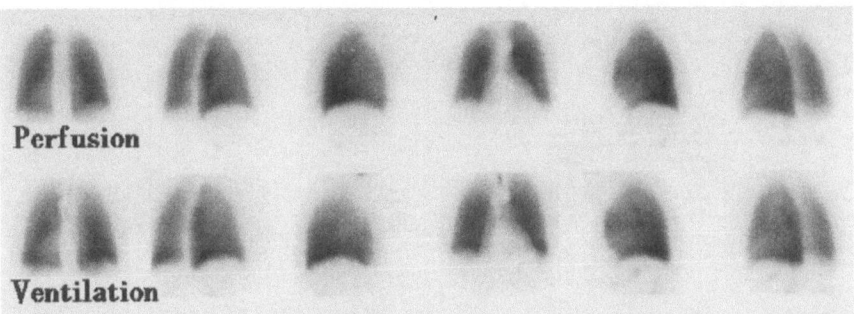

Fig. 3.2. Normal lung scan. *Above*, ^{99m}Tc-MAA perfusion scan. *Below*, ^{99m}Tc-DTPA aersol scan

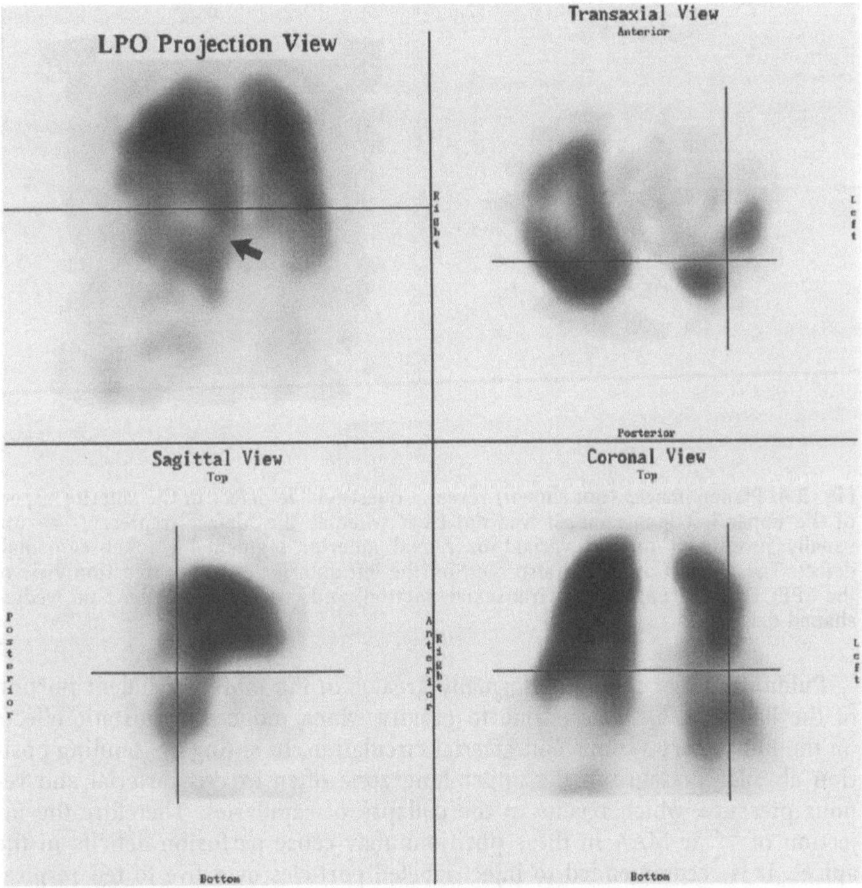

Fig. 3.3. Planar images (not shown) reveal a defect with an equivocal stripe sign in the posterolateral aspect of the left middle lung zone. This defect (*arrows*) is also seen on the left posterior oblique projection view of the SPECT study (*upper left*). Transaxial, sagittal, and coronal views clearly show a pleural based defect

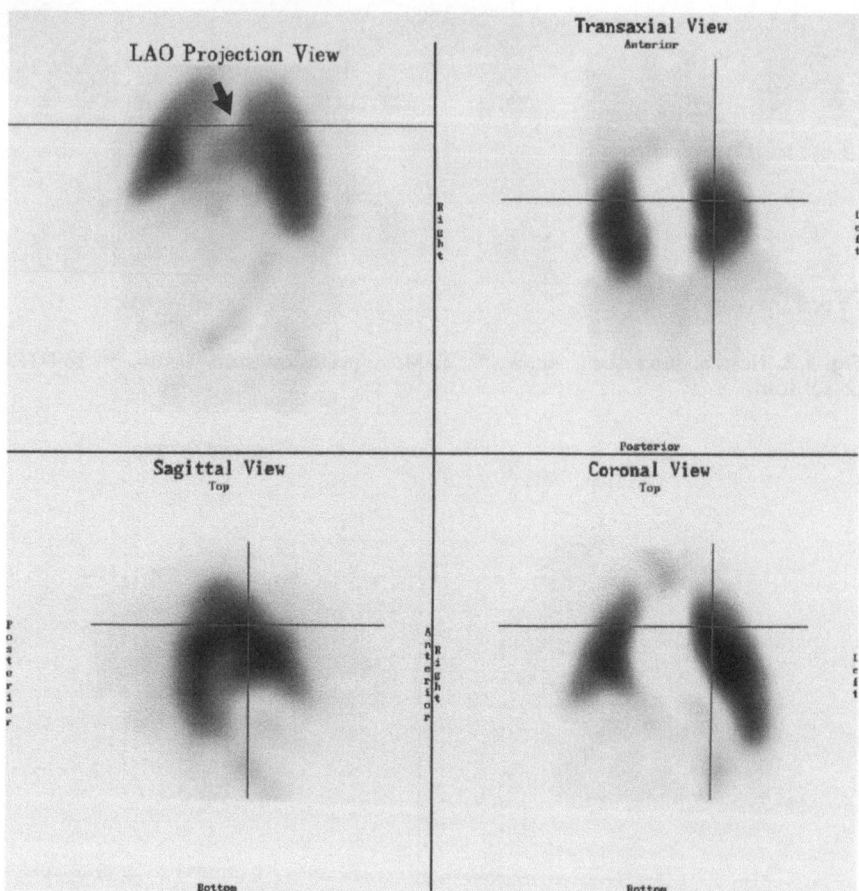

Fig. 3.4. Planar images (not shown) reveal a questionable defect in the anterior aspect of the upper left lung zone. It was not clear whether the "defect" represents an unusually prominent normal variant or a real anterior segmental (or subsegmental) defect. The defect (*arrows*) is also seen on the left anterior oblique projection view of the SPECT study (*upper left*). Transaxial, sagittal, and coronal views show no wedge-shaped defect

Pulmonary blood flow is normally greater in the more dependent portion of the lungs [2, 6]. This is due to gravity which induces hydrostatic effects on the pulmonary venous and arterial circulation. In sitting or standing position alveolar pressure in the upper lung zone often exceeds arterial and venous pressure, which results in the collapse of capillaries. Therefore the injection of ^{99m}Tc-MAA in these positions may cause perfusion deficits in the apices. It is recommended to inject labeled particles over five to ten respiratory cycles with the patient in the supine position, which limits the effect of gravity on regional pulmonary arterial blood flow.

In perfusion scintigraphy at least six views of the lungs should be obtained. These include anterior, posterior, right and left lateral, and right and left posterior oblique views (Fig. 3.2). The most important of these are posterior oblique views because they best demonstrate the lower lobes, the most common site for pulmonary embolism. Additionally, right and left anterior oblique views may be helpful in certain cases. Each image is obtained for a minimum of 500 000 or preferably 1×10^6 counts.

Single photon emission computed tomography (SPECT) imaging, while used by some investigators [3, 5], has not gained wide acceptance for lung scanning. Furthermore, all reported lung scan interpretation criteria are based on planar imaging, which should probably not be extended for SPECT interpretation. However, in selected cases when planar images show equivocal defects SPECT imaging can be helpful in either confirming (Fig. 3.3) or excluding (Fig. 3.4) the presence of defects.

References

1. Alderson PO, Doppman JL, Diamond SS, Mendenhall KG, Barron EL, Girton M (1978) Ventilation-perfusion lung imaging and selective pulmonary angiography in dogs with experimental pulmonary emboli. J Nucl Med 19:164-171
2. Anthonisen NR, Milic-Emili J (1966) Distribution of pulmonary perfusion in erect man. J Appl Physiol 21:760-766
3. Biersack HJ, Altland H, Knopp R, Winkler C (1982) Single photon emission computed tomography of the lung: preliminary results. Eur J Nucl Med 7:166-170
4. Cordova MA, Rhodes BA, Atkins HL et al (1982) Adverse reactions to radiopharmaceuticals, J Nucl Med 23:550-551
5. Donaldson RM, Kahn O, Raphael MJ, Jarritt PH, Ell PJ (1982) Emission tomography in embolic lung disease: angiographic correlations. Clin Radiol 33:389-393
6. Glaister DH (1967) The effect of posture on the distribution of ventilation and blood flow in the normal lung. Clin Sci 33:391-398
7. Haynie TP, Calhoon JH, Nasjleti CE, et al (1963) Visualization of pulmonary artery occlusion by photoscanning. JAMA 185:306-308
8. Heck LL, Duley JW (1975) Statistical considerations in lung scanning with Tc-99m albumin particles. Radiology 113:675-679
9. Rhodes BA, Cordova MA (1980) Adverse reactions to radiopharmaceuticals: incidence in 1978, and associated symptoms. Report of the Adverse Reactions Subcommittee of the Society of Nuclear Medicine. J Nucl Med 21:1107-1110
10. Taplin GV, Johnson DE, Dore EK et al (1964) Suspensions of radioalbumin aggregates for photoscanning the liver, spleen, lung and other organs. J Nucl Med 5:259-275
11. Wagner HN, Sabiston AC, McAfee JG et al (1964) Diagnosis of massive pulmonary embolism in man by radioisotope scanning. N Engl J Med 271:377-384

Cardiac Scan

D. S. LEE

Perfusion Agents

201Tl

^{201}Tl is taken up and retained in myocytes by membrane-bound Na-K ATPase; 94% of ^{201}Tl gamma rays is 69–84 keV; half-life is 73 h. ^{201}Tl is redistributed continuously in tissues, and images can be acquired 4- or 24-h after injection (Table 3.2).

Initial uptake is determined by the product of flow and extraction fraction. The ^{201}Tl extraction fraction in myocardium is 0.85. Some 4% of the injected dose accumulates in myocardium. Myocardial uptake of ^{201}Tl is proportional to blood flow unless blood flow is less than 10%, or twice the normal flow. Relation of uptake and flow is curvilinear.

Redistribution means that ^{201}Tl uptake normalizes at rest in normal myocardium and is maintained in ischemic myocardium as in stress periods. The washout of ^{201}Tl from normal myocardium has a half-life of 4 h. Nothing is washed out from ischemic myocardium if ischemic areas have no reserves, receiving no additional perfusion in stress. The kidney is a critical organ in terms of radiation safety.

^{201}Tl injected at rest is also redistributed 4–24 h after injection. Ischemic myocardium which lacked enough activity after injection has more activity if allowed enough time for redistribution. About one-half of the ischemic segments with decreased uptake obtain more activity over time. Nitrate [1], insulin and glucose [6], and ribose are reported to facilitate redistribution.

99mTc-MIBI

^{99m}Tc-MIBI is a lipophilic cationic (+1) ^{99m}Tc-hexakis compound. ^{99m}Tc-MIBI permeates cellular and mitochondrial membranes and is captured by nega-

Table 3.2. Radiopharmaceuticals for myocardial perfusion scintigraphy

	^{201}Tl	^{99m}Tc-MIBI	^{99m}Tc-tetrofosmin
Energy (keV)	69–83	140	140
Injection dose (MBq)	111	370–1110	370–1110
First-pass extraction fraction	0.85	0.65	0.67
Uptake/ID (%)	4	1–2	1–2
Redistribution	Redistribution	Minimal	No
Mechanism of uptake	NA-K ATPase activity	Mitochondrial membrane potential	Mitochondrial membrane potential

tive membrane potential. The extraction fraction of ^{99m}Tc-MIBI is 0.65. Some 1%–2% is taken up by myocardium. A very slow washout is reported from myocardium, with a half-life of longer than 5 h. A curvilinear relationship is also noted. ^{99m}Tc-MIBI uptake is less linear with myocardial blood flow than ^{201}Tl. Inhibitors of cytochrome c oxidase and drugs that disrupt membranes lower ^{99m}Tc-MIBI uptake in myocytes. Most of the radioactivity is excreted via the bowel, and the large bowel is the critical organ.

^{99m}Tc-Tetrofosmin

^{99m}Tc-Tetrofosmin is a lipophilic cationic compound [2]. It resembles ^{99m}Tc-MIBI in terms of mechanism of uptake and retention in myocardium. Less than 2% is retained in myocardium. No redistribution is reported from the heart. ^{99m}Tc-Tetrofosmin taken up by the liver is excreted somewhat more rapidly than ^{99m}Tc-MIBI. The gallbladder is a critical organ for radiation safety.

Infarct-Avid Agents

^{99m}Tc-Pyrophosphate

^{99m}Tc-Pertechnetate is mixed with stannous pyrophosphate just before injection. If ^{99m}Tc-pertechnetate is in excess, this is bound to red blood cells, and blood-pool images result. Images are acquired 3 h after injection of 740 MBq (20 mCi) ^{99m}Tc-pyrophosphate. Anterior, left lateral, and left anterior oblique images are obtained. Normal findings are similar to those in bone scintigraphy [4].

^{111}In-Antimyosin Antibody

Anti-myosin antibody is mixed with 74 MBq ^{111}In [3]. Antibody is injected after chromatography. Imaging is performed 24 or 48 h after injection, and uptake by liver or kidneys is observed. Intensity is scored as grade 0 (absent), 1 (equivocal), 2 (less than liver), or 3 (equal to liver).

Blood-Pool Agents

^{99m}Tc-labeled red blood cells are used as blood-pool agents. Pertechnetate anion penetrates red cell membranes and is reduced to bind hemoglobin irreversibly. The in vivo method is preferred because it is the simplest and yields fairly good labeling efficiency [5]. Anterior and left lateral images are obtained; the left anterior oblique image is adjusted to reveal the best septal view. The RR interval is divided by 16–32. The 1st–16th frames are collected for more than 300 cycles. List mode acquisition is possible, and acquired images are rearranged afterward in this mode. Cine loop is displayed on the screen. Sixteen frames are enough to evaluate the volume curve and to calculate the ejection fraction. The volume curve is analyzed by obtaining the first derivative of volume over time. Ejection rate and filling rate require 32 frames. Arrhythmia in more than 10% of rhythms renders it difficult to make a smooth closed loop of cine image.

Single-Pass Agents

Most ^{99m}Tc compounds can be used to perform a single-pass study of the heart; the most commonly used are ^{99m}Tc-pertechnetate and ^{99m}Tc-DTPA. The dose is 370–925 MBq (10–25 mCi).

References

1. He Z-X, Darcourt J, Guignier A et al (1993) Nitrates improve detection of ischemic but viable myocardium by thallium-201 reinjection SPECT. J Nucl Med 34:1427–1477
2. Higley B, Smith FW, Smith T et al (1993) Technetium-99m-1,2-bis[bis(2-ethoxyethyl) phophino]ethane: human biodistribution, dosimetry and safety of a new myocardial perfusion imaging agent. J Nucl Med 34:30–38
3. Khaw BA, Beller GA, Habor E et al (1976) Localization of cardiac myosin specific antibody in myocardial infarction. J Clin Invest 58:439–446
4. Parkey RW, Bonte FJ, Meyer SL et al (1974) A new method for radionuclide imaging of acute myocardial infarction in humans. Circulation 50:540–546
5. Pavel D, Zimmer A, Patterson V et al (1977) In vivo labelling of red blood cells with ^{99m}Tc: a new approach to blood pool visualization. J Nucl Med 18:305–308
6. Tartagni F, Fallani F, Corbelli C et al (1995) Detecting hibernated myocardium with SPECT and thallium-glucose-insulin infusion. J Nucl Med 36:1377–1383

Radionuclide Superior Vena Cavography

C. K. KIM

Various ^{99m}Tc agents are currently being used to obtain dynamic studies of the central and peripheral vascular systems, including ^{99m}Tc-labeled pertechnetate, sulfur colloid, DTPA, and macroaggregated albumin (MAA). After an acquisition following the injection into one extremity, the contralateral side is often studied; repeat studies of the same side may also be necessary. Therefore radiotracers that are rapidly removed from the circulation are usually preferred.

^{99m}Tc-MAA particles are removed from the circulation on their first pass through the first capillary bed. This agent is therefore suitable for evaluating vascular structures distant from the chest, for example, leg venous flow and hepatic arterial flow. However, evaluation of superior vena cava (SVC) syndrome and congenital cardiac/great vessel anomalies before or after surgery often requires repeated injections of the tracer into the contralateral or same extremity. Repeat evaluations of the SVC, innominate, and subclavian veins and collaterals which are located within or near the chest are not possible once ^{99m}Tc-MAA is injected because of the pulmonary activity; therefore ^{99m}Tc-MAA is not suitable for this application.

When an isotope with relatively long half-life is used, residual blood-pool and background activity from the first injection may affect the interpretation of subsequent studies. For this reason ^{99m}Tc-pertechnetate is suboptimal; it can be used only if the patient is to undergo a gated blood-pool scan following an SVC study. ^{99m}Tc-DTPA is somewhat better than pertechnetate because of its quite rapid renal clearance. Overall, the ^{99m}Tc-colloid agent is best suited for evaluation of the SVC syndrome because it is removed even more rapidly by the reticuloendothelial system, which results in a sufficiently low background within 10–15 min after first injection. ^{99m}Tc-labeled mercaptoacetyltriglycine (MAG3) is cleared more rapidly by the kidneys than is ^{99m}Tc-DTPA. Also, although not as rapidly removed from the circulation as colloids, there is little or no activity in the liver and spleen, which are closer to the chest and occupy a larger portion of the abdomen. Therefore ^{99m}Tc-MAG3 makes a theoretically attractive agent for evaluation of SVC syndrome. However, the agent should probably not be used for this purpose alone because of its high cost, unless ^{99m}Tc-MAG3 is routinely used for renal scanning so that a vial can be shared with other patients.

The basilic vein together with the brachial vein forms the axillary vein, and the cephalic vein terminates in a more proximal part of the axillary vein. When injected into the cephalic vein, it is possible to miss an obstruction at the distal axillary vein, and therefore the basilic vein is a preferred injection site. However, the radiotracer is usually injected into one of the antecubital veins, which provides the easiest access in some patients, and both veins are often visualized together.

Various techniques are used to achieve rapid delivery of the compact bo-lus to the central venous system, including the Oldendorf technique [1] using a blood pressure cuff that is inflated before the injection and rapidly released after the injection. A three-way stopcock has also been used. Radiotracer is first injected into the tubing which is flushed with a larger volume of saline. However, a compact bolus does not appear to be as critical in SVC study as it is in other studies such as a cardiac first-pass study or renal perfusion curve analysis. Rather, regardless of the injection technique employed, it is very important that the volume of the injectate and duration of injection be consistent when repeated injections are made into the contralateral or same extremity. In passing, we strongly recommend a separate, sequential injec-tion for each arm instead of bilateral simultaneous injection as the latter can obscure a subtle abnormality, especially when the abnormality is located cen-trally.

Most laboratories are now equipped with a large-field-of-view gamma-camera which usually covers the chest and proximal arms. If the camera is not large enough or the patient is too big, the proximal arm and approxi-mately two-thirds of the chest on the abnormal side should be imaged first, and a repeat study of the opposite side can be performed. It is helpful to photograph the two studies on separate films so that they can be superim-posed on each other if necessary.

After injection of the tracer, dynamic acquisition is usually continued for a minimum of 60 s. Digital data should be acquired every 1 or 0.5 s on an appropriate matrix, and images can be viewed on the computer monitor or reformatted on films at any desired frame interval. Particularly the review of dynamic images in a cinematic display often provides useful information. Di-gital acquisition also allows generation of time-activity curves and quantita-tive analysis of transit time [2].

Where digital images of the study are not available, analog images may be obtained at the interval of 2 s per frame. Many multiformatters place up to 16 images on a single film, and consequently a total of 16 images can easily be acquired for studies using 2 s or more per image. For studies using 1 s per image, 16 images may not be enough, necessitating a second piece of film and, possibly, simultaneous digital acquisition.

References

1. Oldendorf WH, Kitano M, Shimizu S (1965) Evaluation of a simple technique for abrupt intravenous injection of radioisotope. J Nucl Med 6:205
2. Klingensmith WC (1986) Evaluation of a physiologic method of interpreting first circulation time-indicator curves. Invest Radiol 21:566–570

Bone Scintigraphy of the Thorax

Y.-W. Bahk

Rationale and Techniques

Bone scintigraphy is a highly sensitive nuclear imaging test, and its specificity can be enormously enhanced by the use of the pinhole magnification technique [1-3] and pinhole-SPECT technique [4, 5]. The bony thorax, comprised of the ribs, clavicles, shoulder bones, sternum, and thoracic spine along with many articulations is one of the important objectives of nuclear bone imaging for one obvious reason: both radiography and computed tomography find only a limited place in diagnosis of the thoracic bones, most of which are thin, flat, irregularly curved, elongated or twisted, and disturbingly overlapping with each other. To be specific, the ribs are thin, elongated and curved; the clavicles are irregularly twisted; the sternum is thin and overlapping with mediastinal structures; the humeri and scapulae are irregular and overlap with each other and the thoracic spine, comprised of many small parts, complexly overshadowed by the mediastinal organs. The radiographic diagnosis becomes still more difficult when the patient's bones are porous due to metabolic or neoplastic diseases, senescence, or menopause.

The range of indications for thoracic bone scintigraphy is very wide, including traumas, operative injuries, infections, inflammation, radiation osteonecrosis, Tietze's disease, sternocostoclavicular hyperostosis, Friedrich's disease, tumors and tumorous conditions, seronegative spondyloarthropathies, and arthritides. In many of these diseases pinhole bone scintigraphy helps greatly in making the specific diagnosis [6-10].

It is standard to begin bone imaging by obtaining both the anterior and posterior views of the whole skeletal system for screening (Fig. 3.5a), followed by the spot view of the region of interest (Fig. 3.5b). As the scrutiny of these basic images dictates the examination, the pinhole magnification technique may further complement the process (Fig. 3.5c). As is well known, the anatomical and pathological details attained by the pinhole technique are indeed comparable to those of radiography (Fig. 3.5d) [1-3, 6-10]. Scanning starts at 3 h after the intravenous injection of 740-925 MBq (20-25 mCi) ^{99m}Tc-methylene disphosphonate (MDP) or 30 min or 1 h earlier when ^{99m}Tc-oxidronate (Osteoscan-HDP) is administered. The dose may be increased minimally in the elderly to compensate for osteoporosis or lowered metabolic turnover. From our experience we strongly advocate that as many seemingly normal whole-body or spot views as possible be subjected to pinhole study if there are any unexplained localizing symptoms or signs such as pain, tenderness, swelling, or heat. This is because pinhole scintigraphy very often reveals unexpected scan signs that are deceptively hidden on planar and even SPECT images (Fig. 3.6) [1]. Moreover, as mentioned above, pinhole scintigraphic findings are specific and unique in many bone and joint diseases (Fig. 3.5c) [1, 3, 6-10].

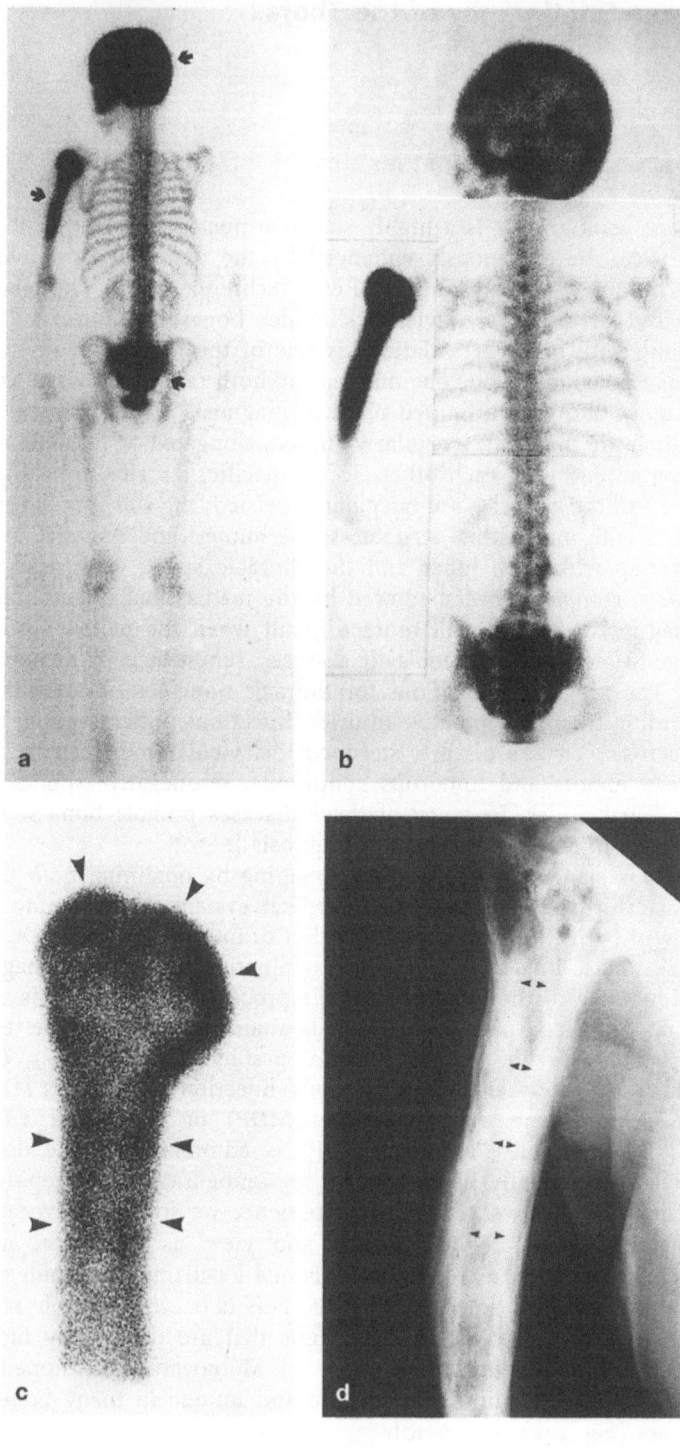

Fig. 3.6a, b. Differences between the sensitivities of different bone scan modes. **a** The ordinary anterior planar bone scan of the chest shows no abnormality. **b** Pinhole magnification view, however, shows a distinct "hot" lesion in the right transverse process of T2, denoting metastasis (*arrow*). The prominent tracer uptake in the costosternal joints and calcified cartilages are physiological

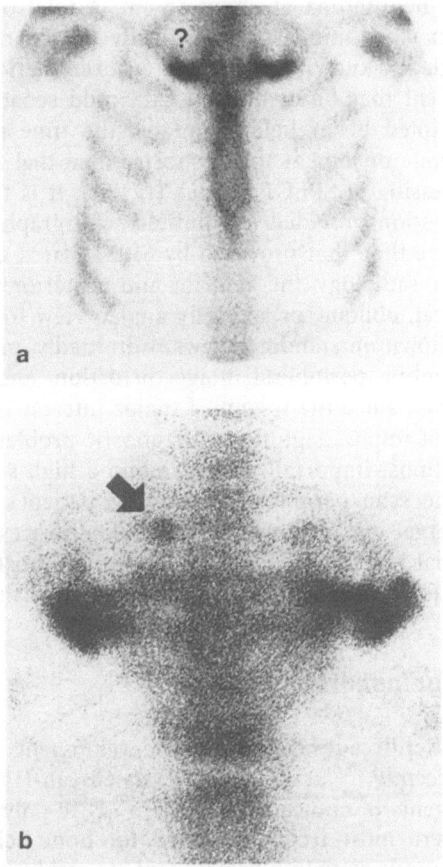

The pinhole aperture sizes commonly employed range from 3 to 6 mm; we have found 4 mm to be an optimal compromise between the scan time and image quality. The aperture-to-skin distances range from 0 cm (contact scan) to 10 cm. The distance depends upon the size of target organs. For example, a few ribs and one clavicle, a few vertebrae with their disc spaces, one shoulder with the scapula can be imaged well by the contact technique, and

Fig. 3.5a–d. Comparison of resolution and diagnostic efficacy of various bone scan modes. **a** Posterior whole-body planar scan of a patient with Paget's disease shows intense tracer uptake in the skull, proximal left humerus, and sacrum (*arrows*). The finding is suggestive of Paget's disease but not specific. **b** Composite spot view shows a bit improved resolution in the skull and sacrum but diagnostic information is still largely limited. **c** Pinhole scan shows incredibly improved resolution, now specifically localizing intense tracer uptake in the bone-end and cortex with narrowed marrow space, characterizing Paget's disease. **d** Anteroposterior radiogram of the left humerus shows classic cortical thickening with pumice bone change and narrowed marrow space (*arrowheads*)

a hemithorax at about 10 cm. A total of 400–450 K counts are accumulated in 15–20 min. Unless critically ill, too old, or too young, patients cooperate gladly, knowing that such an examination is invaluable. If necessary, the patient may be comforted with mild sedatives. Quite in contrast to the unwarranted belief held by many, the time required for pinhole scintigraphy of bone or joint is much shorter than that required for the acquisition and processing of SPECT images [1, 2, 4]. It is to be emphasized that the scan information provided by pinhole scintigraphy is by far more specific and sensitive than that provided by SPECT [1, 2, 4, 5]. As widely practiced in diagnostic radiology, the anterior and posterior views may be supplemented by a lateral, oblique, or specially angled view to delineate the alterations that are not shown on standard views. Admittedly, pinhole scintigraphy suffers from penumbra, peripheral image distortion, and rapid fall-off of count rates. However, since the region of major interest is in the central field of view, they do not impose significant diagnostic problems [1, 4, 5]. Needlness to say, it is of utmost importance to maintain a high standard of image quality by assuring the scan parameters including patient's position, pinhole size, aperture-to-target distance, and photographic processing. It is probably patient's motion that blurs and spoils the scintigram most. The use of an immobilizing device such as sandbag or soft padded-belt is therefore strongly recommended.

Radiopharmaceuticals

After decades of many new developments and selections, ^{99m}Tc-MDP and more recently ^{99m}Tc-oxidronate (Osteoscan-HDP) have emerged as the bone scan agents of choice. Before them ^{99m}Tc-polyphosphate and ^{99m}Tc-pyrophosphate were most frequently used for bone scintigraphy [11, 12]. Phosphate compounds contain plural phosphate residues [P-O-P], the simplest form of which is pyrophosphate which contains two residues. On the other hand, phosphonate compounds contain P-C-P bonds instead of P-O-P bonds, and they are known to have stronger avidity for hydroxyapatite crystal of bone at the site, where new bone is actively formed as in the growing physis, healing fracture, infection, or neoplasm. Following intravenous injection ^{99m}Tc-diphosphonate molecules are rapidly distributed in the extracellular fluid spaces, and almost one-half of them are fixed by bone, with the remainder excreted in the urine by glomerular filtration [13]. The 24-h urinary excretion of ^{99m}Tc-MDP is more complete than that of phosphates. About 40% of injected ^{99m}Tc-MDP activity appears in urine within the 1st h, 60% in 4 h and 70% in 24 h [14]. The amount of tracer deposited in bone 1 h after injection is 58% with MDP and 47% with pyrophosphate [15]. ^{99m}Tc-oxidronate (HDP) is also in wide use (Mallinckrodt Medical, St. Louis). The blood and nonosseous clearance is faster than that of ^{99m}Tc-MDP, reaching a blood level of about 10% of the injected dose after 1 h, and it then rapidly falls to 3% 4 h after injection. Skeletal retention after 24 h is about 50% of the administered dose. A practical advantage of this agent is that with faster build-up of optimum blood level scintigraphy can be begun 1 h earlier without lowering of the image quality.

References

1. Bahk YW (1995) Combined scintigraphic and radiographic diagnosis of bone and joint diseases. Springer, Berlin Heidelberg New York
2. Bahk YW (1995) Pinhole scan and single photon emission computed tomography in the diagnosis of bone and joint diseases. Proceedings of an international symposium on tomography in nuclear medicine. International Atomic Energy Agency, Vienna. IAEA-SM-337/41, pp 197–214
3. Davis RT, Zimmerman RE, Treves ST (1995) Magnification in pediatric nuclear medicine. In: Treves ST (ed) Pediatric nuclear medicine, 2nd edn. Springer, Berlin Heidelberg New York, pp 24–32
4. Bahk YW (1996) Pinhole scan vs SPECT in the diagnosis of bone and joint diseases: an improved scan delineation of structure and physiochemical profile. Syllabus of Educational Lecture, the 6th Asia and Oceania congress of nuclear medicine and biology, Kyoto, pp 1–8
5. Bahk YW, Chung SK, Park YH et al (1997) Pinhole SPECT for the diagnosis of skeletal disorders (abstract). J Nucl Med (in press)
6. Bahk YW, Park YH, Chung SK, Chi JG (1995) Bone pathologic correlation of multimodality imaging in Paget's disease. J Nucl Med 36:1421–1426
7. Yang WJ, Bahk YW, Chung SK (1994) Pinhole skeletal scintigraphic manifestations of Tietze's disease. Eur J Nucl Med 21:947–952
8. Bahk YW, Chung SK, Kim SH (1992) Pinhole scintigraphic manifestations of sternocostoclavicular hyperostosis. Korean J Nucl Med 26:155–159
9. Bahk YW (1994) Friedrich's disease. In: Bahk YW (ed) Combined scintigraphic and radiographic diagnosis of bone and joint diseases. Springer, Berlin Heidelberg New York, p 143
10. Bahk YW (1994) Condensing osteitis of the clavicle. In: Bahk YW (ed) Combined scintigraphic and radiographic diagnosis of bone and joint diseases. Springer, Berlin Heidelberg New York, p 56
11. Fogelman I (1987) The bone scan – historical aspects. In: Fogelman I (ed) Bone scanning in clinical practice. Springer, Berlin Heidelberg New York, pp 1–5
12. Fueger GF, Aigner RM (1990) Grundlagen und Methodik der Skelettszintigraphie mit ^{99m}Tc-Phosphat-Verbindungen. In: Brussatis F, Hahn K (eds) Nuklearmedizin in der Orthopädie. Springer, Berlin Heidelberg New York, pp 1–14
13. Subramanian G, McAffee JG, Bell EG et al (1972) ^{99m}Tc-labeled polyphosphate as a skeletal imaging agent. Radiology 102:701–704
14. Alazraki N (1988) Radionuclide technics. In: Resnick D, Niwayama G (eds) Diagnosis of bone and joint disorders, 2nd edn. Saunders, Philadelphia, pp 460–505
15. Davis MA, Jones AG (1976) Comparison of ^{99m}Tc-labeled phosphate and phosphonate agents for skeletal imaging. Semin Nucl Med 6:19–31

^{201}Tl, ^{99m}Tc-MIBI, and Others

H. S. Bom and J. Lee

^{201}Tl

Mechanism of Uptake

^{201}Tl chloride has biological properties similar to potassium chloride in most biological systems [1-4]. It has been postulated that at least two transport systems, ATPase sodium potassium pump and cotransport system, are involved in the uptake of ^{201}Tl by tumor cells. It is thought that the cotransport system involving transport of potassium and sodium as well as chloride ions into the cell plays a dominant role in the ^{201}Tl uptake by tumor cells [5]. The extent of ^{201}Tl uptake is closely related to tumor viability [6] and cell type [7]. In a review of ^{201}Tl applications in clinical oncology Waxman [8] summarized the factors thought to affect ^{201}Tl uptake by tumor cells: blood flow, ATPase sodium potassium pump, chloride cotransport system, calcium ion channel, and leakage of immature tumor blood vessel.

Techniques of Imaging

The usual dose of ^{201}Tl imaging for lung tumor is 74-111 MBq. Some investigators prefer larger doses to render clear visualization of tumor [9, 10]. However, the administrative dose is often determined under the radiation safety regulations of the individual hospital.

The optimum time for tumor imaging with ^{201}Tl has been studied by Sehweil et al. [11], who found the initial uptake curves of tumor and myocardium are similar. The highest tumor-to-background ratio is achieved between 11 and 20 min after intravenous injection, and imaging can be performed after 20-60 min because there are minimal changes in tumor-to-background ratio during this time. Some investigators prefer early (15 min) or late (3 h) static images after injection of ^{201}Tl to dynamic imaging [9]. The ratio of tumor to normal lung uptake on both early and late images are calculated from region of interests over tumor and contralateral normal lung. The retention index is calculated as follows: retention index=[(delayed ratio-early ratio)/early ratio]×100. A higher uptake ratio and retention index indicate malignancy [9]. Because the blood-pool activity decreases with time, and the tumor/background contrast improves, Tonami et al. [12] recommend delayed ^{201}Tl imaging after 3 h for assessing mediastinal lymph node metastases from lung cancer.

^{99m}Tc-MIBI

Mechanism of Uptake

^{99m}Tc-MIBI uptake in myocardium is proportional to blood flow and comparable to that of ^{201}Tl. Whether ^{99m}Tc-MIBI can serve as a substitute for ^{201}Tl for oncological applications is still under trial. The cellular uptake of ^{99m}Tc-MIBI is related mainly to its lipophilicity and charge distribution [13]. The subcellular site of ^{99m}Tc-MIBI retention is the mitochondrion. Extraction appears to depend both upon the transmembrane potential difference developed by tumors and upon mitochondrial density [13–15]. Tissue viability and vascular permeability may also be related to ^{99m}Tc-MIBI uptake in tumor cells [8]. Recently Piwnica-Worms found that ^{99m}Tc-MIBI is a suitable transport substrate of the 170-kDa p-glycoprotein (Pgp), which is an integral plasma membrane lipoprotein encoded by the human multidrug resistant (*MDR*) gene, and 190-kDa multidrug resistance associated protein (MRP) [16, 17]. Therefore ^{99m}Tc-MIBI uptake is related to multidrug resistance.

Sites of normal uptake in both ^{201}Tl and ^{99m}Tc-MIBI include the salivary glands, thyroid, heart, liver, intestines, and kidneys. With ^{201}Tl there is more relative uptake in the muscles than with ^{99m}Tc-MIBI. There is no bone marrow uptake in either, although minimal uptake may be seen with ^{99m}Tc-MIBI [18].

Techniques of Imaging

The dose of ^{99m}Tc-MIBI is usually 740 MBq. As in ^{201}Tl imaging, imaging may be either early (15 min or 1 h) or late (3 h), and the uptake ratio and the retention index can be calculated from either early or late images. Higher uptake ratios or retention indices is a predictive prognostic factor for response to chemotherapy in small-cell lung cancer patients [19, 20].

[^{111}In-DTPA-D-Phe1]Octreotide

Octreotide, an analogue of somatostatin, is eight amino acids long and has been shown to bind to somatostatin receptors on both tumorous and nontumorous tissues. Because of its relatively long effective half-life, [^{111}In-DTPA-D-Phe1]octreotide can be used to visualize somatostatin receptor bearing tumors efficiently after 24 and 48 h, when interfering background radioactivity is minimized by renal clearance. The usual dose of ^{111}In-octreotide is 185–259 MBq [21].

^{99m}Tc-Pentavalent DMSA

When the dimercaptosuccinic acid (DMSA) is labeled with ^{99m}Tc at an alkali pH and low concentration of SnCl$_2$, it is postulated that the radiotracer obtained holds a pentavalent Tc core and differs from the well-known renal cortical scanning agent [22, 23]. Recently a simple method for preparing ^{99m}Tc-pentavalent DMSA [^{99m}Tc-(V)DMSA] from a commercially available DMSA kit has been used in clinics. The accumulation of ^{99m}Tc-(V)DMSA is observed to accumulate in the medullary carcinoma of thyroid, head and neck tumors, and bone and soft tissue tumors [24, 25]. It has also been applied to target lung cancer. The mechanism responsible for tumoral accumulation is not well understood but is believed to be associated with the volume of blood flow in the lesion, increased protein and phosphate metabolism, pH of the tumors, and tumoral calcification. ^{99m}Tc-(V)DMSA imaging is performed 2–4 h after intravenous injection of 370–740 MBq. One of the drawbacks in ^{99m}Tc-(V)DMSA images is high blood-pool activity in the heart and major vascular structures due to slow blood-pool clearance.

Immunoscintigraphy with Anti-CEA Antibody

Radiolabeled monoclonal antibody to lung cancer tumor-associated antigen provides an attractive new imaging vehicle for cancer detection. Various monoclonal antibodies to carcinoembryonic antigen were labeled with ^{99m}Tc [26, 27] or ^{111}In [28, 29], and were successfully imaged lung tumors. ^{99m}Tc imaging should be done within one day, while ^{111}In imaging can be delayed over several days. The usual dose of ^{99m}Tc is 500–1100 MBq, and of ^{111}In is 150–200 MBq.

References

1. Gehring PJ, Hammond PB (1967) The interrelationship between thallium and potassium in animals. J Pharmacol Exp Ther 155:187–201
2. Lebowitz E, Greene MW, Fairchild R et al (1975) Thallium-201 for medical use, I. J Nucl Med 16:151–155
3. Bradley-Moore PR, Lebowitz E, Greene MW, Atkins HL, Ansari AN (1975) Thallium-201 for medical use. II. Biological behavior. J Nucl Med 16:156–160
4. Atkins HL, Budinger TF, Lebowitz E et al (1977) Thallum-201 for medical use. III. human distribution and physical imaging properties. J Nucl Med 18:133–140
5. Sessler MJ, Geck P, Maul FD et al (1986) New aspects of cellular Tl-201 uptake Tl$^+$Na$^+$-2Cl$^-$ cotransport is the central mechanism of ion uptake. Nuklearmedizin 25:24–27
6. Ando A, Ando I, Katayama M et al (1987) Biodistribution of Tl-201 in tumor bearing animals and inflammatory lesion induced animals. Eur J Nucl Med 12:567–572
7. Waxman AD, Ramanna L, Eller D (1991) Characterization of lymphoma grade using thallium (Tl) and gallium (Ga) scintigraphy. J Nucl Med 32:917–918 (Abstract)
8. Waxman AD (1996) Thallium-201 and technetium-99m methoxyisobutyl isonitrile (MIBI) in nuclear oncology. In: Sandler MP, Coleman RE, Wackers FJT, Patton JA, Gottschalk A, Hoffer PB (eds) Diagnostic nuclear medicine, 3rd edn. Williams and Wilkins, Baltimore, pp 1261–1274
9. Tonami N (1993) Diagnosis of tumor with thallium-201. Kaku Igaku 30:449–55
10. Tonami N, Shuke N, Kunihilo Y et al (1989) Use of thallium-201 single photon emission computed tomography in the evaluation of suspected lung cancer. J Nucl Med 30:997–1004
11. Sehweil A, McKillop JH, Ziada G, Al-Sayed M, Abdel-Dayem H, Omar YT (1988) The optimum time for tumor imaging with thallium-201. Eur J Nucl Med 13:527–529

12. Tonami N, Yokoyama K, Taki J et al (1991) Tl-201 SPECT in the detection of mediastinal lymph node metastases from lung cancer. Nucl Med Commun 12:779–792
13. Maublant JC, Gachon P, Moins N (1988) Hexakis (2-methoxy isobutylisonitrile) technetium-99m and thallium-201 chloride: uptake and release in cultured myocardial cells. J Nucl Med 29:48–54
14. Chiu ML, Kornauge JF, Piwnica-Worms D (1990) Effect of mitrochondrial and plasma membrane potentials on accumulation of hexakis (2-methoxyisobutylisonitrile) technetium (I) in cultured mouse fibroblasts. J Nucl Med 31:1646–1653
15. Delmon-Moingeon LI, Piwnica-Worms D, Van den Abbeele AD, Holman BL, Davison A, Jones AG (1990) Uptake of the cation hexakis (2-methoxyisobutylisonitrile)-technetium-99m by human carcinoma cell lines in vitro. Cancer Res 50:2198–2202
16. Piwnica-Worms D, Chiu ML, Budding J et al (1993) Functional imaging of multidrug-resistant P-glycoprotein with an organiotechnetium complex. Cancer Res 53:977–984
17. Crankshaw C, Piwnica-Worms D (1996) Tc-99m sestamibi may be a transport substrate of the human multidrug resistance-associated protein (MRP). J Nucl Med 37:247P (abstract)
18. Abdel-Dayem HM, Scott AM, Macapinlac HA, El-Gazzar AH, Larson SM (1994) Role of Tl-201 chloride and Tc-99m sestamibi in tumor imaging. In: Freeman LM (ed) Nuclear medicine annals. Raven, New York, pp 181–234
19. Bom HS, Kim YC, Song HC, Kim JY, Park KO (1996) Tc-99m sestamibi uptake in small cell lung cancer: a predictor of response to chemotherapy (abstract). J Nucl Med 37:67P
20. Yamamoto Y, Nishiyama Y, Fukynaga K, Satoh K, Takashima H, Tanabe M (1996) Evaluation of Tc-99m MIBI to predict chemotherapeutic response of patients with small cell lung cancer (abstract). Ann Nucl Med 10 [Suppl]:S137
21. Krenning EP, Kwekkeboom DJ, Reubi JC, Lamberts SW (1994) Somatostatin receptor scintigraphy with [In-111-DTPA-D-Phe1] octreotide. In: Murray IPC, Ell PJ (eds) Nuclear medicine in clinical diagnosis and treatment. Churchill Livingston, New York, pp 757–764
22. Yokoyama A, Saji H, Horiuchi K et al (1985) The design of a pentavalent Tc-99m-dimercaptosuccinate complex as a tumor imaging agent. Int J Nucl Med 12:273
23. Blower PJ, Singh J, Clarke SEM (1991) The chemical identity of pentavalent technetium-99m-dimercaptosuccinic acid. J Nucl Med 32:845–849
24. Endo K, Ohta H, Torizuka K et al (1987) Technetium-99m (V)-DMSA in the imaging of medullary thyroid carcinoma. J Nucl Med 28:252–253
25. Watkinson JC, Lazarus CR, Mistry R et al (1989) Technetium-99m (V)dimercaptosuccinic acid uptake in patients with head and neck squamous carcinoma. Experience in imaging. J Nucl Med 30:174–180
26. Morris JF, Krishnamurthy S, Antonovic R, Duncan C, Turner FE, Krishnamurthy GT (1991) Technetium-99m monoclonal antibody fragment (Fab) scintigraphy in the evaluation of small cell lung cancer: a preliminary report. Int J Rad Appl Instrum B 18:613–20
27. Kramer EL, Noz ME, Liebes L, Murthy S, Tiu S, Goldenberg DM (1994) Radioimmunodetection of non-small cell lung cancer using technetium-99m-anticarcinoembryonic antigen IMMU-4 Fab' fragment. Preliminary results. Cancer 73 [3 Suppl]:890–895
28. Biggi A, Buccheri G, Ferrigno D et al (1991) Detection of suspected primary lung cancer by scintigraphy with indium-111-anti-carcinoembryonic antigen monoclonal antibodies (type Fo23C5). J Nucl Med 32:2064–2068
29. Buccheri G, Biggi A, Ferrigno D, Leone A, Taviani M, Quaranta M (1993) Anti-CEA immunoscintigraphy might be more useful than computed tomography in the preoperative thoracic evaluation of lung cancer. A comparison between planar immunoscintigraphy, single photon emission computed tomography (SPECT), and computed tomography. Chest 104:734–742

Other Techniques

E. E. KIM

Scintimammography and Mammary Lymphoscintigraphy

Several radionuclide imaging techniques have been reported with various radiopharmaceuticals for detecting breast cancer and differentiating benign and malignant breast masses [9]. ^{201}Tl chloride is a myocardial perfusion agent that was first used for breast imaging. ^{201}Tl enters into viable cells using the sodium-potassium pump mechanism [18]. ^{201}Tl is produced by a cyclotron and decays by electron capture, with a half-life of 73 h. A cluster of characteristic X-rays between 69 and 83 keV (94%) are emitted.

^{99m}Tc-sestamibi (MIBI) is a lipophilic cationic complex which accumulates in myocardial tissue in proportion to regional blood flow. It has been very useful in localizing parathyroid adenomas and other tumors, including breast cancer [17]. The exact mechanism of ^{99m}Tc-MIBI uptake is not clearly understood. Approximately 90% of the activity is localized in the mitochondria and the cytoplasm in response to elevated membrane potentials. As with other agents, an adequate blood flow is essential for its delivery to the tumor.

^{99m}Tc-methylene diphophorate (MDP) is a bone scan agent, and its extraskeletal uptake has been observed in various tumors, including breast cancer. The mechanism of its uptake in tumors is unclear, but multiple factors have been postulated. These include increased vascularity, inflammatory changes, modification of local metabolism, collagen deposits, cell membrane damage, and microcalcification [13]. There is no binding of ^{99m}Tc-MDP to tumor cells. Scintimammography using ^{99m}Tc-MDP is an inexpensive study that can be carried out during routine bone scanning.

On the side opposite to that of the known breast lesion 3 or 4 mCi ^{201}Tl or 20–25 mCi ^{99m}Tc-MIBI or MDP is administered intravenously in the arm. Imaging is performed 10 min after injection of ^{99m}Tc-MDP or 5 min after injection of ^{201}Tl or ^{99m}Tc-MIBI. The 10 min anterior image is taken in an upright position with the patient's arms raised for depiction of the axillae and with the face turned away from the side of the known breast lesion. Lateral imaging must be performed in the prone position for 10 min. A plastic table overlay allows the breast being imaged to be freely dependent upon the imaging table without compression but with the force of gravity. A thick styrofoam sheet with two halfmoon-shaped cutouts on each side is laid on the imaging table after installing a 4-mm lead sheet in the midline for both lateral views while the patient is in the prone position [9, 14].

[^{18}F]fluoro-2-deoxyglucose (FDG) is a glucose analog and the most widely used positron radiopharmaceutical in oncology. It is used to monitor the effects of preoperative chemotherapy in patients with locally advanced breast cancer [1]. [^{18}F]fluorotamoxifen also provides useful information for predicting the effect of tamoxifen therapy in patients with estrogen-receptor positive breast cancer [6]. The details about the agents and techniques for positron emission tomography (PET) are in Chap. 3. For mammary lymphoscintigraphy, four injections (each injection contains 0.25–0.5 mCi of ^{99m}Tc-colloids in 0.05–0.1 ml) are usually made into and surrounding the primary breast cancer. Images are recorded immediately and 2–2.5 h using a gamma-camera [16].

SPECT and PET

In contrast to morphological imaging methods, positron emission tomography (PET) produces images that reflect the physiological and biochemical processes of tissues. The most widely used PET radiopharmaceutical is [^{18}F]FDG, which evaluates the glucose metabolic rate of tissues. Because most tumors show high glycolytic rates, FDG is suitable for recurrent active tumors and also monitoring of responses to therapy. FDG is produced by proton irradiation of enriched ^{18}O water in a small-volume titanium target using cyclotron. Under sterile conditions 2-deoxy-D-glucose is labeled with ^{18}F to produce [^{18}F]FDG by the Hamacher method using an automated system [7].

Prior to a PET study patients fast for at least 4 h, at which time normal blood glucose levels are confirmed. PET is performed with a dedicated scanner with multislices, and the reconstructed imaging data acquired with wobling detectors at 40–60 min following the injection of 5–10 mCi [^{18}F]FDG are analyzed by visual inspection and compared to standard uptake values (FDG uptake activity/injected dose/body weight). The standard uptake values of the peak activity in the lesion are usually obtained from the color-coded images.

^{67}Ga Scan

Gallium is a group III element similar to ferric ion. ^{67}Ga is cyclotron produced by bombardment of ^{68}Zn and decays by electron capture. It has a physical half-life of 78 h and emits a complex spectrum of gamma rays ranging from 91 to 391 keV. The lower two or three photopeaks (approximately 100, 200, and 300 keV) are used for imaging. After intravenous injection ^{67}Ga-citrate binds to serum transferrin. It does not interact with protoporphyrins to form heme since it cannot be reduced from its +3 oxidation state. Approximately 20% is excreted by kidneys within 24 h, and its clearance is slow (biological half-life, 25 days) with the colon being the major route of excretion. ^{67}Ga-citrate localizes intracellularly within normal liver, lacrimal and salivary glands, spleen, bone marrow, and bone after binding to transferrin and lactoferrin. Saturation of transferrin with iron overload from repeated transfusion alters the biodistribution, with less hepatic and greater renal uptakes. ^{67}Ga-citrate enters the tumor's extracellular fluid space via the tumor's beaky capillary endothelium. It is also bound to the tumor cell surface by transferrin receptors and then transported into the cell. It localizes intracellularly in the lysosomes of tumor cells and is taken up by actively growing and viable tumors [4].

Larger doses (8–10 mCi) of ^{67}Ga-citrate are administered for tumor imaging than for an infection or inflammation scan. With 10 mCi the large bowel receives about 9.0 cGy, the spleen and bone marrow 5–6 cGy, and the total body 2.6 cGy. Although 500 000 counts per view may be adequate for routine whole-body imaging, higher count images should be obtained with organs of normally high uptake out of the field of view, generally at 48 and 72 h. SPECT should be performed routinely for areas of clinical concern or interest [5]. Because chemotherapy can affect biodistribution of ^{67}Ga-citrate, it is recommended that there be a 3- to 6-week interval from the last complete course of therapy.

Leukocyte Scan

Leukocytes labeled with ^{111}In have been used in the diagnosis of inflammatory disease. Leukocytes are harvested from whole blood and prepared for labeling using the technique modified from that developed by McAffee and Thakur [3]. Studies in leukopenic patients are performed using white cells obtained from ABO-compatible normal donors. In most cases relatively pure granulocyte suspensions are prepared by double-density gradient centrifugation as used in granulocyte kinetic studies [2]. For adult patients 0.3–0.5 mCi ^{111}In-labeled leukocytes are administered by intravenous injection, and imaging is routinely performed approximately 4–6 and 18–24 h after injection, typically including whole-body scans and camera views of selected areas of interest. Each camera image contains 100 000 counts.

The kinetics and distribution of leukocytes labeled with ^{99m}Tc-hexamethylpropylene amine oxime are similar to those of ^{111}In-labeled leukocytes except for nonspecific activity in urine, kidneys, gallbladder, and bowel [12].

Esophageal Scintigraphy

Techniques of nuclear medicine permit the noninvasive evaluation of altered esophageal physiology [11]. Variations in technique allow measurement of the transit time of a single bolus, clearance of a meal, and degree of gastroesophageal reflux. These procedures are useful for detecting early esophageal dysfunction and may assist in defining the specific disorder. Computer-assisted quantification provides an objective method for determining the severity of the dysfunction, assessing the response to therapy, and monitoring the progression of the disease.

Solid (or semisolid) esophageal emptying studies are usually performed in patients with dysphasia [10]. A variety of foods may be radiolabeled with 100–300 μCi ^{99m}Tc-sulfur colloid, which is widely available, nonabsorbable, and relatively acid stable. Other nonabsorbable radiopharmaceuticals, such as ^{99m}Tc-DTPA, would also be satisfactory. The patient usually sits against the camera during ingestion of the meal and for 15–20 min thereafter. Continuous recording permits visual assessment of the speed of emptying, and analysis of activity within regions of interest selected over the esophagus and stomach allows quantification of the data. The percentage of esophageal retention (%ER) is typically made at 1, 5, 10, 15, and 20 min after the meal, using the following equation: $\%ER_t = (E_t/E_1 + G_1) \times 100$, where E_t is counts within the esophagus at time t, and E_1 and G_1 are counts within the esophagus and stomach, respectively, at 1 min after completion of the meal. In normal individuals there is rapid emptying of the esophagus, with less than 5% esophageal retention at 1 min after completion of the meal and a further decline to less than 1% by 20 min.

Esophageal function may also be evaluated by studying the transit of a single swallow of a liquid bolus. A quantity of 10–15 ml water containing 100–300 µCi ^{99m}Tc-sulfur colloid is placed into the mouth of the patient, who is positioned supine beneath a large field-of-view gamma-camera. The patient is instructed to swallow on command, and rapid sequential images (two per s) are acquired for approximately 1 min. Additional 15-s frames may be acquired for up to 10 min. Region-of-interest indications placed over the esophagus allow generation of a variety of indices of the esophageal transit. The percentage clearance can be calculated as follows: $[(E_{max} - E_t) \times 100]/E_{max}$, where E_{max} represents the maximum counts in the esophagus and E_t represents the esophageal counts at time t. In normal volunteers esophageal clearance is rapid, with less than 10% of the activity remaining in the esophagus 15 s after the swallow.

Acidification of the administered material facilitates the detection of gastroesophageal reflux, probably due to lowering the resting pressure of lower esophageal sphincter [15]. The currently recommended liquid test meal consists of a total volume of 300 ml, which includes a mixture of 150 ml orange juice and 150 ml 0.1 N HCl that contains up to 300 µCi ^{99m}Tc-sulfur colloid. ^{99m}Tc-pertechnetate, when administered orally, is rapidly absorbed from the gastrointestinal tract and actively secreted by the salivary glands. Detection of mucosal tracer accumulation by Barett's epithelium after intravenous administration of 10 µCi ^{99m}Tc-pertechnetate has been suggested as a potentially useful test [8].

References

1. Bassa P, Kim EE, Inoue T, Wong FCL, Korkmaz M, Yang DJ, Wong W-H, Hicks KW, Buzdar AU, Podoloff DA (1996) Evaluation of preoperative chemotherapy using PET with F-18 fluorodeoxyglucose in breast cancer. J Nucl Med 37:931–938
2. Datz FL (1994) In-111 labeled leukocytes for the detection of infection: current status. Semin Nucl Med 24:92–109
3. Datz FL, Morton KA (1991) Radionuclide detection of occult infection. Current strategies. Cancer Invest 9:691–698
4. Front D, Israel O (1995) The role of Ga-67 scintigraphy in evaluating the results of therapy of lymphoma patients. Semin Nucl Med 25:60–71
5. Front D, Israel O, Epelbaum R (1990) Gallium-67 SPECT before and after treatment of lymphoma. Radiology 175:515–521

6. Inoue T, Kim EE, Wallace S, Yang DJ, Wong FCL, Bassa P, Cherif A, Delpassand E, Buzdar A, Podoloff DA (1966) Positron emission tomography using F-18 fluoro-tamoxifen to evaluate therapeutic responses in patients with breast cancer. Cancer Biother Radiopharm 11:235–245

7. Inoue T, Kim EE, Komaki R, Wong FCL, Bassa P, Wong W-H, Yang DJ, Endo K, Podoloff DA (1995) Detecting recurrent or residual lung cancer with FDG-PET. J Nucl Med 36:788–793

8. Karvelis KC, Drane WE, Johnson DA, Silverman ED (1987) Barret's esophagus: decreased esophageal clearance shown by radionuclide esophageal scintigraphy. Radiology 162:97–99

9. Khalkhali I, Cutrone JA, Mena IG, Diggles LE, Venegas RJ, Vargas HI, Jackson BL, Khalkhali S, Moss JF, Klein SR (1995) Scintimammography: the complementary role of Tc-99m sestamibi prone breast imaging for the diagnosis of breast carcinoma. Radiology 196:421–426

10. Klein HA (1995) Esophageal transit scintigraphy. Semin Nucl Med 25:306–317

11. Parkman HP, Miller MA, Fisher RS (1995) Role of nuclear medicine in evaluating patients with suspected gastrointestinal motility disorders. Semin Nucl Med 25: 289–305

12. Peters AM (1994) The utility of Tc-99m HMPAO-leukocytes for imaging infection. Semin Nucl Med 24:110–127

13. Piccolo S, Lastoria S, Mainolfi C, Muto P, Bazzicalupo L, Salvatore M (1995) Tc-99m methylene diphosphonate scintimammography to image primary breast cancer. J Nucl Med 36:718–724

14. Taillefer R, Robidoux A, Lambert R, Turpin S, Laperriere J (1995) Tc-99m sestamibi prone scintimammography to detect primary breast cancer and axillary lymph node involvement. J Nucl Med 36:1758–1765

15. Urbain J-L, Charkes ND (1995) Recent advances in gastric emptying scintigraphy. Semin Nucl Med 25:318–325

16. Uren RF, Howman-Giles RB, Thompson JF, Malouf D, Ramsey-Stewart G, Niesche FW, Renwick SB (1995) Mammary lymphoscintigraphy in breast cancer. J Nucl Med 36:1775–1780

17. Villanueva-Meyer J, Leonard MH, Cesani BF, Ali SA, Rhoden S, Hove M, Cowan D (1996) Mammoscintigraphy with Tc-99m sestamibi in suspected breast cancer. J Nucl Med 37:926–930

18. Waxman AD, Ramanna L, Memsic LD (1993) Thallium scintigraphy in the evaluation of mass abnormalities of the breast. J Nucl Med 34:18–23

Clinical
Applications

4 Ventilation/Perfusion Scan in the Diagnosis of Acute Pulmonary Embolism

D. F. WORSLEY and C. K. KIM

Introduction

Pulmonary embolism (PE) is a relatively common and potentially fatal disorder, for which treatment is highly effective and improves patients' survival. The accurate and expeditious diagnosis of acute PE can be difficult because of nonspecific clinical, laboratory, and radiographic findings [26, 48]. In 1975 it was estimated that 600 000 cases of PE occur in the United States annually and approximately 10% of patients with PE die within 1 h of the event [5]. For those who survive beyond the 1st h following PE, anticoagulation with heparin or thrombolytic agents is an effective therapy [1, 5]. Mortality in patients with PE who are not treated has been reported to be as high as 30% [5]. In contrast, correct diagnosis and appropriate therapy significantly lowers mortality to between 2.5% and 8% [1, 2]. Although anticoagulant therapy is effective in treating PE and reducing mortality, it is not without some risk. The prevalence of major hemorrhagic complications has been reported to be as high as 10%–15% among patients receiving anticoagulant therapy [23, 25]. One study found heparin to be responsible for the majority of drug-related deaths in noncritically ill hospital patients [28]. Accurate diagnosis of PE is therefore essential not only to prevent excessive mortality but also to avoid complications related to unnecessary anticoagulant therapy.

The ventilation/perfusion (V/Q) lung scan has been shown to be a safe noninvasive technique to evaluate regional pulmonary perfusion and ventilation. The technique has been widely used in the evaluation of patients with suspected PE. Perfusion scintigraphy is sensitive but not specific for diagnosing PE. Virtually all parenchymal lung diseases (including tumors, infections, chronic obstructive pulmonary disease, or asthma) can cause decreased pulmonary arterial blood flow within the affected lung zone. Consequently shortly after the introduction of perfusion scintigraphy Wagner et al. [45] and DeNardo et al. [7] combined ventilation and perfusion scintigraphy to improve the specificity for diagnosing PE. The pathological basis for combining ventilation and perfusion scintigraphy is that PE characteristically causes abnormal perfusion with preserved ventilation (mismatched defects; Fig. 4.1, 4.2), whereas parenchymal lung disease generally causes both ventilation and perfusion abnormalities in the same lung region (matched defects; Fig. 4.3).

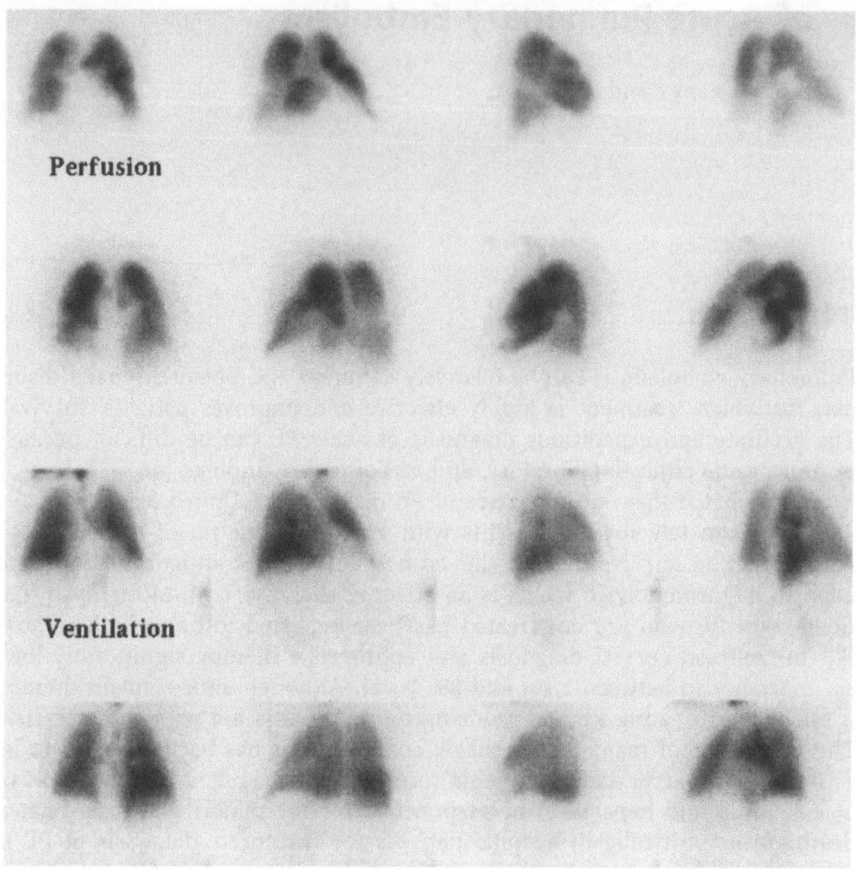

Fig. 4.1. A case of PE. Perfusion images (*top two rows*) show multiple wedge-shaped defects in both lungs, whereas ventilation (*bottom two rows*) is only mildly heterogeneous without segmental defects

Pleural effusion, acute or chronic airway obstuction, mucous plug, atelectasis, and pneumonia often cause a ventilation abnormality significantly worse than the perfusion abnormality (reverse mismatch) [3]. Some of these conditions may coexist. In these conditions the ventilation scan may show virtual absence of activity in the affected area, and perfusion can be decreased to a much lesser degree or near normal (Fig. 4.4–4.6). In patients with atelectasis or pneumonia, positive pressure respiratory support can even cause higher perfusion in the affected lobes than in the rest of the lung [20, 47]. Patients with metabolic alkalosis or limited pulmonary vascular and those treated with inhaled albuterol may also experience failure or inhibition of hypoxic pulmonary vasoconstriction which results in reverse mismatch. Perfusion images from patients with thrombophlebitis and from those in whom too few particles have been injected show an inhomogenous distribu-

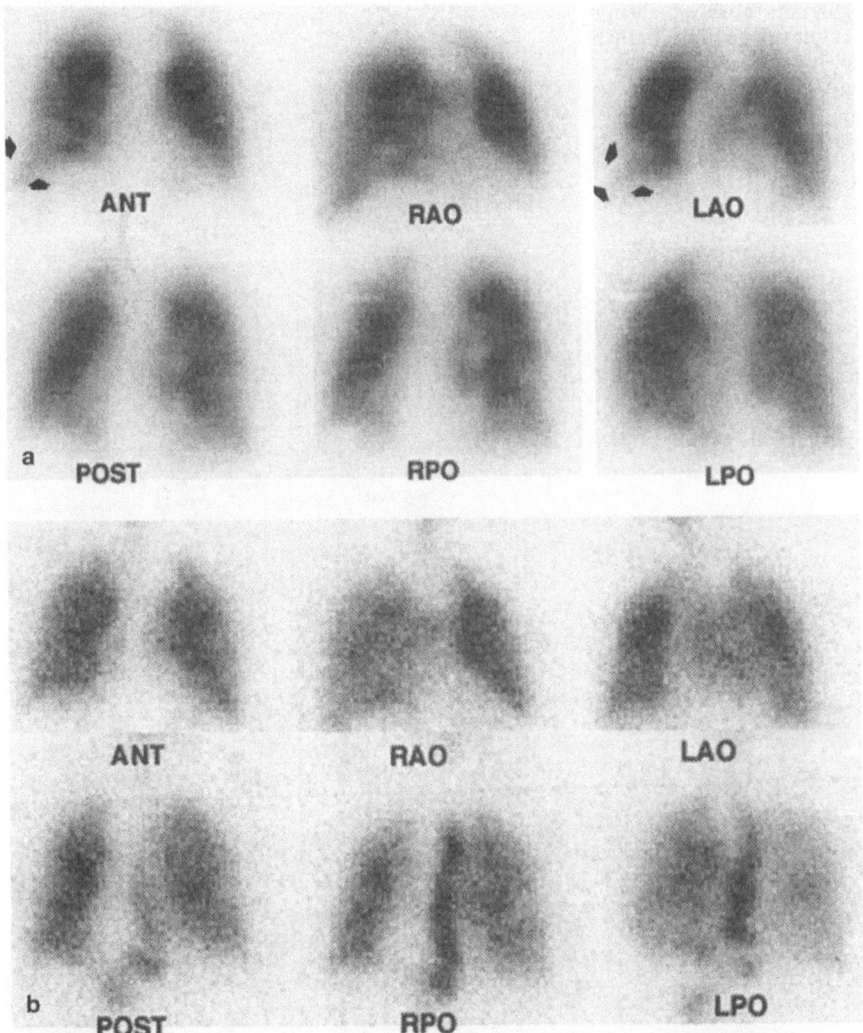

Fig. 4.2 a–b. Perfusion (**a**) and ventilation (**b**) images show a mismatched defect (*arrows*) in the lateral segment of the right middle lobe

tion of activity with focal hot spots in both lungs (Fig. 4.7). Alternatively, injection of large particles or blood clots may also yield a similar pattern within the lungs.

Despite studies suggesting the underdiagnosis of PE, critics have suggested that V/Q scanning is overutilized and has minimal impact on patient management [14, 30, 31]. The first large-scale study using perfusion lung scanning as a screening test for the diagnosis of PE was the Urokinase Pul-

Fig. 4.2 c. Subsequent angiogram (**c**) shows abrupt
cutoff (*arrow*) in a branch
of the right middle lobe
pulmonary artery

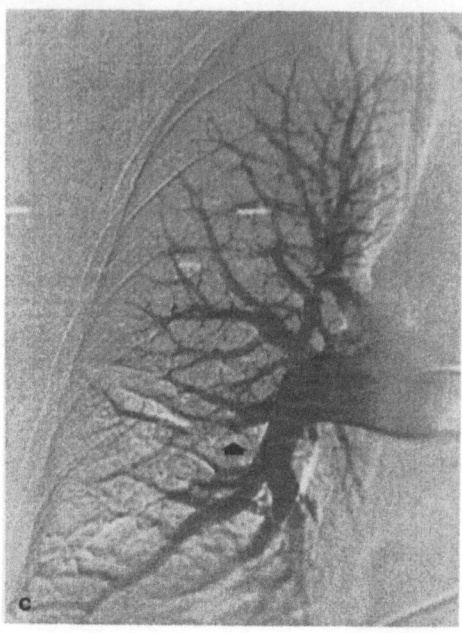

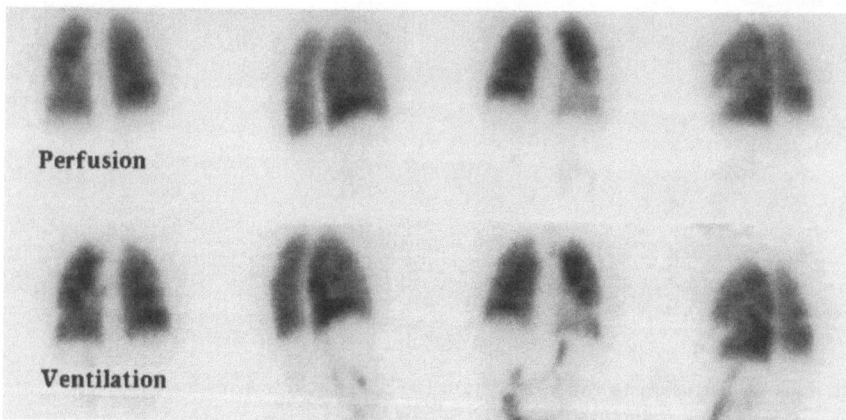

Fig. 4.3. A lung scan of a patient with known sarcoidosis shows moderately heterogeneous perfusion and ventilation with multiple, small defects (matched)

monary Embolism Trial (UPET). In more than 90% of the patients perfusion
lung scanning was performed following the intravenous administration of
^{131}I-labeled macroaggregated albumin. Perfusion scanning was carried out
with rectilinear scanner, and therefore no ventilation imaging was performed. Despite the use of radiopharmaceuticals and instrumentation that
would be judged as suboptimal by today's standards, this study established

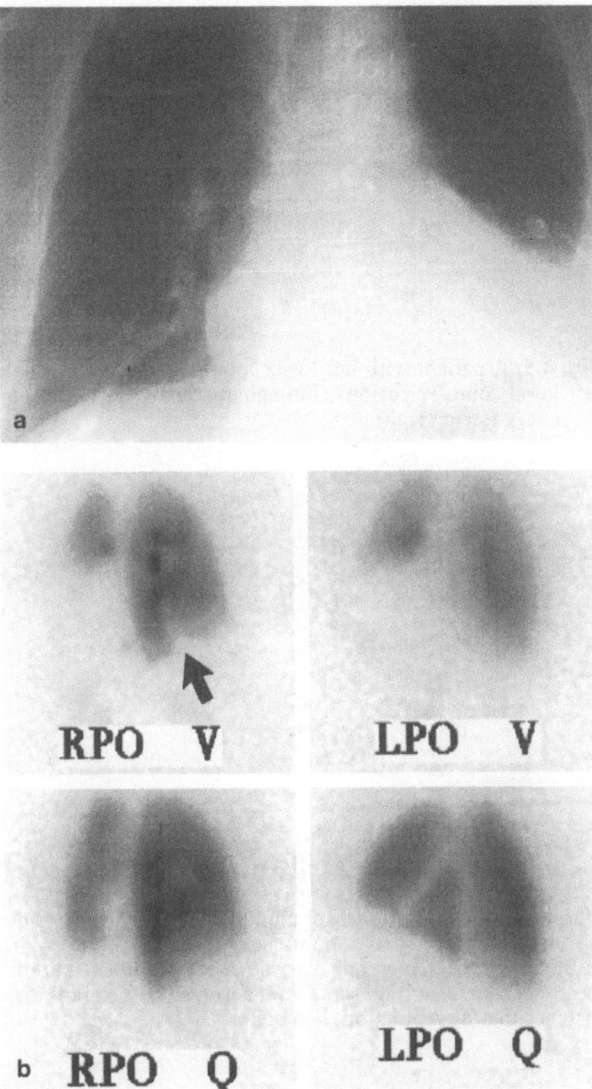

Fig. 4.4a. Chest radiograph shows pleural effusion in the left chest and atelectasis in the right lung base. **b** Selected ventilation images show lack of activity in the left lower lobe and a small defect in the right base (*arrow*). Perfusion is significantly better than ventilation both in the left lower lobe and in the right base, although the left lower lobe appears small with a photopenic defect along the left major fissure due to pleural effusion

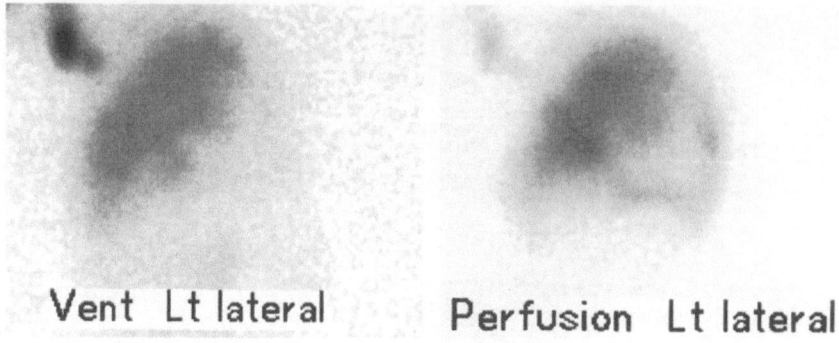

Vent Lt lateral   Perfusion Lt lateral

Fig. 4.5. A patient with left lower lobe pneumonia. Ventilation is almost absent in the left lower lobe. Perfusion, although markedly decreased, is noted, particularly in the periphery (stripe sign)

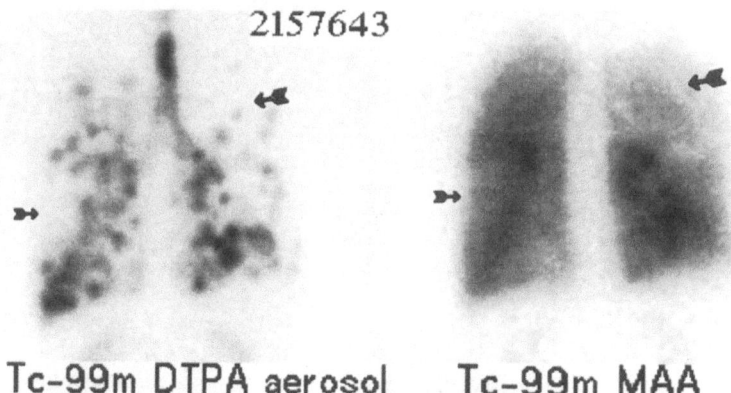

2157643

Tc-99m DTPA aerosol   Tc-99m MAA

Fig. 4.6. Marked radioaerosol clumping is noted throughout the lungs, which is typical of chronic obstructive pulmonary disease. There is particularly decreased activity in the right upper lung and lateral aspect of the left middle lung. Perfusion is moderately decreased in the same areas (*arrows*). Overall the distribution of perfusion matches that of ventilation, but better

perfusion lung scanning as an effective technique both for the diagnosis of PE and for assessing restoration of pulmonary blood flow following an embolic event [43].

Most patients with acute PE either completely lyse their thrombus or partially recanalize their pulmonary arteries. Approximately 75%–80% of perfusion defects in the UPET study resolved by 3 months. Perfusion defects which did not resolve by 3 months were generally still present at 1-year follow-up. However, the proportion of clot resolution observed in the UPET is likely an underestimate, since ventilation scanning was not performed. It is likely that many of the unresolved perfusion defects were due to preexisting chronic obstructive lung disease rather than persistent PE. Therefore,

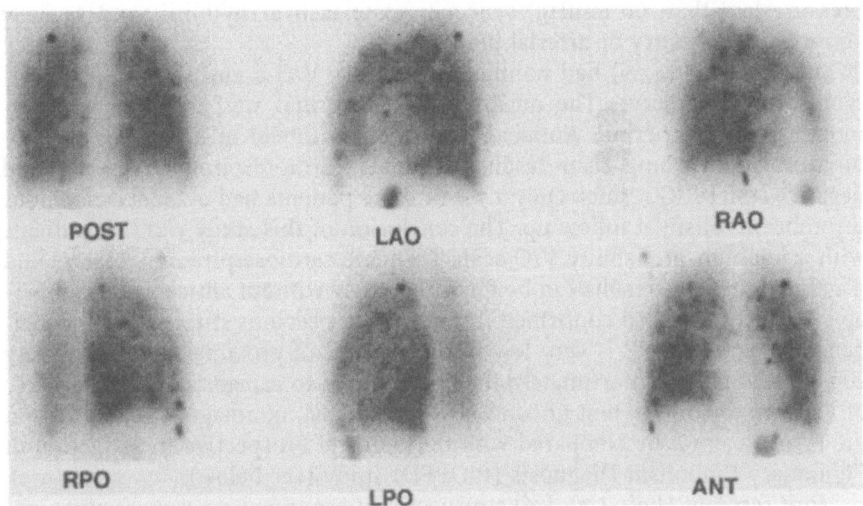

Fig. 4.7. The patient had a partially infiltrated injection of ^{99m}Tc-labeled macroaggregated albumin. Consequently only a fraction of the particle made it to the lungs, which resulted in an inhomogenous distribution of activity with focal hot spots within both lungs. A repeat scan (not shown) following a second injection demonstrated a normal distribution of activity

although chronic thromboembolism is a well-documented cause of a false-positive high probability V/Q scan interpretation, the overall diagnostic performance of the V/Q scan does not appear to be affected by the past history of venous thromboembolism [53]. Based on the data from the UPET we nevertheless still recommend performing a repeat perfusion lung scan approximately 3 months following the initial diagnosis of PE to evaluate clot resolution and to serve as a baseline for future comparisons.

Three large studies using modern imaging agents and instrumentation have reported more recent data on the efficacy of V/Q scanning in patients suspected of having acute PE [15, 16, 27]. A prospective study by Hull et al. [15] enrolled 874 patients suspected of having PE, and V/Q scan results were grouped into three diagnostic categories; normal, nonhigh probability, and high probability (mismatch defect involving at least 75% of a segment). The purpose of the study was to determine whether anticoagulation can be withheld in patients with a nonhigh probability V/Q scan, adequate cardiorespiratory reserve, and absent proximal vein thrombosis as determined by negative serial impedance plethysmography (IPG). This diagnostic approach emphasizes the importance of the basic pathophysiological concept of venous thromboembolism as a systemic disease process and PE as merely its respiratory manifestation. High-probability and normal V/Q scans were found in 8% and 36% of patients, respectively. In 9% of patients there were nonhigh-probability V/Q scans and inadequate cardiorespiratory reserve, defined by the presence of pulmonary edema, right ventricular failure, systolic blood pressure less than 90 mmHg, syncope, acute tachyarrhythmia, and severely abnormal spirometry or arterial blood gases.

Most patients (47%) had nonhigh-probability V/Q scans and adequate cardiorespiratory reserve. The outcome in each group was assessed over a 3-month follow-up period. Anticoagulants were withheld in patients with non-high-probability lung scan results, adequate cardiorespiratory reserve, and negative serial IPG results. Only 2.7% of these patients had evidence of venous thromboembolism at follow-up. The conclusion of this study was that patients with a nonhigh-probability V/Q scan, adequate cardiorespiratory reserve, and negative serial IPG results can be managed safely without anticoagulation therapy. These results also confirmed findings from previous studies that the incidence of recurrent PE is very low in the absence of proximal lower extremity venous thrombus. Unfortunately, the criteria used to categorize the probability of PE were to some extent unconventional (normal, nondiagnostic, high), and the results cannot be compared with those of the Prospective Investigation of Pulmonary Embolism Diagnosis (PIOPED) study (see below).

More recently Hull et al. [16] prospectively examined 1564 consecutive patients with suspected PE who underwent both V/Q scanning and IPG of the lower extremities. In 40% of cases (627/1564) V/Q scans were interpreted as nondiagnostic and serial IPG results as negative. All of these patients had adequate cardiorespiratory reserve and were managed without anticoagulation. Using this algorithm, only 1.9% (12/627) had evidence of either deep venous thrombosis or PE on follow-up.

Prospective Investigation of Pulmonary Embolism Diagnosis Study

The most comprehensive prospective study to date addressing the role of V/Q scanning in the diagnosis of PE has been the PIOPED study [27], a multicenter study evaluating the efficacy of various conventional methods for diagnosing acute PE and in particular the sensitivity and specificity of V/Q lung scanning. In addition, the relative contributions of clinical assessment, chest radiograph, and other routine studies were assessed, and the study also provided an opportunity to assess the validity of pulmonary angiography for diagnosing acute PE and to determine the incidence of complications related to this procedure.

Clinical Diagnosis of PE

The PIOPED study found risk factors, clinical signs, and symptoms suggestive of PE to be similar in men and women [29]. Clinical findings in patients with no preexisting cardiac or pulmonary disease were evaluated in a subset of PIOPED patients by Stein et al. [39], including 117 patients with PE and 248 patients in whom PE was excluded. The prevalence of immobilization (strict bed rest for more than 3 continuous days) and surgery (incision under regional or general anesthesia) within 3 months prior to enrollment were more common in patients with PE than in those without PE [39]. The frequency of other risk factors was approximately the same regardless of the presence or absence of PE. The most common symptoms of patients with PE and no preexisting cardiac or pulmonary disease were shortness of breath, pleuritic chest pain, and cough [39]. However, the prevalence of these symptoms was not significantly different than in patients in whom PE was excluded. Shortness of breath, tachypnea, or pleuritic chest pain alone or in combination was present in 97% of patients with PE [38]. Based on this observation Stein et al. concluded that only very few patients do not have at least one of the important clinical manifestations of PE. While this statement is valid for patients evaluated in the PIOPED study, selection bias due to the study design should be taken into consideration, as the entry criteria included only patients with risk factors, signs, symptoms, or laboratory findings that were unexplained and were suggestive of acute PE. Therefore it is not surprising that very few patients had no important clinical manifestations of acute PE.

Although the clinical signs of PE are seldom diagnostic, the results of the PIOPED study emphasize the importance of incorporating the clinical assessment when evaluating patients suspected of having acute PE (Table 4.1). As expected, combining clinical assessment with V/Q scan interpretation improved the diagnostic accuracy. The prevalence of PE was only 4% in patients with low or very low probability on V/Q scan interpretation and no history of immobilization, recent surgery, trauma to the lower extremities, or central venous instrumentation [52]. On the other hand, the prevalences was 12% and 21%, respectively, in patients with low or very low probability on V/Q lung scan interpretation and one or more of the above risk factors. However, the majority of patients in the PIOPED study had intermediate-probability V/Q scans and an intermediate clinical likelihood of PE. For these patients the combination of clinical assessment and V/Q scan interpretation did not provide adequate information for patient management, and further investigations with peripheral venous studies or pulmonary angiography were usually required.

Table 4.1. Value of combining selected risk factors (immobilization, recent surgery, trauma to lower extremities, central venous instrumentation) and V/Q scan probability in determining the posttest likelihood of PE (modified from [49])

V/Q interpretation	0 risk factors		1 risk factor		2 risk factors	
	n	%	n	%	n	%
High	63/77	82	41/49	84	56/58	97
Intermediate	52/207	25	40/107	37	77/173	45
Low/very low	14/315	4	19/155	12	37/179	21
Normal	0/28	0	0/7	0	0/39	0

Table 4.2. Value of V/Q scanning in detecting acute PE (modified from [49])

V/Q Interpretation	Sensitivity	Specificity	Positive prediction
High	40%	98%	87%
High, intermediate	82%	64%	49%
High, intermediate, low	98%	12%	32%

V/Q Scan in the Diagnosis of Acute PE

The sensitivity and specificity for V/Q scanning for detecting acute PE are presented in Table 4.2. The sensitivity, specificity, and positive and negative predictive values of V/Q scanning did not differ significantly between women and men [29]; the overall diagnostic performance of the V/Q scan was also similar among patients in different age groups [37, 53]. The diagnostic utility of V/Q scanning for detecting PE was similar among those with preexisting cardiac or pulmonary disease and those without underlying cardiac or pulmonary disease [36, 53]. In a subset of patients with chronic obstructive pulmonary disease the sensitivity of V/Q scan for the diagnosis of PE (when a high-probability interpretation is considered as positive) was significantly lower than in patients without preexisting cardiopulmonary disease [22]. However, the positive predictive value of a high-probability V/Q scan interpretation was 100% and the negative predictive value of a low- or very low-probability V/Q scan interpretation was 94%.

The most common cause of V/Q mismatch in patients who did not have acute PE was related to chronic or unresolved PE; other causes included: compression of the pulmonary vasculature (mass lesions, adenopathy, mediastinal fibrosis), vessel wall abnormalities (pulmonary artery sarcoma, vasculitis), intraluminal obstruction (tumor emboli, foreign body emboli), and congenital vascular abnormalities (pulmonary artery agenesis or hypoplasia).

Interpretation Criteria and Amendments of Original PIOPED Criteria

Several diagnostic criteria, including those of McNeil, Biello, and PIOPED, have been suggested for the interpretation of V/Q lung scans. All criteria rely on determining whether perfusion defects are segmental or nonsegmental, and whether corresponding ventilation abnormalities are present. In a study comparing the various interpretation algorithms the original PIOPED criteria had the highest likelihood ratio for predicting the presence of PE on pulmonary angiography [46]. However, the PIOPED criteria also had the highest proportion of V/Q scans interpreted as representing an intermediate probability of acute PE. Several revisions of the original PIOPED criteria have been made based on the observations from the PIOPED study. Using a number these revisions makes it possible to decrease the number of intermediate

V/Q scan interpretations and to interpret them correctly as low probability of acute PE. The use of revised PIOPED criteria has already been shown to provide a more accurate assessment of angiographically confirmed PE than the original criteria [9, 35].

The modified PIOPED criteria are as follows:

- High probability
- Two or more large (>75% of a segment) segmental perfusion defects with smaller corresponding ventilation or chest-radiographic abnormalities
- One large segmental perfusion defect and more than two moderate (25%–75% of a segment) segmental perfusion defects with smaller corresponding ventilation or chest-radiographic abnormalities
- Four or more moderate segmental perfusion defects with smaller corresponding ventilation or chest-radiographic abnormalities
- Intermediate probability
- One moderate to two large segmental perfusion defects with smaller corresponding ventilation or chest-radiographic abnormalities
- Corresponding V/Q defects and chest-radiographic parenchymal opacity in lower lung zone
- Single moderate matched V/Q defects with normal chest-radiographic findings
- Corresponding V/Q defects and small pleural effusion
- Difficult to categorize as normal, low or high probability
- Low probability
- Multiple matched V/Q defects, regardless of size, with normal chest-radiographic findings
- Corresponding V/Q defects and chest-radiographic parenchymal opacity in upper or middle lung zone
- Corresponding V/Q defects and large pleural effusion
- Any perfusion defects with substantially larger chest-radiographic abnormality
- Defects surrounded by normally perfused lung (stripe sign)
- More than three small (<25% of a segment) segmental perfusion defects with a normal chest radiograph
- Nonsegmental perfusion defects (cardiomegaly, aortic impression, enlarged hila)
- Very low probability
- Three or fewer small (<25% of a segment) segmental perfusion defects with a normal chest radiograph
- Normal
- No perfusion defects and perfusion outlines the shape of the lung as shown on chest radiograph

Multiple matched V/Q defects which involve more than 50% of one lung or more than 75% of one lung zone were classified as having intermediate probability for acute PE, according to the original PIOPED criteria. Matching V/Q defects of less extent were classified as representing a low probability of acute PE. The prevalence of PE in patients with extensive matched V/Q defects and no chest-radiographic evidence of pleural effusion or parenchymal abnormality was 14% [11]. In patients with a single matched V/Q defect the prevalence of PE was 26%, although this was a relatively uncommon finding [11]. Therefore multiple matched V/Q abnormalities (regardless of size) may be categorized as entailing low probability of acute PE in the absence of a pleural effusion or parenchymal abnormality.

Patients with single matched segmental V/Q defects with a normal chest X-ray had a 26% prevalence of PE and therefore should probably be classified as having intermediate probability of acute PE.

The original PIOPED criteria classified a single, moderate segmental V/Q mismatch as representing a low probability of PE. However, 36% of patients with a moderate segmental V/Q mismatch had PE. Therefore this finding represents an intermediate probability for acute PE [11].

Ventilation study results are usually normal in patients with PE without infarction or hemorrhagic edema, and perfusion to the affected segment may be absent or decreased depending upon the degree of vascular occlusion, which results in a classic V/Q mismatch. When PE is complicated by infarction or hemorrhagic edema, findings of the ventilation, perfusion, and chest radiography in the affected segment are usually abnormal (triple matches). The overall prevalence of PE in a zone with triple matches was 26% [51]. Triple matches within the upper and middle lung zones have a lower prevalence of PE than triple matches in the lower lung zones. When triple matches are present within the upper and middle lung zones, the prevalence of PE is 11% and 12%, respectively, whereas PE is present in 33% of lower lung zones with triple matches [51]. Based on the hypothesis that patients with PE complicated by infarction or hemorrhagic edema are more likely to lack perfusion than to have decreased perfusion to the affected segment, Kim et al. [21] further examined the prevalence of PE by dividing the triple matches into two subgroups on the basis of whether perfusion was absent or only decreased. They found that triple matches with decreased perfusion and triple matches with no perfusion in the upper/middle lung zones were associated with a prevalence of 0% and 25%, respectively. The prevalence of PE in areas of triple matches with decreased perfusion and triple matches with no perfusion in the lower lung zone was 18%, and 61%, respectively. The prevalence of PE associated with all triple matches varied from very low to upper-intermediate (61%) depending on whether perfusion was decreased or absent and also on the location of the triple matches.

Among patients with no previous cardiopulmonary disease none with PE had radiographic evidence of a pleural effusions that occupied more than one-third of the hemithorax [39]. Therefore V/Q defects with large pleural effusion represent a low probability of acute PE. In contrast, the majority of patients with PE and   ural effusions had small effusions, which caused blunting of the costophrenic angles. The prevalence of PE within the lower lung zones in patients with small pleural effusions was 32% in the right hemithorax and 25% in the left hemithorax [50]. Therefore matching V/Q defects with a small effusion represent an intermediate probability of acute PE. In patients with pleural effusion, performing the perfusion scan with the patient in lateral decubitus or prone position may be helpful; this can shift pleural fluid and provide optimum visualization of the costophrenic angles [33].

The stripe sign is defined as a rim of perfused lung tissue between the perfusion defect and the adjacent pleural surface (Fig. 4.5). The presence of the sign excluded the diagnosis of PE within the effected zone in 93% of cases [34]. Perfusion defects which demonstrate a stripe sign are thus unlikely to be due to PE and in the absence of perfusion defects elsewhere should be interpreted as representing a low probability of PE.

The nuclear-medicine physician's subjective estimate of the likelihood of PE (without using specific interpretation criteria) was well correlated with the proportion of patients with angiographic evidence of PE. Thus experienced physicians (such as the PIOPED investigators) can accurately estimate the probability of PE based on radiographic and scintigraphic findings.

Pulmonary Angiography in Pulmonary Embolism

Although associated with nonfatal and fatal complications, pulmonary angiography remains the "gold standard" test for diagnosing acute PE. In the PIOPED study pulmonary angiography was performed in 99% of patients (1099/1111) consenting to the procedure [40]. Nondiagnostic pulmonary angiograms were obtained in only 3% (35/1111). The angiographic diagnosis of acute PE was based on the identification of an intraluminal filling defect or the trailing edge of a thrombus obstructing a vessel. Using these strict criteria, interobserver agreement in patients who had angiographic evidence of PE was 86% (331/383). In patients with angiograms interpreted as negative or uncertain for PE, interobserver agreement was only 80% (544/681) and 40% (14/35), respectively [49]. The validity of pulmonary angiography was assessed by the outcome classification committee (Fig. 4.8). Of 681 patients

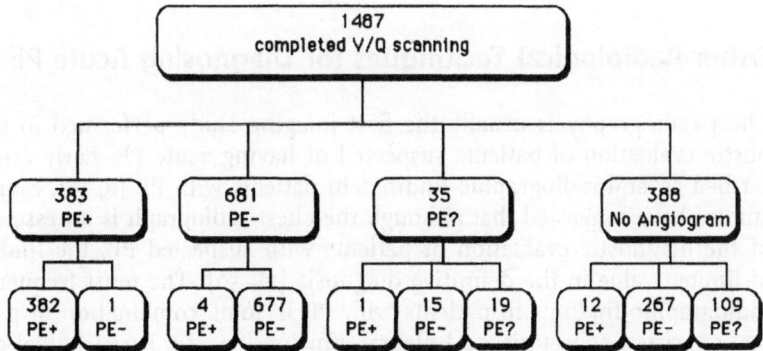

Fig. 4.8. The validity of pulmonary angiography assessed by the outcome classification committee. +, Presence of PE; –, absence of PE. *Middle row*, assessment based on angiography; *bottom row*, assessment by outcome classification committee

whose angiograms were interpreted as being negative for PE only four had their diagnosis reversed by the outcome classification committee. Thus a negative pulmonary angiogram excluded the diagnosis of acute PE in 99% of cases (667/681). Patients with suspected PE and a negative pulmonary angiogram should therefore be investigated for an alternative diagnosis. Since angiography was considered the gold standard in the PIOPED study, the validity of a positive angiogram representing PE could not be assessed.

The complications related to pulmonary angiography during the PIOPED study have been well documented by Stein et al. [40]. In the majority of patients in whom angiography was not performed a complication was encountered during the procedure, death was attributed to pulmonary angiography in 0.5% of patients (5/1111). Nonfatal major complications including respiratory distress, severe renal failure, and hematoma requiring transfusion occurred in 1% (14/1111). The frequency of major complications was higher in those from the medical intensive care unit than in those from other wards. Minor complications that were not life threatening and responded promptly to pharmaceutical therapy occurred in 5% (60/1111). The most common minor complications were urticaria or pruritus and mild renal dysfunction. The frequency of complications caused by pulmonary angiography was not related to patient age, the presence of PE, or pulmonary artery pressure.

Outcome of Patients with Acute PE

Of the 399 patients in the PIOPED study with confirmed PE treatment was initiated for 94% (375/399). Only 2.5% of patients with PE (10/399) died as a result of the PE [2]. Patients were far more likely to die from comorbid conditions than from PE itself. Of the ten patients who died of PE only one was untreated, and the other nine were due to clinically suspected recurrent PE. Therefore, when properly diagnosed and treated, death attributed to PE was relatively uncommon.

Other Radiological Techniques for Diagnosing Acute PE

Chest radiography is usually the first imaging study performed in the diagnostic evaluation of patients suspected of having acute PE. Early reports described several radiographic findings in patients with PE [8, 19]. More recent studies have suggested that although the chest radiograph is an essential part of the diagnostic evaluation of patients with suspected PE, the findings are of limited value in the definitive diagnosis [12, 50]. The most frequent chest-radiographic findings in patients with PE is some combination of parenchymal opacities, atelectasis, and pleural effusion [39, 50]. Parenchymal opacities associated with PE are often ascribed to pulmonary infarction; however, their generally rapid resolution suggest that these infiltrates are hemorrhagic edema and not the tissue necrosis that would be present in the case of true infarction [6]. Pleural effusion in patients with PE is usually small and causes only blunting of the costophrenic angles [39, 50]. The findings of hypovascularity within a lung segment (Westermark's sign), especially when associated with an ipsilateral enlarged pulmonary artery (Fleischner's sign), should raise the suspicion of PE and prompt further investigation. Similarly, a wedge-shaped pleural-based opacity (Hampton's hump) or a normal chest radiograph in the setting of dyspnea and pleuritic chest pain may also suggest the presence of PE. However, none of these findings provide adequate information for either confirming or excluding the diagnosis of PE [50]. Chest radiographs are used primarily to exclude diseases which clinically mimic PE and are required for interpretation of the V/Q scan.

Both conventional computed tomography (CT) and magnetic resonance imaging have proven useful in the diagnosis of centrally located PE [4, 32]. However, prolonged acquisition times, poor proton signal from air-filled lung, and motion artifacts have detracted from their usefulness in diagnosing peripheral PE. Recent advances in CT technology, contrast-enhanced electron-beam and spiral CT (Fig. 4.9), and magnetic resonance angiography have led to their use in the diagnosis of acute PE [10, 13, 41, 42, 44]. Both helical and electron-beam CT have improved temporal resolution over that in conventional CT and are capable of visualizing thrombus within segmental arteries. Currently the spatial resolution of helical CT is better compared than that of electron-beam CT or magnetic resonance angiography. Because of the rapid acquisition times with helical CT the timing between the contrast injection and scanning must be controlled. In addition, thrombus within the imaging plane (right middle lobe and lingular arteries) may be particularly difficult to identify. Although some authors recommend the routine use of helical or electron-beam CT in screening patients with suspected PE, more clinical experience and outcome-based studies are required before these recommendations can be adopted in clinical practice [10, 24]. Because of familiarity and validation with outcome-based studies V/Q scanning remains the most effective and the most frequent study for the noninvasive diagnosis of acute PE.

Diagnostic and Management Strategies

The combination of V/Q scan findings and peripheral venous studies can be very useful in selecting patients who have not had substantial PE, and in whom there is no evidence of proximal lower extremity venous thrombi. In these patients the risk of recurrent embolic events is low, and anticoagulation may not be required [15–18]. Based largely on these results, current investigative strategies for hemodynamically stable patients with suspected PE have appropriately included both V/Q scanning and an evaluation of the deep venous system of the lower extremities (Fig. 4.10). A normal V/Q scan interpretation excludes the diagnosis of clinically significant PE (Fig. 4.10a). Patients with low- or very low-probability V/Q scan interpretation and low

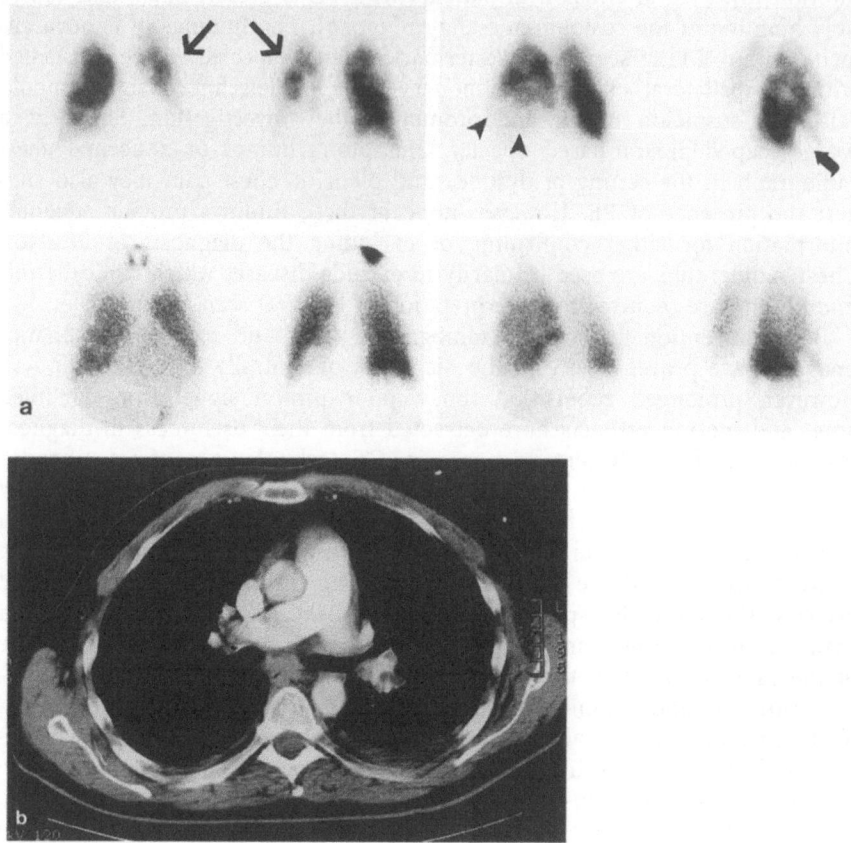

Fig. 4.9 a. Perfusion (*top row*) and per-Technegas ventilation (*bottom row*) images. There is decreased perfusion in the entire left lung (*arrows*), with virtually no activity in the basal segments of the lower lobe as well as lingula, which is predominantly mismatched (*arrowheads*). A matched defect is noted in the right lung base anteriorly (*curved arrow*). **b** A selected slice of the spiral CT reveals intraluminal filling defects in the left lower lobe pulmonary artery

clinical likelihood of PE do not require angiography or anticoagulation (Fig. 4.10 a, b). In patients with low- or very low-probability V/Q scan interpretation the intermediate or high clinical likelihood of PE and negative serial noninvasive venous study results of the lower extremities do not require anticoagulation or angiography. If serial noninvasive venous study results of the lower extremities are positive, patients should be treated. Clinically stable patients with intermediate-probability V/Q scan interpretation require noninvasive venous studies of the legs and negative venogram may require angiography or spiral CT (Fig. 4.10 c). Clinically stable patients with a high-probability V/Q scan interpretation and a high clinical likelihood of PE require treatment and need no further diagnostic tests to confirm the diagnosis

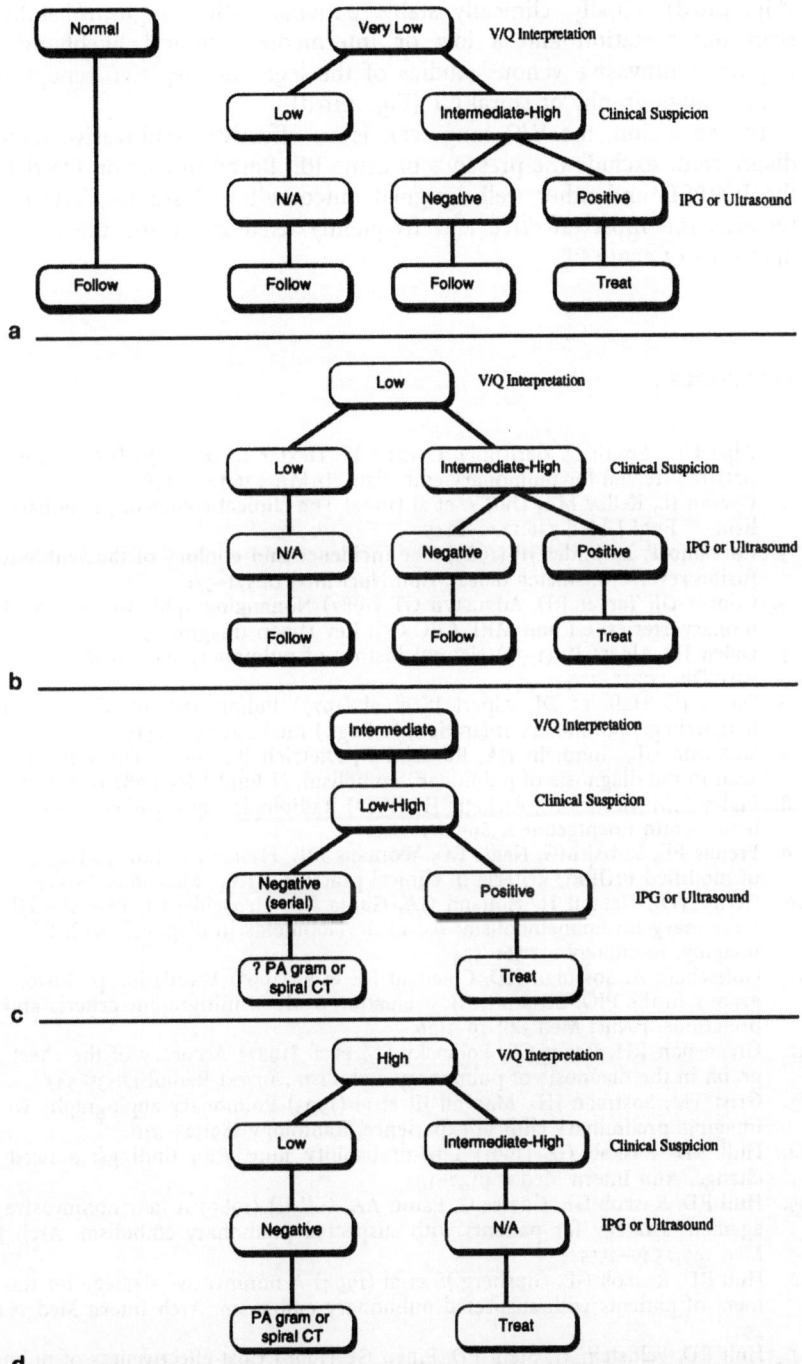

Fig. 4.10a–d. Diagnostic and management strategies depending on V/Q scan interpretation and variable degree of clinical suspicion

(Fig. 4.10 d). Finally, clinically stable patients with a high-probability V/Q scan interpretation and a low or intermediate clinical likelihood of PE require noninvasive venous studies of the legs and negative venogram may require angiography or spiral CT (Fig. 4.10 d).

In conclusion, the V/Q lung scan is an effective, noninvasive method to diagnose or exclude the presence of acute PE. Based in part on the data from the PIOPED and other well-designed outcome-based studies, V/Q scanning remains the most effective and frequently used study for the noninvasive diagnosis of acute PE.

References

1. Alpert JS, Smith R, Carlson J, Ockene IS, Dexter L, Dalen JE (1976) Mortality in patients treated for pulmonary embolism. JAMA 236:1477–1480
2. Carson JL, Kelley MA, Duff A et al (1992) The clinical course of pulmonary embolism. N Engl J Med 326:1240–1245
3. Carvalho P, Lavender JP (1989) The incidence and etiology of the ventilation/perfusion reverse mismatch defect. Clin Nucl Med 14:571–576
4. Conces DJ, Tarver RD, Augustyn GT (1987) Nonangiographic imaging of the pulmonaryarteries: CT and MRI. CRC Crit Rev Diagn Imaging 27:237–246
5. Dalen JE, Alpert JS (1975) Natural history of pulmonary embolism. Prog Cardiovasc Dis 17:257–270
6. Dalen JE, Haffajec DI, Alpert JS et al (1977) Pulmonary embolism, pulmonary hemorrhage, pulmonary infarction. N Engl J Med 296:1431–1435
7. DeNardo GL, Goodwin DA, Ravasini R, Dietrich PA (1970) The ventilatory lung scan in the diagnosis of pulmonary embolism. N Engl J Med 282:1334–1336
8. Figley MM, Gerdes AJ, Ricketts HJ (1967) Radiologic aspects of pulmonary embolism. Semin Roentgenol 2:389–405
9. Freitas FE, Sarosi MG, Nagle CC, Yeomans ME, Freitas AE, Juni JE (1995) The use of modified PIOPED criteria in clinical practice. J Nucl Med 36:1573–1578
10. Gefter WB, Hatabu H, Holland GA, Gupta KB, Henschke CI, Palevsky HI (1995) Pulmonary thromboembolism: recent developments in diagnosis with CT and MR imaging. Radiology 197:561–574
11. Gottschalk A, Sostman HD, Coleman RE et al (1993) Ventilation-perfusion scintigraphy in the PIOPED study. II. evaluation of the scinitigraphic criteria and interpretations. J Nucl Med 34:1119–1126
12. Greenspan RH, Ravin CE, Polonsky SM et al (1982) Accuracy of the chest radiograph in the diagnosis of pulmonary embolism. Invest Radiol 17:535–543
13. Grist TM, Sostman HD, MacFall JR et al (1993) Pulmonary angiography with MR imaging: preliminary clinical experience. Radiology 189:523–530
14. Hull RD, Raskob GE (1991) Low-probability lung scan findings: a need for a change. Ann Intern Med 114:142–143
15. Hull RD, Raskob GE, Coates G, Panju AA, Gill GJ (1989) A new noninvasive management strategy for patients with suspected pulmonary embolism. Arch Intern Med 149:2549–2555
16. Hull RD, Raskob GE, Ginsberg JS et al (1994) A noninvasive strategy for the treatment of patients with suspected pulmonary embolism. Arch Intern Med 154:289–297
17. Hull RD, Feldstein W, Stein PD, Pineo GF (1996) Cost-effectiveness of pulmonary embolism diagnosis. Arch Intern Med 156:68–72
18. Kelley MA, Carson JL, Palevsky HI, Schwatz JS (1991) Diagnosing pulmonary embolism: new facts and strategies. Ann Intern Med 114:300–306

19. Kelley MJ, Elliott LP (1975) The radiographic evaluation of the patient with suspected pulmonary thromboembolic disease. Med Clin North Am 59:3–36
20. Kim CK, Heyman S (1989) Ventilation/perfusion mismatch caused by positive pressure ventilatory support. J Nucl Med 30:1268–1270
21. Kim CK, Worsley DF, Alavi A (1993) "Ventilation (V)/perfusion (Q)/chest xray" match is less likely to represent pulmonary embolism if Q is only "decreased" rather than "absent." J Nucl Med 34:17P
22. Lesser BA, Leeper KV Jr, Stein PD et al (1992) The diagnosis of acute pulmonary embolism in patients with chronic obstructive pulmonary disease. Chest 102:17–22
23. Mant MJ, O'Brien BD, Thong KL, Hammond GW, Birtwhistle RV, Grace MG (1977) Haemorrhagic complications of heparin therapy. Lancet 1:1133–1135
24. Matsumoto AH, Tegtmeyer CJ (1995) Contemporary diagnostic approaches to acute pulmonary emboli (review). Radiol Clin North Am 33:167–183
25. Nelson PH, Moser KM, Stoner C, Moser KS (1982) Risk of complications during intravenous heparin therapy. West J Med 136:189–197
26. Palevsky HI (1991) The problems of the clinical and laboratory diagnosis of pulmonary embolism (review). Semin Nucl Med 21:276–280
27. PIOPED Investigators (1990) Value of the ventilation/perfusion scan in acute pulmonary embolism. JAMA 263:2753–2759
28. Porter J, Jick H (1977) Drug-related deaths among medical inpatients. JAMA 237:879–881
29. Quinn DA, Thompson BT, Terrin ML et al (1992) A prospective investigation of pulmonary embolism in women and men. JAMA 268:1689–1696
30. Robin ED (1977) Overdiagnosis and overtreatment of pulmonary embolism: the emperor may have no clothes. Ann Intern Med 87:775–781
31. Robinson PJ (1989) Lung scintigraphy-doubt and certainty in the diagnosis of pulmonary embolism. Clin Radiol 40:557–560
32. Shah HR, Buckner B, Purness GL et al (1989) Computed tomography and magnetic fesonance imaging in the diagn. Computed tomography and magnetic fesonance imaging in the diagnosis of pulmonary thrombotic disease. J Thorac Imaging 4:58–61
33. Solomon RW, Palestro C, Kim CK, Goldsmith SJ (1989) Effect of patient position on interpretation of lung images complicated by chest radiograph opacities. Clin Nucl Med 14:261–263
34. Sostman HD, Gottschalk A (1992) Prospective validation of the stripe sign in ventilation-perfusion scintigraphy. Radiology 184:455–459
35. Sostman HD, Coleman RE, DeLong DM, Newman GE, Paine S (1994) Evaluation of revised criteria for ventilation-perfusion scintigraphy in patients with suspected pulmonary embolism. Radiology 193:103–107
36. Stein PD, Coleman RE, Gottschalk A, Saltzman HA, Terrin ML, Weg JG (1991a) Diagnostic utility of ventilation/perfusion lung scans in acute pulmonart embolism is not diminished by pre-existing cardiac or pulmonary disease. Chest 100:604–606
37. Stein PD, Gottschalk A, Saltzman HA, Terrin ML (1991b) Diagnosis of acute pulmonary embolism in the elderly. J Am Coll Cardiol 18:1452–1457
38. Stein PD, Saltzman HA, Weg JG (1991c) Clinical characteristics of patients with acute pulmonary embolism. Am J Cardiol 68:1723–1724
39. Stein PD, Terrin ML, Hales CA et al (1991d) Clinical, laboratory, roentgenographic, and electrocardiographic findings in patients with acute pulmonary embolism and no pre-existing cardiac or pulmonary disease. Chest 100:598–603
40. Stein PD, Athanasoulis C, Alavi A et al (1992) Complications and validity of pulmonary angiography in acute pulmonary embolism. Circulation 85:462–468
41. Teigen CL, Maus TP, Sheedy PF, Johnson CM, Stanson AW, Welch TJ (1993) Pulmonary embolism: diagnosis with electron-beam CT. Radiology 188:839–845
42. Teigen CL, Maus TP, Sheedy PF et al (1995) Pulmonary embolism: diagnosis with contrast-enhanced electron-beam CT and comparison with pulmonary angiography. Radiology 194:313–319

43. UPET Investigators (1973) The urokinase pulmonary embolism trial. A national cooperative study. Circulation 47 [Suppl 2]:46–50
44. van Rossum AB, Treurniet FE, Kieft GJ, Smith SJ, Schepers-Bok R (1996) Role of spiral volumetric computed tomographic scanning in the assessment of patients with clinical suspicion of pulmonary embolism and an abnormal ventilation/perfusion lung scan. Thorax 51:23–28
45. Wagner HN Jr, Lopez-Majano V, Langan JK, Joshi RC (1968) Radioactive xenon in the differential diagnosis of pulmonary embolism. Radiology 91:1168–1174
46. Webber MM, Gomes AS, Roe D, La Fontaine RL, Hawkins RA (1990) Comparison of Biello, McNeil, and PIOPED criteria for the diagnosis. AJR Am J Roentgenol 154:975–981
47. Wegner WA (1990) Hyperperfusion of a lower-lobe pneumonia by positive pressure ventilatory support. J Nucl Med 31:125–126 (letter)
48. Wigton RS, Hoellerich VL, Patil KD (1986) How physicians use clinical information in diagnosing pulmonary embolism: an application of conjoint analysis. Med Decis Making 6:2–11
49. Worsley DF, Alavi A (1995) Comprehensive analysis of the results of the PIOPED diagnosis. J Nucl Med 36:2380–2387
50. Worsley DF, Alavi A, Aronchick JM, Chen JT, Greenspan RH, Ravin CE (1993a) Chest radiographic findings in patients with acute pulmonary embolism: observations from the PIOPED study. Radiology 189:133–136
51. Worsley DF, Kim CK, Alavi A, Palevsky HI (1993b) Detailed analysis of patients with matched ventilation-perfusion defects and chest radiographic opacities. J Nucl Med 34:1851–1853
52. Worsley DF, Palevsky HI, Alavi A (1994) Clinical characteristic of patients with pulmonary embolism and low or very low probability lung scan interpretations. Arch Intern Med 154:2737–2741
53. Worsley DF, Alavi A, Palevsky HI, Kundel H (1996) Comparison of the diagnostic performance of ventilation/perfusion lung scanning in different patient populations. Radiology 199:481–483

5 ^{99m}Tc-Phytate Aerosol Scan of Nonembolic Pulmonary Diseases: A Pattern Analysis with Radiographic Correlation

Y.-W. BAHK and S.-K. CHUNG

Introduction

The modern clinical concept of ventilatory function in normal and pathological conditions owes much to nuclear pulmonary imaging. Indeed pulmo-
nology was first implemented with an objective noninvasive assay in 1955
when Knipping et al. [1] ingeniously applied radioactive ^{133}Xe to *Isotopen-
Thorakographie*, a surface γ-counting test of the heart and lung function. Until then the laboratory test for evaluating pulmonary ventilation was spirometry, which was very limited in the information that it could provide, particularly concerning regional ventilatory function. Nuclear imaging differs basically in that it can accurately and simultaneously assess both the regional
and integrated overall ventilatory states of the lung from any desired angles,
assisting both visual and digital diagnosis of many bronchopulmonary diseases [2–6]. Moreover its diagnostic scope has been remarkably broadened
by the addition of perfusion scan in pairs, which permits a matched assessment of pulmonary aeration and blood flow.

Over the past four decades the initial ^{133}Xe scan has been substantially
modified through new radiopharmaceuticals, advanced technology, and mod-
ernized instrumentation. The result is a highly refined ventilation scan at
reasonable expense. In the early 1960s, in addition to ^{133}Xe and ^{81m}Kr gas, a
number of cyclotron-generated positron emitters such as ^{11}C, ^{13}N, and ^{15}O
were tried for lung scans in the form of ^{11}CO$_2$, ^{11}CO, ^{13}N, ^{13}NNO, ^{15}O$_2$, and
H$_2$^{15}O [7–9]. However most agents failed because of extremely short half-life
and restricted availability. It was fortunate that in 1965, 10 years after Kip-
pling's publication, Taplin et al. [10] and Pircher et al. [11] introduced aerosol
preparations of ^{198}Au-colloid and ^{131}I-labeled human serum albumin (HSA),
respectively, as ventilation scan agents. ^{99m}Tc-labeled diethylene triamine
pentaacetate (DTPA) was another important aerosol agent developed for the
same purpose [12].

Most recently a number of generator systems have become widely available for convenient house production of excellent microaerosols and ultrafine
particles. Among these are the Bhabha Atomic Research Centre (BARC) jet
nebulizer that produces microaerosols with an activity median aerodynamic
diameter (AMAD) of 0.84 µm and a geometric standard deviation (GSD) of
1.57 [13]; the Technegas generator system that creates ultrafine microaerosols
with a size of 0.01–0.02 µm by combusting, under an argon gas atmosphere,

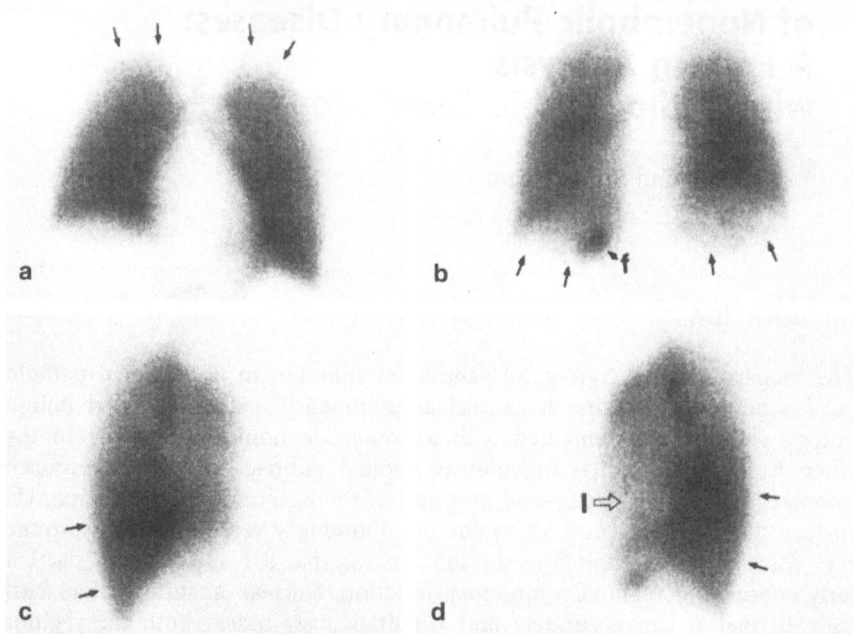

Fig. 5.1 a–d. Normal ^{99m}Tc-phytate aerosol deposition pattern of the lung. Anterior (**a**), posterior (**b**), right lateral (**c**), and left lateral (**d**) lung scans in a normal female nonsmoker show airspace aerosol deposition to be uniform with minimal aberration in the apex and peripheries where the lung is thin (*arrows*). **c,d** Aerosol depositions are more prominent in the lower lung because of large lung volume (*arrows*). Note ingested radioactivity in the gastric fundus (*f*) and cardiac defect in the lingular division (*l*)

^{99m}Tc-pertechnetate in carbon crucible at 2500 °C [14]; and the Mistogen EN-142 ultrasonic nebulizer that generates aerosols with an AMAD of 1.64 μm and GSD of 1.39 with reservoir and of 1.93 μm with GSD of 1.52 without reservoir utilizing HSA [15]. The microaerosols thus produced behave much like a gaseous agent, readily penetrating normal lung peripheries to produce excellent airspace ventilation images [16] (Fig. 5.1).

Characteristically and importantly, when these preparations are used, there is no visible aerosol deposition in the normal bronchial tree or airways, although some trivial aerosol deposition may occur in the trachea [5]. The scan reproducibility is excellent and imaging can be repeated even hours after the initial study (Fig. 5.2). At this point, a short remark on pulmonary perfusion scan seems indicated. As is well known, perfusion scan is highly informative [17], making an indispensable partner of ventilation scan. As discussed in much greater detail in Chap. 3, perfusion scan makes use of macro-aggregated human serum albumin (MAA), previously labeled with ^{131}I [18, 19] and more recently with ^{99m}Tc, or HSA microspheres labeled with ^{99m}Tc [20]. Being noninvasive and easy to perform, it is well suited for the diagnosis not only of pulmonary embolism but also a number of nonembolic pulmonary

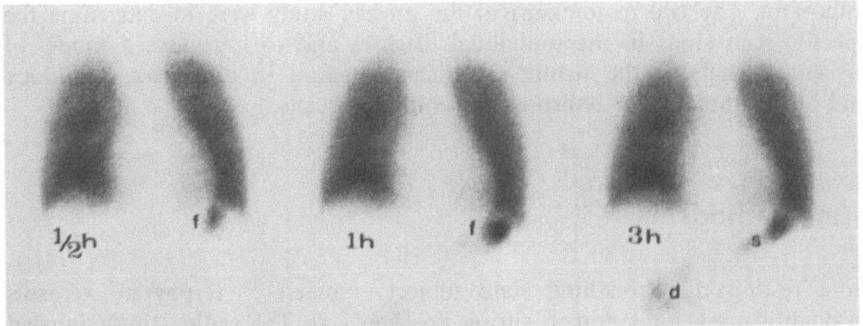

Fig. 5.2. Excellent reproducibility of ^{99m}Tc-phytate aerosol lung scans. Serial scans of a normal lung obtained 30 min, 1 h, and 3 h postinhalation show uniform airspace deposition with minor apical aberration. *f*, gastric fundus; *s*, stomach body; *d*, duodenum. Note excellent reproducibility of scan images regardless of the time elapsed

diseases, as described below. Its usefulness is enhanced enormously when combined with ventilation scans, and their results are assessed in terms of "match" or "mismatch."

Since 1987 we have used ^{99m}Tc-phytate aerosols produced with a BARC jet nebulizer for the study of various bronchopulmonary diseases. The size of aerosols is 0.84 μm in AMAD, which is larger than 0.2 μm of Technegas. Nevertheless ^{99m}Tc-phytate aerosols are well comparable with the Technegas in clinical performance [21]. In this chapter we describe our clinical experience with ^{99m}Tc-phytate aerosol scanning in the diagnosis of chronic obstructive pulmonary disease (COPD) and similar bronchopulmonary diseases, emphasizing the diagnostic scan features of the individual diseases. First, technical aspects of ^{99m}Tc-phytate aerosol scanning and its image quality and reproducibility are discussed. A general presentation of scan alterations of the normal lung, smoker's lung, and a variety of bronchopulmonary diseases follows. In most instances, aerosol scan alterations are compared with those of simple radiography, bronchography, and computed tomography (CT).

The clinical materials for normal study were pooled from ten nuclear-medicine laboratories in Asia that participated in a coordinated research project sponsored by the International Atomic Energy Agency in Vienna [5]. Some of the cases included in the present analysis were also derived from this source, but they were examined exclusively by us. Where necessary, more information concerning materials is provided in detail in the presentation of the individual diseases. The diseases that we have studied are pulmonary emphysema, chronic bronchitis, bronchial asthma, bronchiectasis, bronchial obstruction, compensatory overinflation, acute pulmonary edema, diffuse panbronchiolitis, focal tuberculous lung fibrosis, diffuse idiopathic pulmonary fibrosis, acute lobar pneumonia, lung abscess, tuberculosis, and primary and metastatic lung cancers.

A substantial portion of the discussion is allocated to COPD because this disorder is clinically prevalent, academically interesting, and sociomedically important. The two major aims of the present study were to determine the specific scan signs in the individual diseases and to introduce a model of piecemeal analysis, the firmly established method in diagnostic radiology and histopathology, for interpreting ventilation scans.

Scan Methods

In a resting tidal-breathing state subjects inhaled ^{99m}Tc-phytate aerosols through a mask for 5 min in sitting position [13]. The radioactivity inhaled was approximately 3 mCi (111 MBq). Aerosols were prepared afresh each time by using a BARC nebulizer with the instillation of 15 mCi (555 MBq) ^{99m}Tc-phytate. After rinsing the esophagus with water the anterior, posterior, and both lateral views were taken with the subject lying on a scan couch. The cumulative radioactivity was 500–600 K counts depending on the size of lung. This number of counts was almost twice as high as the recommended 300 K counts. This was intended to obtain the best possible images by suppressing the detector sensitivity by setting the filter at a near-baseline level. The acquisition time was 10–15 min per view. With a dual-head camera system two views were taken simultaneously, shortening acquisition time by one-half. The gamma-camera systems which we previously used was the Siemens Scintiview II (Model ZLC 7500S) and Orbiter (Model 6601) and the most recent one is Multi-SPECT.

Pattern Analysis of Scan Manifestations

Both normal and pathological scans were analyzed element by element, including the size or extent, shape, location, number, internal architecture, and radioactivity as they were depicted on the scan. The altered findings were then patterned out where possible. The analysis focused first on whether there was aerosol deposition in the airways and defective or increased airspace deposition. The airways were normally free of aerosol deposition or "clean"; hence positive aerosol deposition was the sign of abnormality. It was assessed in terms of intensity, location, appearance, and shape. The intensity was mild, moderate, or marked; location was central, middle, or peripheral; shape was clubbed, bulbous, or withered-bough-like; and appearance was dilated, narrowed, or occluded. On the other hand, the abnormal deposition in airspace was either increased, normal, or decreased, and it could be assessed in a similar way with an addition of extent. Airspace deposition was either decreased, normal, or increased; intensity was mild, moderate, or marked; location was either in the upper, middle, or lower lung; distribution was diffuse or local; and extent was either segmental, lobar, or entire lung. Additionally, nonsegmental distribution was recognized as such as a separate category.

A semiquantitative assessment of scan alterations was possible using the traditional criteria: grade I for an area of involvement less than 25% of the total lung, grade II between 25% and 50%, and grade III more than 50%. However, as this seemingly simple method was found to be difficult in practice, we introduced a modification: the lesional extent was graded according to a division that trisects the lung vertically into the central, intermediary, and peripheral thirds by two laterally curved equidistant lines drawn parallel to the lateral chest wall. By this division, the central third contained the mainstem and lobar bronchi about the hilum, the intermediary third the segmental bronchi, and the peripheral third alveolar airspaces.

Clinical Applications

Normal Nonsmoker Controls

As noted above, a total of 100 normal aerosol scans were pooled from ten nuclear-medicine laboratories in Asia to establish normal criteria. All were from young and middle-aged subjects without health problems. None was sampled from the geriatric (over 65 years) or pediatric age (under 15 years) group.

In most cases the airspace deposition was uniform and the bronchial tree was completely free of deposition – a "clean airway" (Figs. 5.1, 5.2). A small proportion of cases showed subtle or minimal tracheal deposition. There were also subtle focal airspace defects in the lung apices, presumably due to the combined effects of gravity and small lung at the apex. Similar defects, attributable to relatively limited respiratory excursion, were seen in the lung bases. Such peripheral defects were partially remedied by having the subject inhale aerosols in a lying position. On the lateral views a reduced deposition was produced in the middle and lingular lobes by the heart. Image reproducibility was superb, and satisfactory scanning was possible 3 h after aerosol inhalation (Fig. 5.2).

Asymptomatic and Symptomatic Smokers

Smokers were divided into two groups, those with clinical symptoms and those without. The asymptomatic smoker group consisted of 13 volunteers with a history of smoking more than one pack of cigarettes per day for more than several years. They were in the third to sixth decades of life. Those with symptoms included 12 men with a history of smoking more than one pack of cigarettes per day for many years. They were volunteers recruited from house staffs and ambulatory patients who visited us for pulmonary scans, chest radiography, and spirometric tests. All had coughing with or without expectoration, dyspnea, and/or chest pain. They were in the third and fifth decades of life. For the present study we adopted the protocol used by Barter et

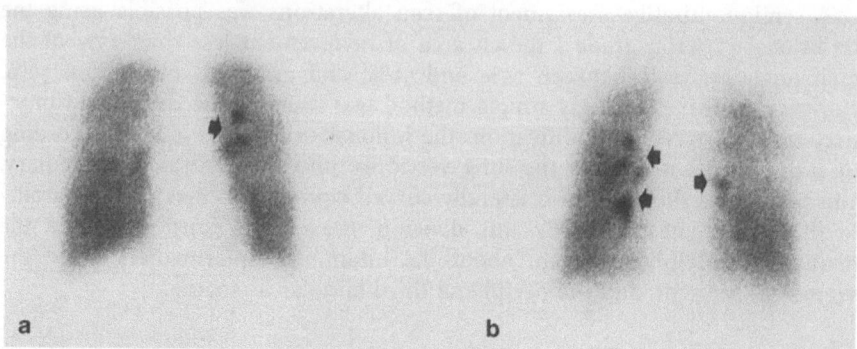

Fig. 5.3a,b. Aerosol scans in asymptomatic smoker (mild case). A Anterior lung scan in a smoker who had smoked an average of one pack of cigarettes per day for 5 years shows minimal airway deposition in hilar areas, more prominently on the left (*arrow*). Airspace deposition is irregularly reduced in the upper and middle lungs. B Posterior lung scan shows the airway deposition and airspace aberration to be more prominent (*arrows*)

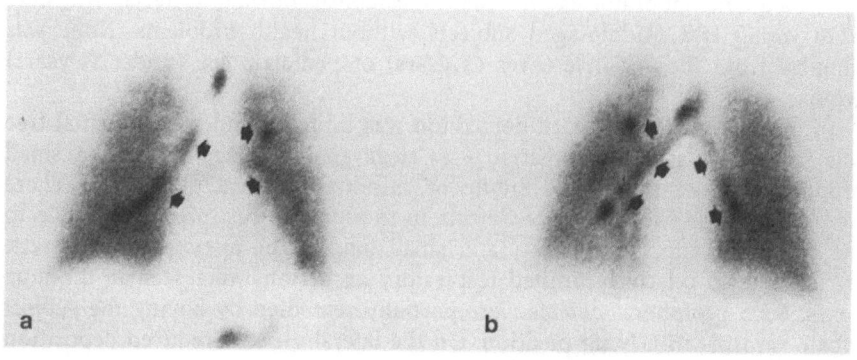

Fig. 5.4a,b. Aerosol scans of symptomatic smoker (moderate case). **a** Anterior lung scan in a man with productive cough who had smoked a half pack of cigarettes per day for 30 years shows the classic arboriform aerosol deposition in the lower trachea and central airway (*arrows*) and intensified airspace defects. Findings strongly resemble chronic bronchitis that can be the case in this subject (Figs. 5.12, 5.13). **b** Posterior lung scan shows both airway deposition and airspace change to be much more prominent

al. [22], who carried out a similar clinical survey study on middle-aged smokers using ^{81m}Kr gas.

Airspace deposition in the asymptomatic group was uniform, as in normal smokers, but with slightly more than trivial peripheral airspace aberration. The aerosol scans in ten cases in this group showed mild airway deposition, suggesting mild chronic bronchitis or smoker's lung change (Fig. 5.3). On the other hand, the aerosol scans of the symptomatic smokers showed typical arboriform airway deposition that was more than minimal in intensity, along with some patchy airspace defects (Fig. 5.4). Generally the scan alterations were more marked in the symptomatic group than in the asymptomatic. Although we did not perform a systematic analysis, there seemed to exist a rough parallel between aerosol scan alterations and clinical symptoms, particularly cough and expectoration. In addition, it is to be noted that the ^{99m}Tc-phytate aerosol scan was superior in portraying alterations not only in the airspaces but also in the airways.

Using the ^{81m}Kr scan, Barter et al. performed a classic study in normal nonsmokers and life-long smokers [22]. The scan that they used was obviously suitable for the imaging of airspace alteration but apparently not airway alteration. Their ^{81m}Kr scans in 46 nonsmokers showed airspace deposition to be uniform, although three cases had minimal defects. They noted airspace defects in 19 of 46 current smokers but did not mention airway alteration. The airspace alteration in our series of smokers was basically the same as that found by Barter et al. [22]. Interestingly, however, unlike ^{81m}Kr scans, the aerosol scans in the present series showed the characteristic arboriform deposition in the airways that, we believe, indicates chronic bronchitis (Fig. 5.4).

Chronic Obstructive Pulmonary Disease and Similar Lung Diseases

The usefulness and sensitivity of ventilation-perfusion scans in the diagnosis of COPD and their superiority to chest radiography in milder cases of COPD have been well documented [23, 24]. The present study demonstrates that the aerosol scan using the microaerosols that have good penetrability produces highly informative *bronchopulmonary* images in many pulmonary diseases, particularly COPD and similar diseases. We present below the results of analytical studies on aerosol scan manifestations in 103 cases of COPD and 25 cases of similar diseases. COPD included pulmonary emphysema ($n=32$), simple chronic bronchitis ($n=23$), chronic bronchitis with asthmalike or bronchiectatic complication ($n=17$), bronchial asthma ($n=18$), and bronchiectasis ($n=13$). The diseases similar to COPD were bronchial obstruction ($n=13$) and compensatory pulmonary overinflation ($n=12$).

Pulmonary Emphysema

Pulmonary emphysema is defined as permanent abnormal distension of the airspaces (acini) distal to the terminal bronchiole with the destruction of their walls, and without obvious fibrosis [25, 26]. Based on the distribution pattern of the main pathological changes the disease can be classified into centriacinar, panacinar, and other types [26, 27]. Clinical symptoms include productive cough, dyspnea, and cyanosis.

Chest radiography may show hyperlucency with overinflation, vascular attenuation and diversion, bulla formation, small heart, flattened or ventroverted diaphragm, and the barrel-chest deformity (Fig. 5.5). As with patholo-

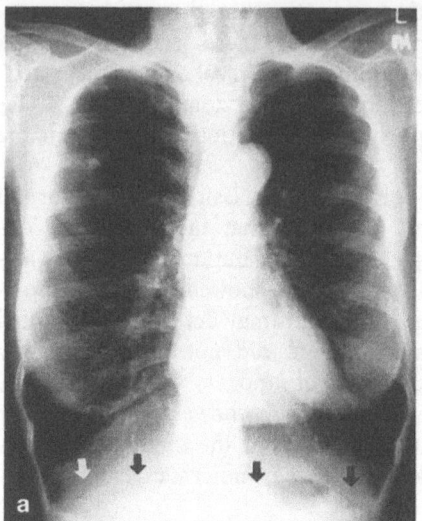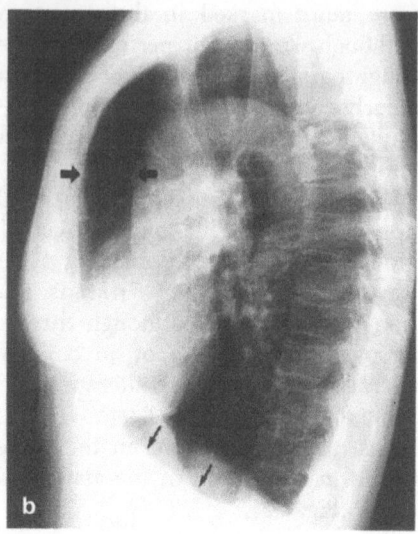

Fig. 5.5 a, b. Typical radiographic signs of pulmonary emphysema. **a** Posteroanterior chest radiograph shows pulmonary overdistension, increased translucency, and attenuated vasculature. In addition, both hemidiaphragms are flattened and ventroverted (*arrows*). **b** Right lateral chest shows widened anteroposterior diameter and retrosternal space (*thick arrow*), ventroverted hemidiaphragms (*thin arrows*), and kyphosis, creating the "barrel chest" deformity

gical categorization, pulmonary emphysema can be classified radiographically into the panacinar, centriacinar, and "increased markings" types depending on intrapulmonary location of dominant hyperlucency and diverted or redistributed pulmonary vasculature [26, 27]. The panacinar type is featured by the lower-lung hyperlucency with cranialized vasculature (Fig. 5.6 a), the centrilobular type by the upper-lung hyperlucency with caudalized vasculature (Fig. 5.6 b), and the "increased markings" type by the midlung hyperlucency with increased vasculature in the middle lung [26, 27] (Fig. 5.6 c).

Aerosol scan alterations of pulmonary emphysemas vary with the type and severity of disease. Relatively mild emphysema manifests nonsegmental patchy airspace defects in the upper and middle lung fields with little or no airway deposition (Fig. 5.7), strongly resembling bronchial asthma although asthmatic involvement is usually uniform (Fig. 5.16). The predilection of airspace defects for the upper lung in pulmonary emphysema may be due to relatively high vulnerability of the upper lung [28]. In contrast, severe emphysemas manifest quite prominent airspace defects and bizarre airway depositions (Figs. 5.8). The bronchi are tubular, bulbous, or withered-bough-like in appearance. The aerosol scan alterations in different types of emphysemas seem to closely reflect the radiographic manifestations, distinguishing one type of disease from the other in classic cases (Fig. 5.6). For example, panacinar emphysema is characterized by dominant airspace defects in the lower

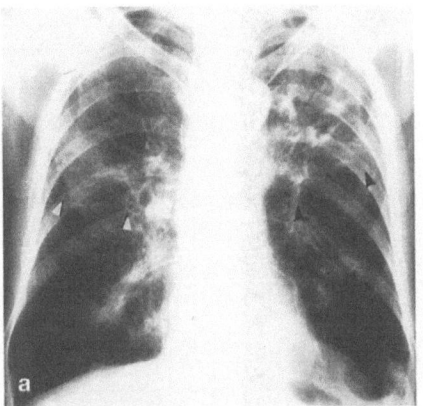
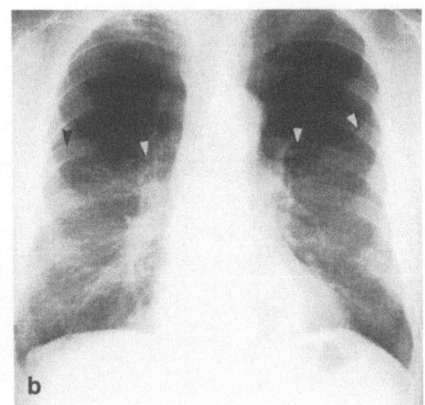
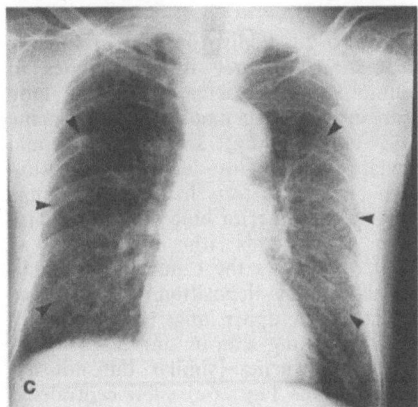

Fig. 5.6a–c. Vascular redistribution in three different types of emphysema. **a** Posteroanterior chest radiograph of panacinar emphysema shows cranialized vasculature with lower lung hyperlucency (*arrowheads*). **b** Posteroanterior chest radiograph of centriacinar emphysema shows caudalized vasculature with upper lung hyperlucency (*arrowheads*). **c** Posteroanterior chest radiograph of increased-markings emphysema shows centralized vasculature with a generalized hyperlucency (*arrowheads*)

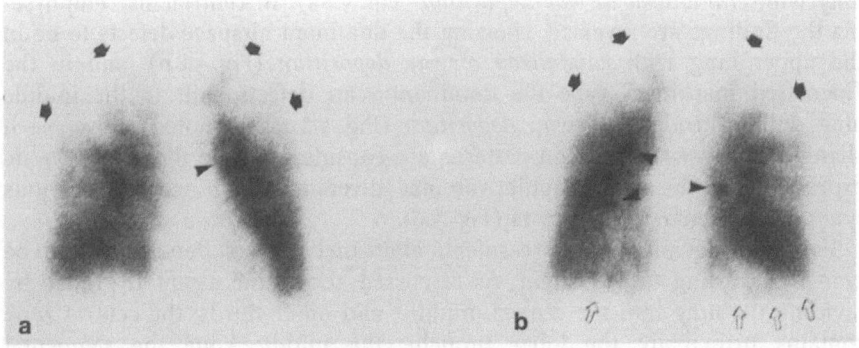

Fig. 5.7a, b. Aerosol scans in pink-puffer emphysema. Anterior (**a**) and posterior (**b**) lung scans show prominent airspace defects in the upper lungs (*arrows*). No significant airway deposition is seen (*arrowheads*). Note the classic "stripe" sign in the basal lung (*open arrows*)

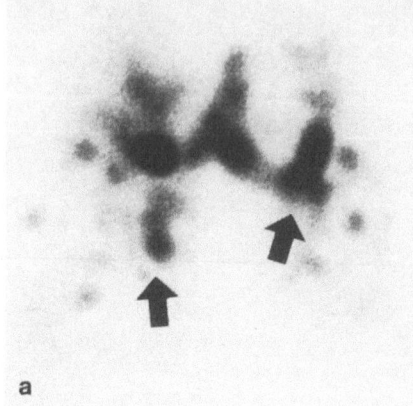
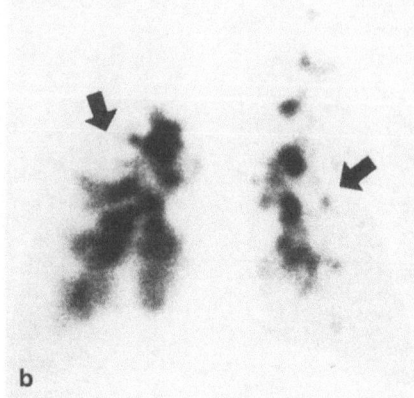

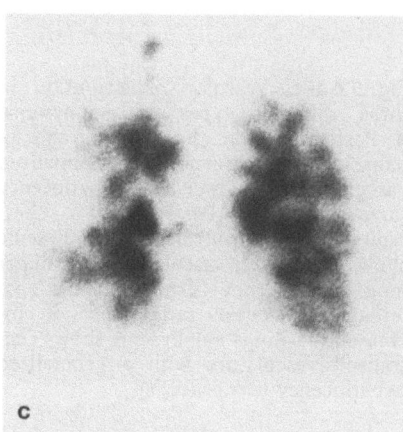

Fig. 5.8a–c. Redistribution of airway deposition in three different types of pulmonary emphysema. **a** Anterior lung scan in panacinar emphysema (the same case as Fig. 5.6a) shows the cranial deviation of intense airway deposition with airspace defects in the lower lungs (*arrows*). **b** Anterior lung scan in centriacinar emphysema (the same case as Fig. 5.6b) shows the caudal deviation of intense airway deposition with airspace defects in the upper lungs (arrows). **c** Anterior lung scan in "increased markings" emphysema (similar but not the same case as Fig. 5.6c) show centralized intense airway deposition with generalized airspace defects

lung with *cranialized airway deposition* (Fig. 5.8a). In centriacinar emphysema the findings are reversed, showing the dominant airspace defects to be in the upper lung with *caudalized airway deposition* (Fig. 5.8b), and in the "increased markings" type the dominant scan defects shift to the middle lung with *centralized airway deposition* (Fig. 5.8c). As noted above, such changes in airway deposition patterns are considered to be the scintigraphic expression of the radiographic vascular diversions that occur in various types of pulmonary emphysema (Fig. 5.6).

For a semiquantitative assessment, abnormal aerosol deposition can be graded according to the extent. As discussed above, the extent is graded by dividing the lung into the central, middle, and outer thirds: the central zone contains principally the lobar bronchi, the middle zone the segmental bronchi, and the outer zone alveolar airspaces. Analysis of scan alterations in emphysema using this criteria showed a direct correlation between the severity of illness and scan alterations, and an inverse correlation between the airway deposition and airspace deposition – the more prominent the airway deposition the less the airspace deposition and vice versa (Figs. 5.7, 5.8). These findings indicate that when more aerosol deposits in the airways, less aerosol reaches the lung peripheries and vice versa.

Reports on the value of ventilation scan in the diagnosis of COPD have been published. For example, Alderson et al. [23] emphasized that ^{133}Xe scan is more sensitive than radiography in detecting COPD and, more recently Lavender and Finn [29] described the value of ^{81m}Kr scan in the study of nonthromboembolic diseases, including COPD. However, they were concerned principally with airspace scan alterations in COPD and not with airway change. Interestingly Isawa et al. [30] published aerosol patterns in COPD. Using ^{99m}Tc-HSA aerosols, they portrayed both airspace and airway alterations in emphysema and chronic bronchitis and ascertained two different scan patterns – central deposition in the former and peripheral deposition in the latter. This observation was significant but received little attention probably because most workers use gaseous agents that are not suitable for the airway imaging and naturally are interested in the airspace alterations.

Our ^{99m}Tc-phytate aerosol scan study amply confirmed the diagnostic importance of airway deposition in emphysema. We also noted that airspace deposition is as important as airway change. In fact, the intrapulmonary distribution patterns of both the airway and airspace depositions are of special diagnostic value, as described above. It was indeed peculiar that different types of emphysemas show different patterns of airway deposition and airspace defects: *cranialization, caudalization,* and *centralization*. Interestingly Cunningham and Lavender [31] also noted that airspace defects in panacinar emphysema involve predominantly the lower lung on ^{81m}Kr scans: however they did not discuss airway deposition. A plausible account of the specific diversion of the airway deposition in different emphysemas is that, as with pulmonary blood flow, inhaled aerosols seek the area of least resistance for easier penetration: the upper lung in panacinar emphysema, the lower lung in centriacinar emphysema, and the middle lung in "increased markings" emphysema. Pathogenetically aerosol deposition in dilated bronchi in pulmonary emphysema is considered to be related to chronic bronchitis and bronchiectasis, two common complications of pulmonary emphysema [32].

Chronic Bronchitis

One of the most widely quoted definitions of chronic bronchitis is that of the Ciba Guest Symposium, which regards it as the presence of "chronic or excessive mucus secretion in the bronchial tree" [33]. Pathological changes include increased goblet cells in the bronchial mucosa and mucous gland hypertrophy in the bronchial walls [34]. The diagnostic criterion of chronic bronchitis is productive cough for months over more than 2 consecutive years without wheeze or other pulmonary disease [35]. IgE levels may be normal or mildly increased, and forced expiratory volume (FEV) normal or minimally decreased.

Fig. 5.9. Radiographic signs of chronic bronchitis. Posteroanterior chest radiograph shows "tram-line" sign of thickened bronchial wall in the medial aspect of the right lower lobe (*open arrows*)

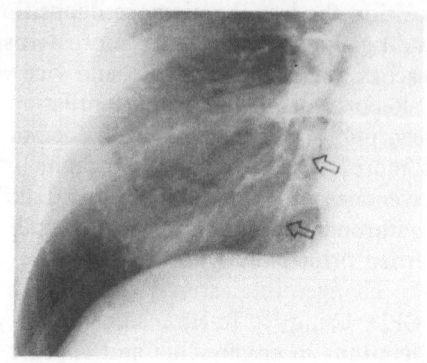

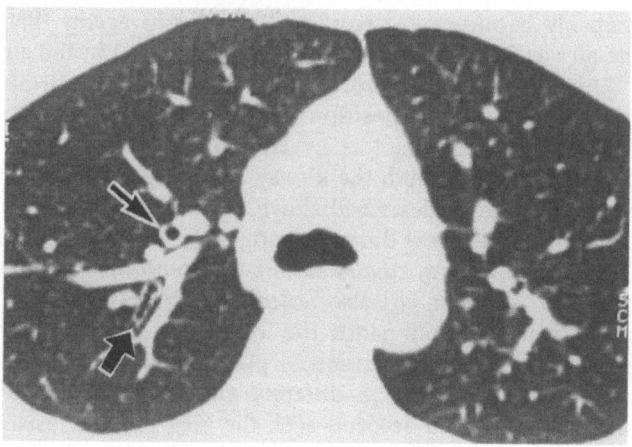

Fig. 5.10. CT demonstration of thickened bronchial wall sign in chronic bronchitis. Transaxial CT of the hilum shows a ringlike shadow of thickened bronchial wall seen on end (*long arrow*) and a tubular shadow seen longitudinally (*short arrow*), explaining the bronchial cuff sign and the "tram-line" sign, respectively

Radiography may present the tram-line shadow, bronchial cuff, dirty lung sign, and overinflation with vascular attenuation (Fig. 5.9), but these signs are not regularly seen. CT is useful to delineate a thickened bronchial wall which accounts for tram-line and bronchial cuff (Fig. 5.10). Bronchography is very specific, directly visualizing hypertrophied bronchial glands in addition to bronchial narrowing and deformity and small patches in the terminal bronchi (Fig. 5.11). Most cases are simple bronchitis but some are "asthmatic bronchitis" which is accompanied by bronchiectatic complication and wheeze [36].

The aerosol scan finding in simple chronic bronchitis of mild grade is characterized by minimal to moderate perihilar bronchial deposition, giving rise to an arboriform appearance (Fig. 5.12). It is indistinguishable from that of symptomatic smoker's lung (Fig. 5.4). Occasionally the "stripe" sign is

Fig. 5.11. Bronchographic demonstration of hypertrophic bronchial glands in chronic bronchitis. Anteroposterior bronchogram of the left hilum shows the "sawtooth" sign of hypertrophic glands in the proximal lingular bronchus (*arrowheads*)

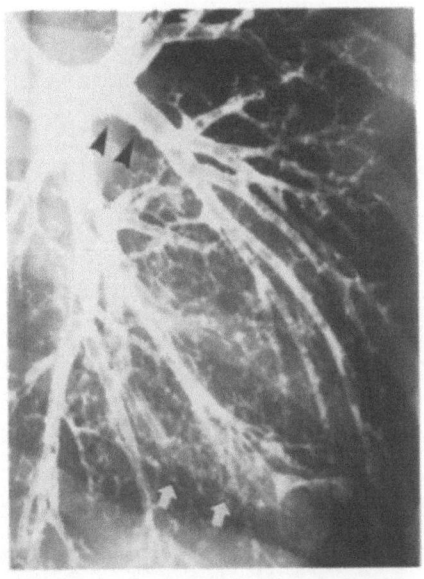

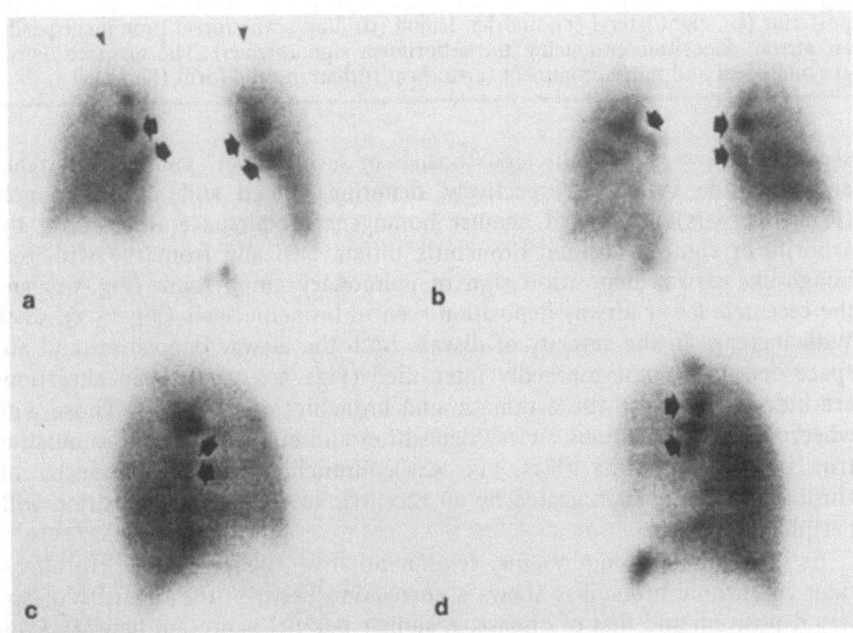

Fig. 5.12 a–d. Mild aerosol scan alterations in chronic bronchitis. Anterior (**a**), posterior (**b**), right lateral (**c**), and left lateral (**d**) lung scans reveal minimal hilar airway deposition (*arrows*) with irregular apical airspace defects (*arrowheads*)

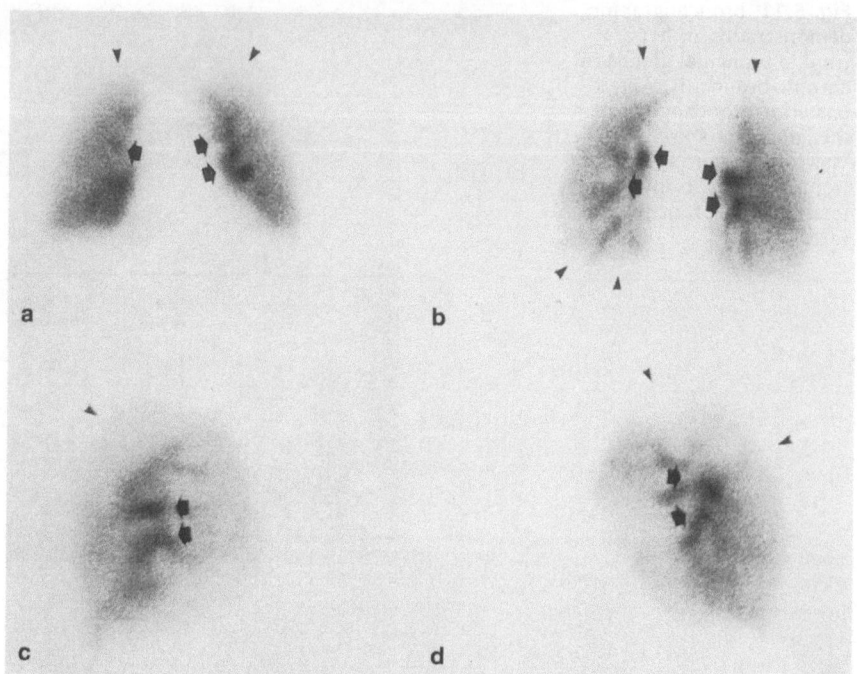

Fig. 5.13a–d. Moderate aerosol scan alterations in chronic bronchitis. Anterior (**a**), posterior (**b**), right lateral (**c**), and left lateral (**d**) lung scans reveal prominent perihilar airway deposition producing the arboriform sign (*arrows*). The airspace defects are multifocal and more prominent (*arrowheads*) than in mild form (Fig. 5.12)

seen in the lower lung. The sign consists of several "hot" and "cold" streaks arranged side by side, respectively, denoting dilated and spastic bronchi (Figs. 5.14, 5.15). Portrayed against homogeneous airspace deposition, the arboriform sign of chronic bronchitis differs basically from the withered-bough-like airway deposition sign of pulmonary emphysema (Fig. 5.8) and the eccentric lower airway deposition seen in bronchiectasis (Figs. 5.23, 5.24). With increase in the severity of disease both the airway deposition and airspace defects become markedly intensified (Figs. 5.13, 5.15). Scan alterations are indeed bizarre in the asthmatic and bronchiectatic variants. Those with wheeze show conspicuous airway deposition and airspace defects, simulating true bronchial asthma (Figs. 5.13, 5.14). Bronchiectasis superimposed on chronic bronchitis is indicated by an eccentric lower airway deposition with peripheral defects.

As in pulmonary emphysema, semiquantitative assessment of scan alterations in chronic bronchitis shows a correlation between the intensity of airway deposition and that of disease. A similar parallel is present between scintigraphic and radiographic alterations and between airway deposition and airspace defect. The high sensitivity of aerosol scan in the diagnosis of COPD has been described by Alderson et al. [23], and we have confirmed

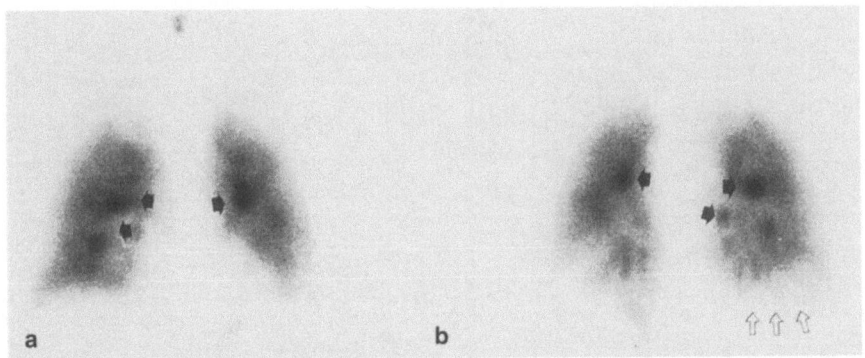

Fig. 5.14a, b. Central airway deposition and the "stripe" sign in chronic bronchitis. Anterior (**a**) and posterior (**b**) lung scans show moderate airway deposition in the central lung (*arrows*) and irregular airspace defects. A classic stripe sign can be seen in the left posterior basal lung (*open arrows*)

Fig. 5.15. The stripe sign in severe chronic bronchitis. Posterior lung scan of a long-standing chronic bronchitis reveals a classic stripe sign in both lung bases (*open arrows*). The stripes appear more distinctly on the posterior scan. Note that the prominent hilar airway deposition (*solid arrow*) is connected with the stripes, an evidence that the stripes denote dilated and spastic or occluded bronchi that are arranged side by side (*solid arrows*)

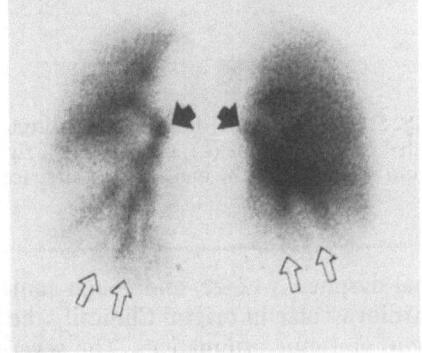

their result in both chronic bronchitis and smoker's lung. Indeed it is not rare to observe an arboriform airway deposition in the absence of a radiographic abnormality. In a ^{99m}Tc-HSA aerosol scan study on COPD Isawa et al. [21] noted peripheral scan defects in bronchitis and central or airway depositions in emphysema. However, they did not observe airway deposition in bronchitis.

Bronchial Asthma

Bronchial asthma is a clinical condition characterized by diffuse reversible spasm of airways in an increased response to various extrinsic and intrinsic stimuli [37]. During attacks smooth muscle spasm, mucus plug, and mucosal edema may easily occlude the airways from the segmental bronchi to as far distally as the respiratory bronchioles. With chronicity bronchiectasis may supervene, but true emphysema is rare [38]. Symptoms may include paroxys-

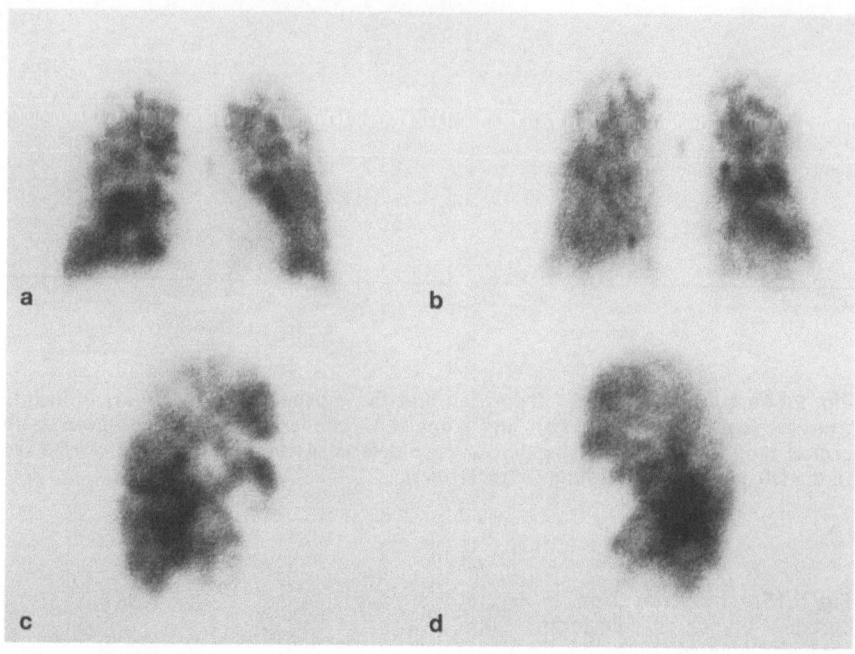

Fig. 5.16a–d. Aerosol lung scans of bronchial asthma in an attack (fresh, uncomplicated case). Anterior (**a**), posterior (**b**), right lateral (**c**), and left lateral (**d**) lung scans show irregular patchy and mottled airspace defects with little airway deposition

mal dyspnea, wheeze, and cough sometimes with sputum. They must not be cardiovascular in origin. Clinically the patient may be either in attack, remission, or status asthmaticus. The severity of disease may change rapidly over a short period either spontaneously or in response to treatment [33].

Radiographic manifestations include hyperlucency, which is usually severe, lung overdistension, and vascular attenuation with prominent perihilar vessels. Frequently the tram-line shadow and peribronchial cuff sign can be seen, denoting axial connective edema (Figs. 5.9, 5.10). The "staghorn" shadow of mucus plug is not rare. Focal lung disease must not be present [37].

Aerosol scan manifestations vary according to the stage and type of disease [39]. During a paroxysmal attack of uncomplicated asthma, aerosol scan shows widespread irregular nonsegmental defects in the entire lung, with generalized decrease in airspace deposition representing air trapping (Fig. 5.16). An important scan feature of simple asthma is the absence of airway deposition, the "clean" airway sign. This contrasts sharply to the arboriform airway deposition of chronic bronchitis. However, in addition to prominent nonsegmental airspace defects, long-standing asthma with bronchitic complication manifests the typical arboriform deposition resembling and in fact denoting bronchitic complication (Fig. 5.17). Severe emphysemic complication causes prominent airway deposition, creating the characteristic

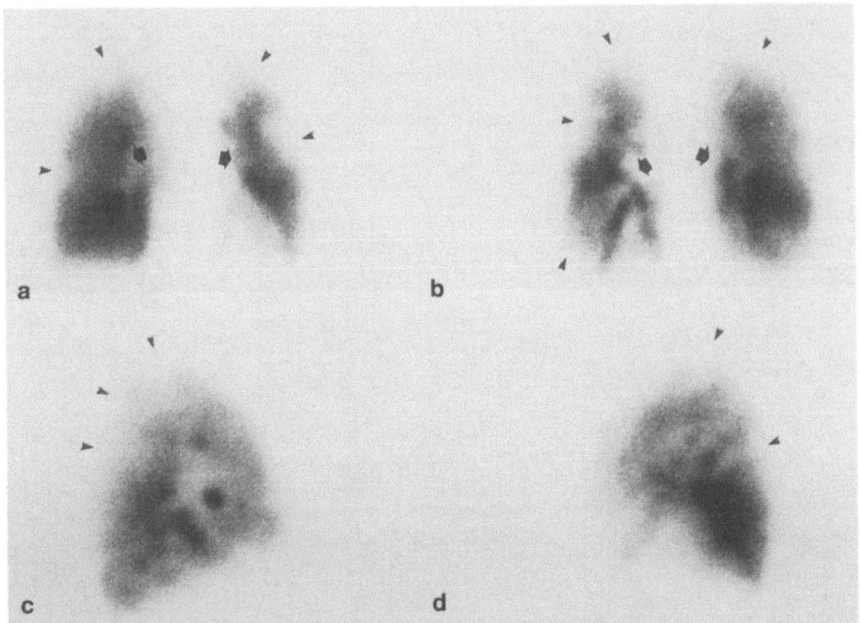

Fig. 5.17 a–d. Aerosol lung scans in bronchial asthma with chronic bronchitis (moderate case). Anterior (**a**), posterior (**b**), right lateral (**c**), and left lateral (**d**) lung scans show nonsegmental patchy airspace defects (*arrowheads*) and moderate central airway deposition (*arrows*)

"withered-bough" sign (Fig. 5.18). At this stage airspace defects become markedly intensified. In status asthmaticus the airspace alterations are tremendously exaggerated (Fig. 5.19) and resemble panbronchiolitis (Fig. 5.37). Even in status asthmaticus the airway deposition remains inconspicuous unless the disease is complicated by bronchitis or bronchiectasis (Fig. 5.19). As one can anticipate, ^{99m}Tc-phytate aerosol scan is an efficient means for assessing and documenting dramatic improvement of a severe ventilation defect after a bronchodilator treatment (Fig. 5.20).

Bronchiectasis

Bronchiectasis is defined as an abnormal and frequently permanent dilatation of bronchi [40]. The dilatation may be cylindrical, varicose, and saccular, or cystic; in most cases different types coexist. It is a common sequela of childhood diseases such as the lower respiratory tract infection, measles, pertussis, tuberculosis, and cystic fibrosis. In adults it occurs as a complication of asthma, lung carcinoma, pulmonary tuberculosis, allergic aspergillosis, and bronchostenosis. Simple bronchiectasis is asymptomatic, but with infection the disease becomes distressful and produces coughing with copious

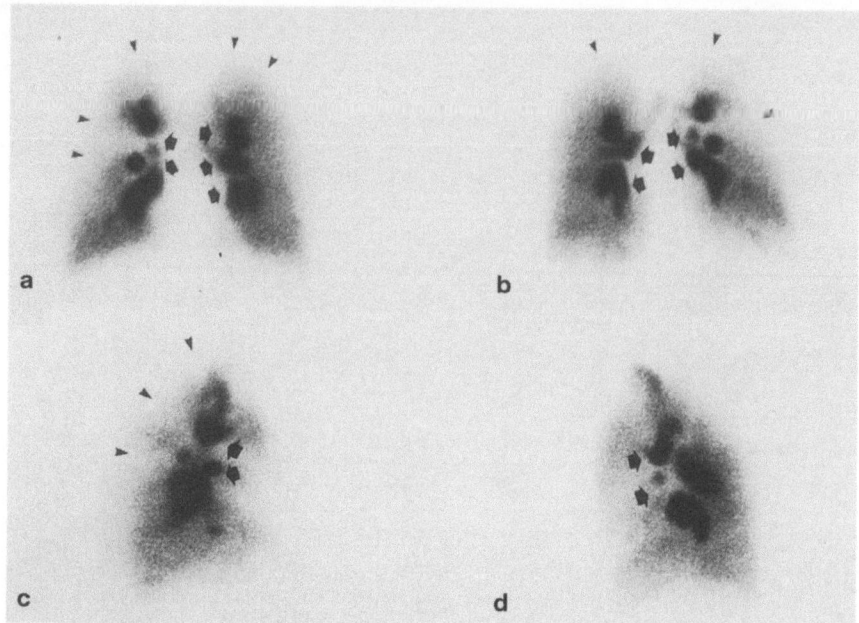

Fig. 5.18 a–d. Aerosol lung scans in long-standing bronchial asthma with obstructive pulmonary disease (severe case). Anterior (**a**), posterior (**b**), right lateral (**c**), and left lateral (**d**) lung scans reveal marked central airway deposition (*arrows*) and irregular airspace defects in the upper and middle lungs (*arrowheads*)

sputum, which is purulent, bloody, and foul-smelling. In established cases the diagnosis can be made without difficulty using the high kV technique. However bronchography, conventional tomography, or CT may be necessary to detect mild or obscure cases and to plan surgery.

Radiographic findings include crowding of vascular markings and tubular or cystic shadows sometimes with air-fluid levels and lung collapse, typically in the middle and lower lung (Fig. 5.21). Conventional tomography, bronchography, and CT provide specific information regarding topography, bronchial dilatation or narrowing, lung collapse, and concurrent bronchitis (Figs. 5.22, 5.23).

The scan manifestation of bronchiectasis has been described as a matched defect in the lower lung [41] and trapping of ^{133}Xe with delayed washout [42]. These features are nonspecific and common to many lung diseases. ^{99m}Tc-phytate aerosol scans in the present series showed an interesting manifestation that directly indicates the disease; irregular aerosol deposition in the dilated, crowded, and eccentrically located bronchi in the lower lung (Figs. 5.23, 5.24). Typically the bronchial alteration is accompanied by the airspace defect of collapsed lung. Similar airway deposition is seen in smoker's lung, chronic bronchitis, asthma, and pulmonary emphysema. Unlike in bronchiectasis, however, the airway deposition in these diseases is typically

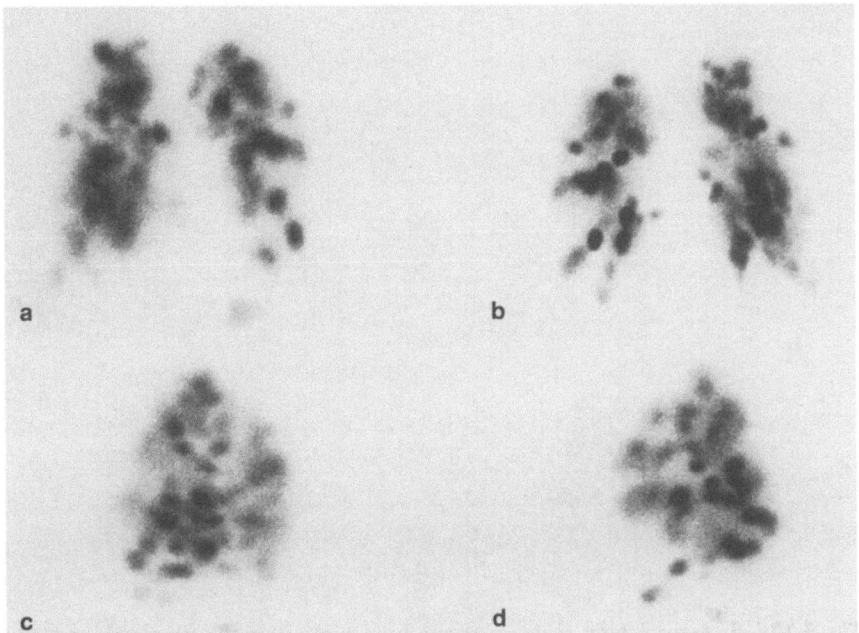

Fig. 5.19 a–d. Aerosol lung scans in status asthmaticus. Anterior (**a**), posterior (**b**), right lateral (**c**), and left lateral (**d**) lung scans show intense aerosol deposition in the dilated airways in both lungs with conspicuous airspace defects. The findings are much similar to those of increased-markings emphysema (Fig. 5.8 c)

in the central and upper lungs (Figs. 5.4, 5.12–5.15, 5.18, 5.20). In some mild cases aerosol alterations are obvious, but radiographic findings are not. This is particularly true when disease is hidden behind the heart (Fig. 5.24).

Understandably, when bronchiectasis is generalized and diffuse, the localizing sign is no longer valid (Fig. 5.25). A good correlation is noted between scintigraphic and radiographic alterations in established cases. Aerosol scans are useful in detecting bronchial obstruction in bronchiectasis (see below).

Bronchial Obstruction

Bronchial obstruction is an important airway pathology, imposing diagnostic problems both clinically and radiographically. This is particularly the case when the obstruction is associated with a bizarre lung disease such as advanced tuberculosis or carcinoma because of overlap and concealment (Figs. 5.26, 5.27). Obstruction may be complete or incomplete and the site peripheral, segmental, lobar, or in the mainstem bronchus. The causes vary, including inflammation, tuberculosis, tumors, trauma, foreign bodies, scar, and congenital malformations. Of these, tuberculosis and tumor are probably the two most common causative diseases in adults.

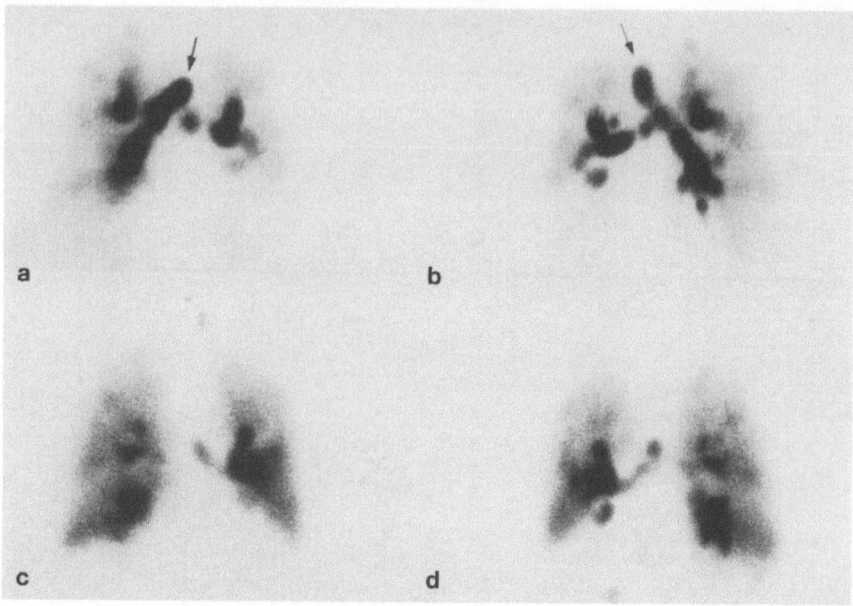

Fig. 5.20 a–d. Aerosol lung scans in severe bronchial asthma in an attack and after bronchodilator treatment. **a,b** Anterior and posterior lung scans obtained during an attack show very intense aerosol deposition in the dilated tracheobronchial tree (*arrow*) and gross airspace defects. **c,d** Anterior and posterior lung scans obtained after the use of bronchodilator show remarkably improved scan alterations with reduced airway deposition and restored airspace defects

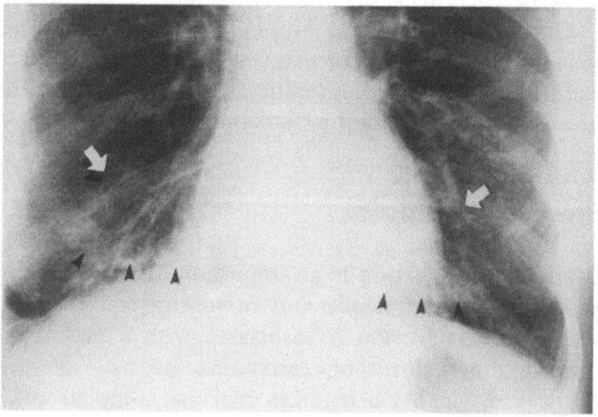

Fig. 5.21. Radiographic sings of bronchiectasis. Posteroanterior chest radiograph demonstrates multiple irregular cystic shadows and bronchial thickening in basal lungs (*arrowheads*). Vascular markings are crowded denoting pulmonary collapse (*arrows*)

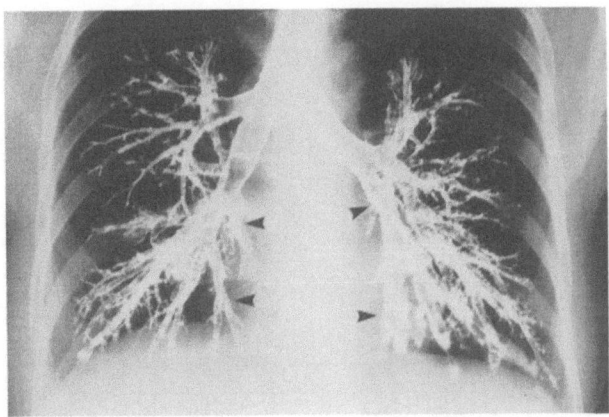

Fig. 5.22. Bronchographic signs of bronchiectasis. Posteroanterior bronchogram shows irregularly dilated clubbed and crowded bronchi in the lower and middle and lingular lobes. Note the sawtooth sign of glandular hypertrophy (*arrowheads*)

Radiographic evidences are either direct or indirect. The only direct sign is an abrupt or gradual termination of bronchial air shadow, which can be visualized on high-penetration radiography (Fig. 5.27), conventional X-ray tomography, and CT. Diagnosis may not be difficult when the mainstem or a large bronchus is occluded, but most lobar and segmental obstructions are hard to detect on plain radiograph (Fig. 5.26). The indirect radiographic signs include increased density, reduced lung volume, crowded vascular markings, and retracted anatomical landmarks, indicating lung collapse. Occasionally an incomplete obstruction causes a check-valve mechanism, creating regional emphysema that masks the obstruction.

Earlier applications of ventilation scan for the diagnosis of bronchial obstruction have been reported by Alderson et al. [23] and Lavender and Finn [43] using ^{133}Xe gas and ^{87m}Kr gas, respectively. The former group found the scan to be superior to radiography in detecting COPD, and the latter showed that bronchial obstruction can be indicated by airspace defect. Clearly, however, airspace defect cannot be a specific finding, occurring in a variety of lung diseases such as pneumonia, tuberculosis, edema, emphysema, asthma, and tumor. It seems that these authors did not attempt to visualize the obstruction site directly, probably for two reasons: the small dimension of airway obstructions in COPD and the radiogases used being not adequate for the imaging of diseased airways. Fortunately the aerosol scan that we performed was very effective in visualizing the bronchial tree when diseased. We performed aerosol scans in more than a dozen cases of confirmed bronchial obstruction. All cases showed scan signs of obstruction, although the radiographic finding was obscure or indirect at best. Indeed airway obstructions as far distal as the segmental bronchi were clearly shown as a small spotty aerosol deposition in the prestenotic bronchus, the prestenotic bronchial deposition sign [44] (Figs. 5.26–5.28). Pathogenetically it has been postulated

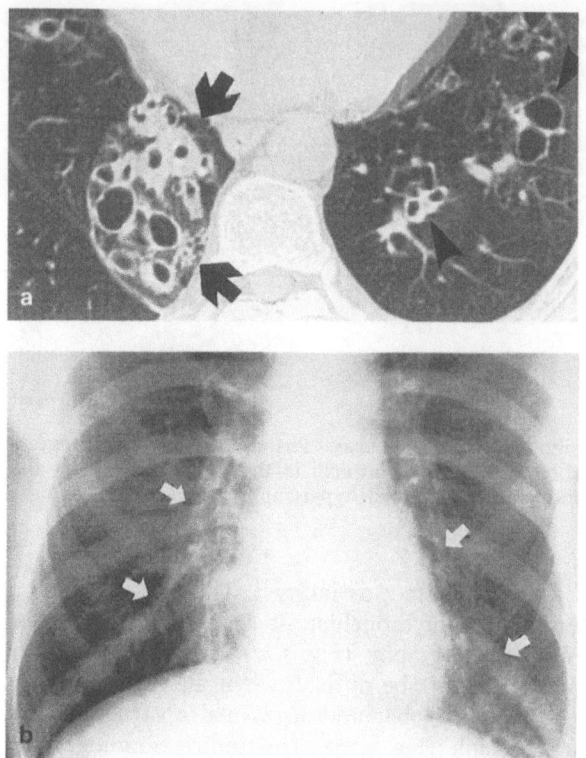

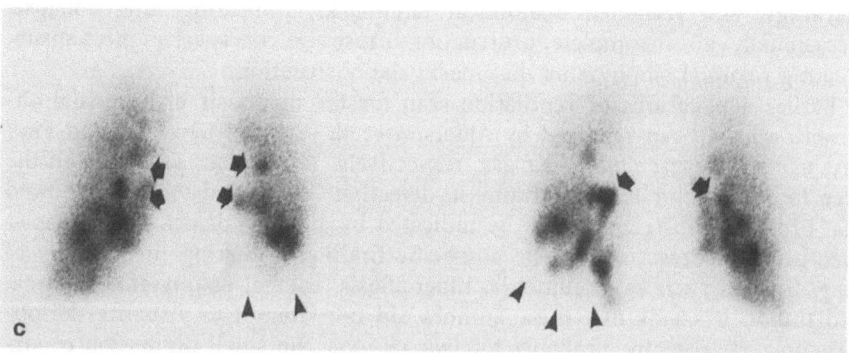

Fig. 5.23 a–c. CT, radiographic, and aerosol scan alterations of bronchiectasis. **a** CT of the lower lungs shows dilated and crowded bronchi in the right lower lobe (*arrows*) and some cystic change in the left lung (*arrowheads*). **b** Posteroanterior chest radiograph shows dilated crowded bronchi with thickened wall sign in both lower lobes (*arrows*). **c** Anterior (*left*) and posterior (*right*) lung scans reveal moderate aerosol deposition in the dilated hilar and lower lobe bronchi (*arrows*) and a large airspace defect in the collapsed left lower lobe (*arrowheads*)

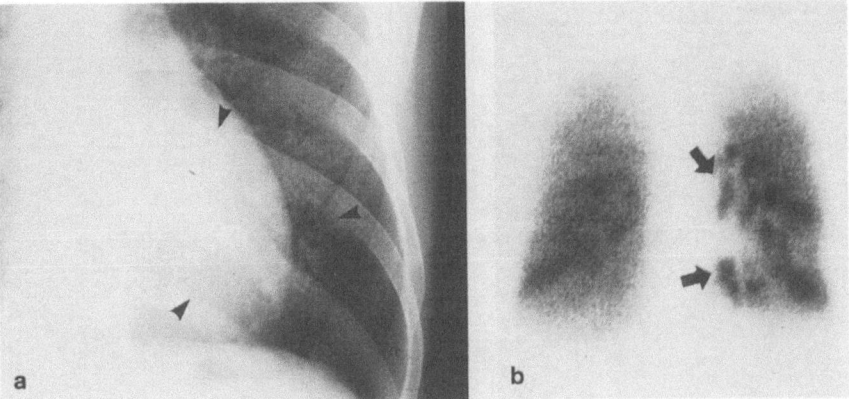

Fig. 5.24a, b. Obvious aerosol scan alteration in radiographically ambiguous bronchiectasis. **a** Posteroanterior chest radiograph shows suspicious bronchial abnormality in the left retrocardiac lung (*arrowheads*). **b** Posterior lung scan reveals obvious aerosol deposition in the dilated left lower lung bronchi, indicating bronchiectasis (*arrows*). Note that the lesion typically involves the lower lung

that bronchial mucosal damage created by inflammation or neoplasm abolishes mucociliary transport function resulting in the holding of aerosols at the obstruction site. Such a spotty deposition is attended by airspace defect, generally reflecting lung collapse and rarely focal emphysema.

Compensatory Emphysema or Overinflation of the Lung

The term compensatory emphysema describes an overinflated state of the lung without structural destruction or air trapping [45]. It may occur in compensation for reduced or lost lung volume such as collapse, surgical resection, and hypoplasia. Involvement may be segmental, lobar, or in an entire lung. Diagnosis is easy when volume loss and resultant overinflation are prominent. However segmental or small lobar overinflation is difficult to detect.

Radiographic features include hyperlucency and stretched vascular markings. Unlike in true emphysema with air trapping, hyperlucency subsides during expiration unless the condition is complicated by secondary COPD. The expiratory deflation can be confirmed by double-exposure inspiratory-expiratory radiography. In most cases the cause of overinflation such as lung collapse, fibrothorax, or missing lobe is readily recognized.

No study has yet been carried out in this condition using the ventilation scan. Based on the aerosol scans in our series of seven cases, simple overinflation can be characterized by increased lung size with a uniform airspace deposition, the intensity of which is either unaltered or increased. The intensity depends upon the magnitude of overinflation, which in turn depends upon the volume of the lung lost. Aerosol deposition is thus unaltered in

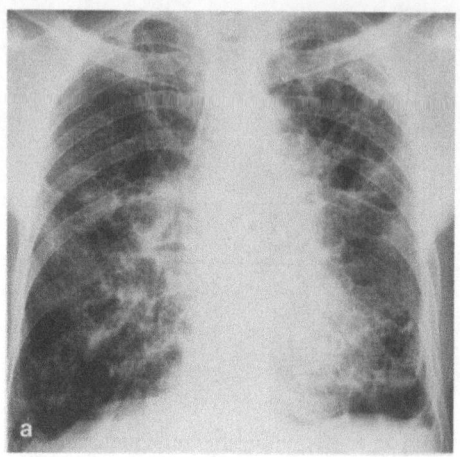

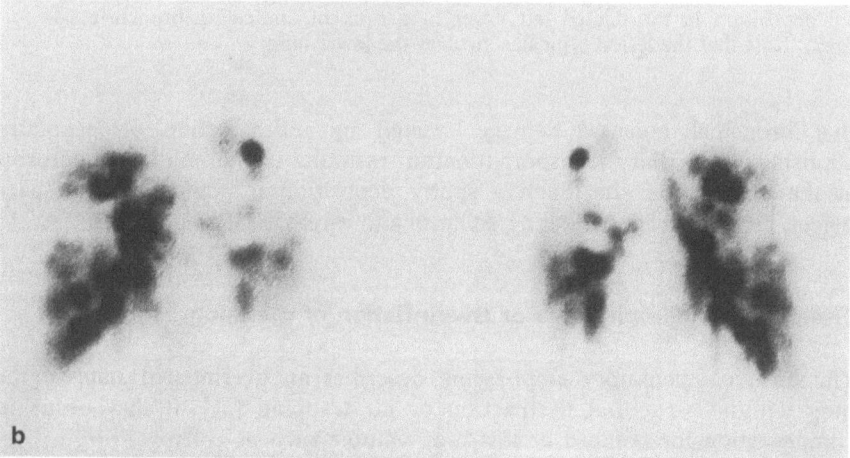

Fig. 5.25 a, b. Invalidation of lower-lung localizing sign in diffuse cystic bronchiectasis. **a** Posteroanterior chest radiograph shows extensive cystic change throughout both lungs. Some contain air-fluid level. **b** Anterior (*left*) and posterior (*right*) lung scans reveal intense aerosol deposition in irregularly dilated bronchi with bizarre airspace defects. Note that the lower lung localizing sign is no more applicable

minimal overinflation in segmental or small lobar collapse (Fig. 5.26) and moderately increased in moderate to marked overinflation in large lobar or multiple lobar collapse (Figs. 5.28, 5.29). The intensity of the aerosols deposited in the overinflated lung depends largely upon the amount of aerosols available in excess after the lung collapse or resection. Unlike true emphysema, compensatory overinflation shows no significant airway deposition unless complicated by COPD. We have observed two such cases of overinflation occurring in one lung in compensation for diffuse fibrothorax in the oppo-

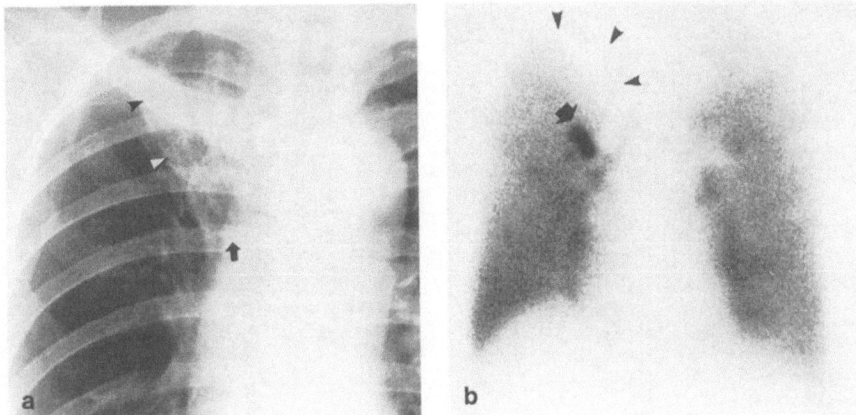

Fig. 5.26a, b. Prestenotic bronchial deposition sign in tuberculous bronchial obstruction. **a** Posteroanterior chest radiograph shows the marked collpase of the right upper lobe (*arrowheads*) and compensatory overinflation in the remaining lung. The bronchial obstruction cannot be detected. **b** Anterior lung scan reveals a large airspace defect in the right upper lobe (*arrowheads*) and an intense aerosol deposition in the prestenotic bronchus, denoting obstruction (*arrow*)

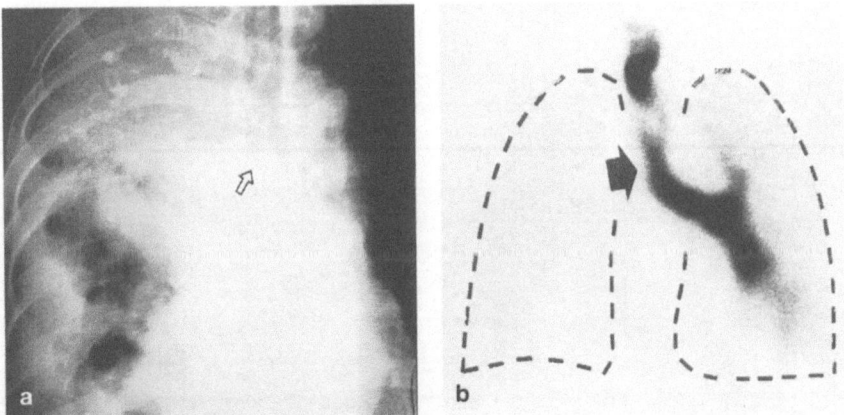

Fig. 5.27a, b. Obstruction of the right mainstem bronchus. **a** High kV posteroanterior chest radiograph shows an abrupt cutoff of the right mainstem bronchus (*open arrow*) that is occluded by carcinoma arisen from tuberculous lung. **b** Anterior lung scan shows marked aerosol deposition in the dilated trachea and left hilar bronchus, a modified prestenotic aerosol deposition sign (*arrow*)

site hemithorax. Both cases manifested increased airspace deposition but little airway deposition (Fig. 5.29). The airspace deposition in the fibrosed and contracted lung was generally decreased with patchy defects but, again, with a "clean" airway. However, once COPD or bronchial infection supervened, the airway deposition became notable (Figs. 5.26–5.28).

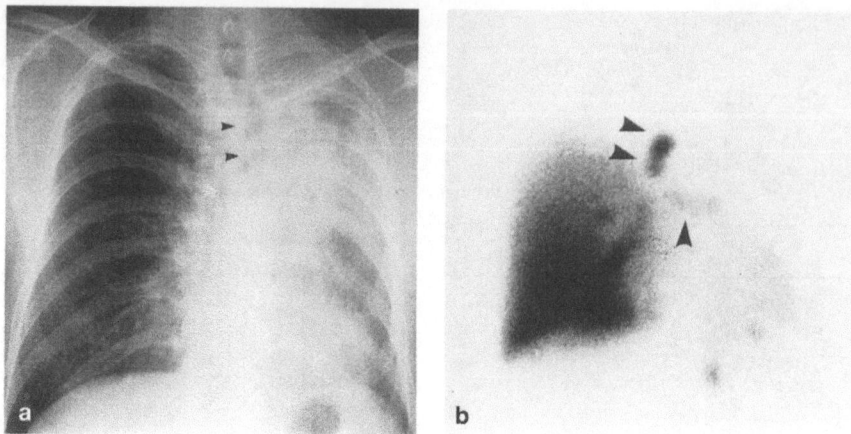

Fig. 5.28a, b. Prestenotic bronchial deposition sign and increased aerosol deposition in overinflated lung in tuberculosis. **a** Posteroanterior chest radiograph shows collapsed left upper lobe along with tracheal and hilar dislocation (*arrowheads*). The site of obstruction cannot be made out. The contralateral lung shows overinflation. **b** Anterior lung scan demonstrates intense aerosol deposition in the tracheal end (*upper arrowheads*), denoting left mainstem bronchus stenosis (*lower arrowhead*). The overinflated right lung reveals increased aerosol deposition

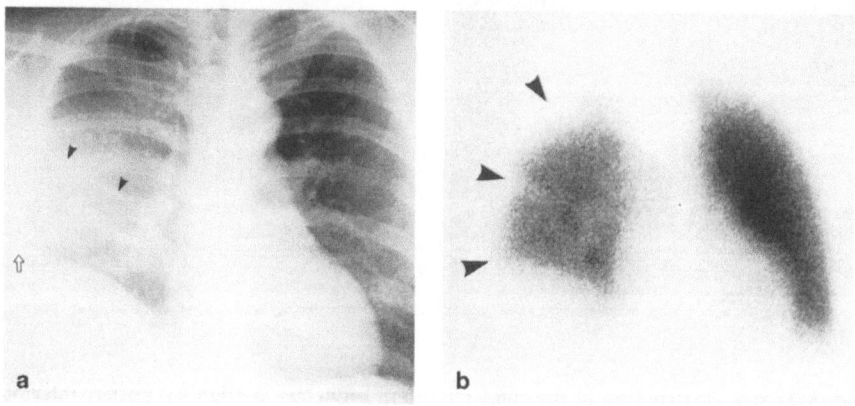

Fig. 5.29a, b. Diminished airspace deposition in passive pulmonary collapse. **a** Posteroanterior chest radiograph shows diffuse pleural thickening in the right hemithorax including the minor interlobar fissure (*arrowheads*) resulting in rib cage contraction and diaphragmatic elevation (*open arrow*). The left lung is overinflated in compensation. **b** Anterior lung scan shows reduced airspace deposition in the contracted right lung (*arrowheads*) and conversely increased deposition in the overinflated left lung

Common and Interesting Nonembolic Pulmonary Diseases

The nonembolic pulmonary diseases of clinical and scintigraphic interest we studied include acute pneumonia, pulmonary tuberculosis, diffuse interstitial fibrosis, diffuse panbronchiolitis, pulmonary edema, and primary and metastatic tumors. The diagnostic guidelines and pathological and radiographic criteria of the individual diseases are freely quoted from the standard textbooks, basically those of Dunnill [46] and Heitzman [47].

Acute Pneumonia and Synpneumonic Abscess

Acute bacterial or viral pneumonia with a lung consolidation and tuberculosis are probably the two most common infectious lung diseases. Micrococcal and *Klebsiella* pneumonias are prone to necrosis and cavity formation. In most cases chest radiography suffices for the diagnosis not needing a scan. Nevertheless an aerosol scan is indicated in some selected cases of pneumonia to distinguish it from other lung diseases such as infarction and edema that produce the same radiographic density but different aeration and perfusion pattern. Airway patency in lung abscess can be established by this means.

Kjellman [48] and Lavender et al. [49] have published ventilation-perfusion scan findings of pneumonias, respectively, using ^{133}Xe and ^{89m}Kr along with ^{99m}Tc-MAA. Another popular nuclear imaging technique for pneumonia is the ^{67}Ga scan which can image inflammatory tissue more or less directly. Lavender et al. [49] reported that the demonstration of well-demarcated ventilation defect with preserved perfusion, a reverse mismatch, is characteristic of acute pneumonic consolidation. However in chronic pneumonia the perfusion becomes deprived and results in a matched defect. We performed ^{99m}Tc-phytate aerosol scans in two cases of acute lobar pneumonia, including a case with synpneumonic abscess, and in four cases of segmental pneumonia, confirming that such pneumonias produce sharply demarcated defects (Figs. 5.30–5.31). In one case with segmental pneumonia in the middle lobe, the radiographic diagnosis was equivocal whereas aerosol scan was convincing (Fig. 5.31). In another case with *Klebsiella* pneumonia, again involving the middle lobe, aerosols penetrated into the cavity, denoting the patency of draining bronchus (Fig. 5.32). The cavity was bilocular with a small connecting neck and the medial loculus was visualized. In three cases we saw increased aerosol deposition in the lung adjacent to pneumonia, the nature of which could not be determined. Interestingly there was no airway deposition in pneumonia suggesting that the airways were not significantly damaged (Figs. 5.30–5.32).

Pneumonia in the posterior segment of the upper lobe and the superior segment of the lower lobe is best visualized on the posterior view. The lateral view is useful for delineating pneumonia in the middle and lingular lobes (Fig. 5.31).

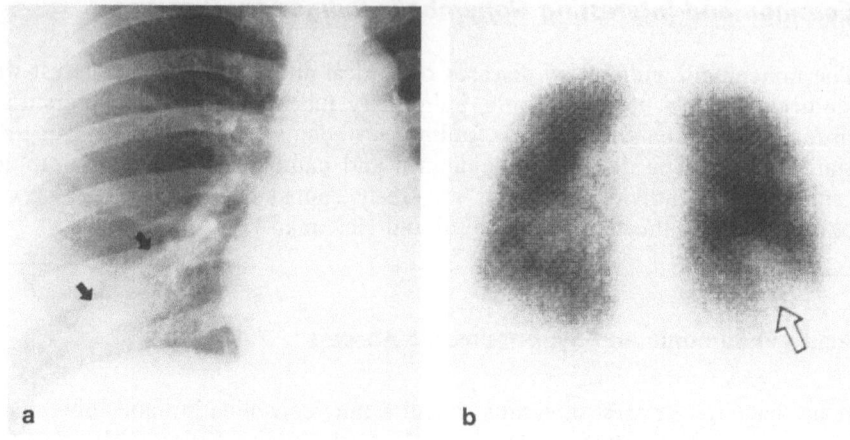

Fig. 5.30a,b. Aerosol scan alteration of acute segmental pneumonia. **a** Posteroanterior radiograph of the right lung shows a segmental consolidation in the central aspect of the lung base (arrows). **b** Posterior lung scan reveals a well-demarcated airspace defect in the lateral basal segment (*open arrow*)

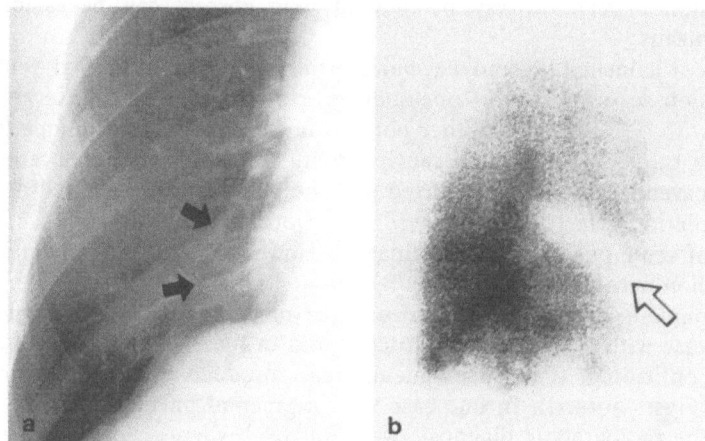

Fig. 5.31a,b. Usefulness of aerosol scan in the study of equivocal acute segmental pneumonia. **a** Posteroanterior chest radiograph of the right lower lung shows an ill-defined density in the right paracardiac area that is unimpressive (*arrows*). **b** Right lateral lung scan clearly portrays an airspace defect involving the medial segment of the middle lobe (*arrows*)

Pulmonary Tuberculosis

As with pneumonia, pulmonary scanning is not a primary diagnostic means of tuberculosis. Nevertheless it is useful for assessing the ventilation and perfusion states and airway complications, especially in advanced cases in which the residual pulmonary function is often critical in the clinical management

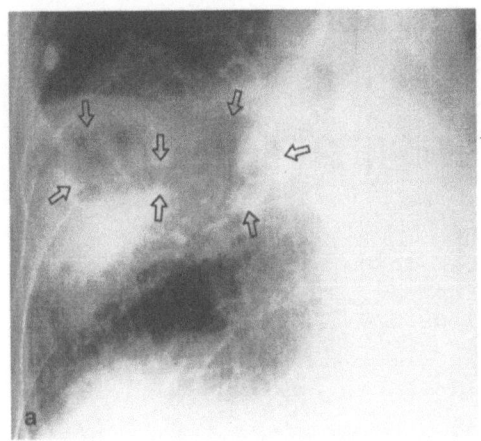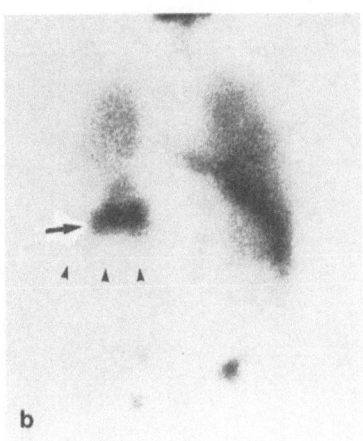

Fig. 5.32 a, b. Aerosol scan delineation of synpneumonic abscess cavity in *Klebsiella* pneumonia. **a** Posteroanterior radiograph of the right lower lung shows a large consolidation with a bilocular cavity in the middle lobe (*arrows*). **b** Anterior lung scan reveals the demonstration of medial loculus (*arrow*). Aerosol deposition is reduced in the upper lobe and totally absent in the lower lobe (*arrowheads*)

of disease (Figs. 5.26–5.28, 5.33). The tuberculosis included in the present series varied from minimal exudative and/or fibroproductive type through moderate chronic pneumonic and productive type with pulmonary consolidation to advanced bizarre pleomorphic type with bronchial obstruction and bronchiectasis and lung collapse (Figs. 5.26–5.28, 5.33, 5.34).

Scintigraphically the ^{67}Ga scan can be used in tuberculosis. It is a highly sensitive but not specific test. A classic study by Siemsen et al. showed a 97% positivity in active tuberculosis [50]. As mentioned above, ventilation-perfusion scans may be of use for assessing residual pulmonary functions in advanced tuberculosis. Moreover the ventilation scan is probably the most readily available noninvasive means of diagnosing bronchitis, bronchiectasis, bronchostenosis, and atelectasis which are common yet diagnostically challenging complications of tuberculosis. There has been no systematic documentation of aerosol scan manifestations in pulmonary tuberculosis. We performed ^{99m}Tc-phytate aerosol scans in 15 instances of various types of pulmonary tuberculosis in 12 patients.

Aerosol scan can efficiently portray airway and airspace changes in tuberculosis. Minimal fibrotic tuberculosis is imaged as an ill-defined airspace defect (Fig. 5.34), tuberculous consolidation and collapse as a large defect (Figs. 5.26, 5.34), and advanced lesions as bizarre scan alterations (Figs. 5.28, 5.33). The airspace defect in minimal fibrosis is usually more prominent than the radiographic alteration (Fig. 5.34). The pleomorphic lesions of advanced tuberculosis with airway involvement and pulmonary collapse produce large airspace defect, irregular airway deposition and pulmonary and mediastinal distortion (Figs. 5.28, 5.33). The discrepancy between the findings of aerosol

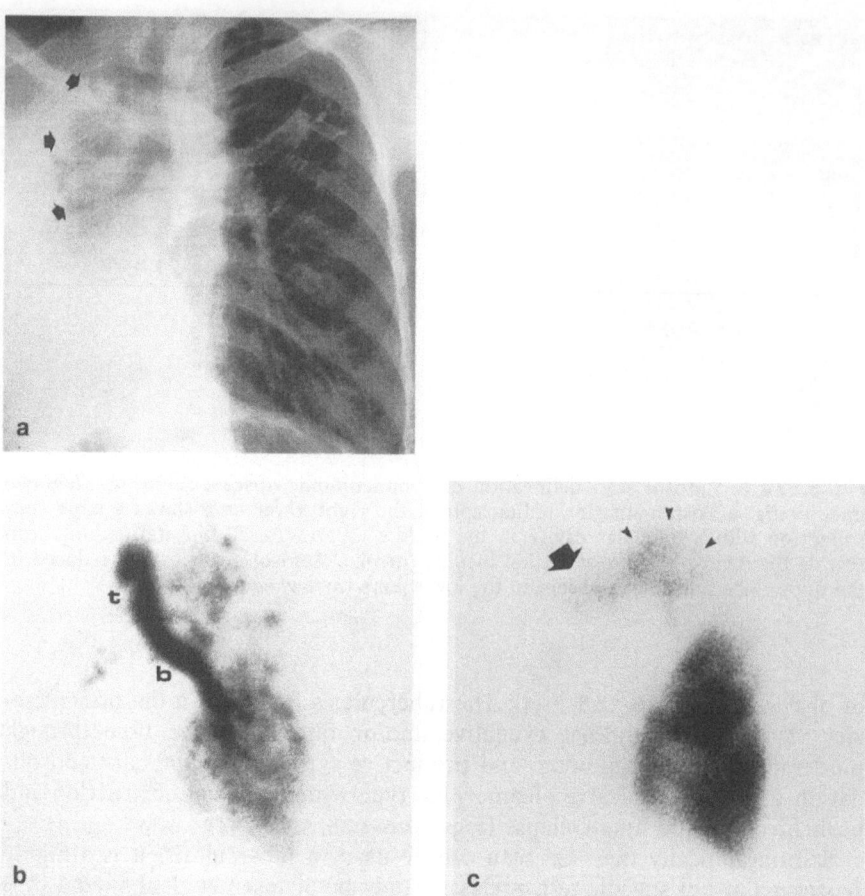

Fig. 5.33a–c. Prominent scan defect and *partial reverse mismatch* in chronic pneu-monialike tuberculosis. **a** Posteroanterior chest radiograph shows marked opacity of the collapsed right lower lung and dislocated heart shadow and less intense opacity of chronic tuberculous pneumonia in the upper lobe (*arrows*). The left lung is over-inflated in compensation and minimal calcifications are seen in the upper aspect. **b** Anterior *aerosol* scan shows virtually complete airspace defect in the right lung. In contrast, intense aerosol deposition occurs in the trachea (*t*) and the left mainstem bronchus (*b*) as well as in the overinflated left lower lung. The upper lung is underaer-ated. **c** Posterior *perfusion* scan portrays a small perfusion in the right upper lobe (*arrow*). The mismatch is considered to be related with increased bronchial arterial supply and bronchopulmonary shunts. As with aeration, perfusion is also reduced in the left upper lobe (*arrowheads*) but the lower lobe is overperfused in compensation

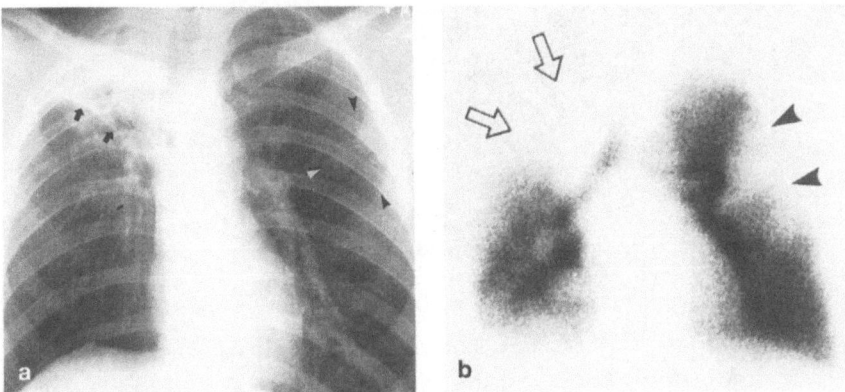

Fig. 5.34 a, b. Disparity between radiographic and aerosol lung scan findings in focal tuberculous fibrosis. **a** Posteroanterior chest radiograph shows minimal fibrosis in the posterior segment of the left upper lobe (*arrowheads*). The right upper lobe is collapsed due to advanced tuberculosis (*arrows*). **b** Anterior aerosol scan reveals a large airspace defect in the fibrosed left upper lung in question (*arrowheads*). The scan defect is disproportionately large compared to unimpressive fibrosis shown on radiograph. The collapsed right upper lobe is portrayed as another large scan defect (*open arrows*)

scan and radiography in fibrotic tuberculosis is probably the result of microatelectasis and paracicatricial emphysema [51].

Unlike COPD, which affects the lung in a diffuse manner, adult-type tuberculosis tends to localize in the upper lung. On the other hand, we observed a case of *partial reverse mismatch* in chronic tuberculous pneumonia that involved the right upper lobe (Fig. 5.33). The aerosol scan in this case showed virtually complete absence of aeration, but the perfusion scan portrayed a small imageable perfusion in the medial aspect. Such a partial reverse mismatch contrasted with the matched defect reported in chronic pneumonia by Lavender et al. [49], and it was considered to be related to abnormally increased bronchial arterial supply and bronchopulmonary capillary anastomoses that commonly occur in tuberculosis, bronchiectasis, and tumors [52].

Acute Pulmonary Edema

Pulmonary edema is defined as the presence of excessive fluid in the extravascular compartment of lung due to increased capillary pressure and increased capillary permeability [51]. The edema may involve interstitial tissue, alveolar spaces or both, and may be local or diffuse. Clinically the pressure type manifests heart failure and venous congestive syndrome, and the permeability type is related to uremia, infection, or noxious gas inhalation.

Radiographic manifestations include vascular haze, Kerley's lines, acinar shadows, and confluent opacity with air bronchogram sign, typically in the lower peripheral lung (Figs. 5.35, 5.36). The "butterfly" shadow is a well-

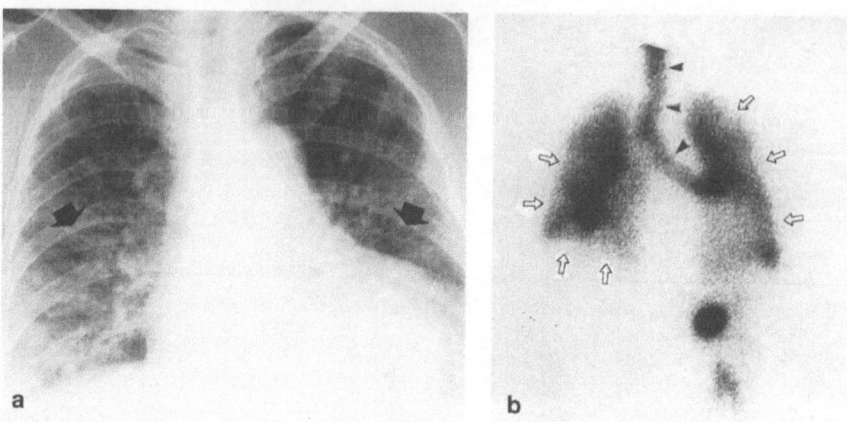

Fig. 5.35a,b. The "hot center and cool periphery" sign in pulmonary edema. **a** Posteroanterior chest radiograph shows irregular patchy densities in both lower lungs (*arrows*). The heart is moderately enlarged. **b** Anterior aerosol scan reveals intense tracer deposition in the central lungs surrounded by undulated decreased peripheral deposition (*open arrows*), giving rise to a "hot center and cool periphery" appearance. The trachea and left mainstem bronchus also reveal moderate aerosol deposition (*arrowheads*)

known sign of acute pulmonary edema. The finding of cardiomegaly helps establish the diagnosis of an edema of cardiac origin.

Ventilation-perfusion scans are useful for assessing the aeration and blood flow pattern in pulmonary edema, which is characterized by a reverse mismatch – preserved perfusion in the absence of ventilation. Lavender and Finn found the ^{81m}Kr scan unsuited for imaging of pulmonary edema [53], and Kim and Haynie have reported that ^{133}Xe scan changes in pulmonary edema are not consistent [54]. Although limited to two cases, our observations are at variance with theirs in that the aerosol scan proved unique in portraying the gravitational change in acute pulmonary edema. The etiology in one case was renal failure with secondary cardiopathy and cardiac failure (Fig. 5.35) and in the other acute adult respiratory distress syndrome (Fig. 5.36). In both cases the supine aerosol scans revealed diffuse intense airspace deposition in the central lung. It was surrounded by irregular nonsegmental peripheral defects, creating a "hot" central lung surrounded by rugged "cool" peripheral defects (Figs. 5.35, 5.36). The radiographic correlation showed that the "hot" central deposition represented the edema-free frontal lung which was independent of the supine position whereas the peripheral defects corresponded to the edemas in the dependent dorsal lung. Such a discriminative distribution of edema is likely due to gravitation, as shown by rapid change in the aerosol deposition pattern when the subject turned from the supine to prone position (Fig. 5.36). There was a close correlation between scintigraphic and radiographic alterations so long as their imaging positions were identical. Interestingly, unlike ^{81m}Kr and ^{133}Xe gas scans [53, 54], ^{99m}Tc-phytate aerosol scans showed marked aerosol deposition in the central airway, especially in the trachea and mainstem bronchi

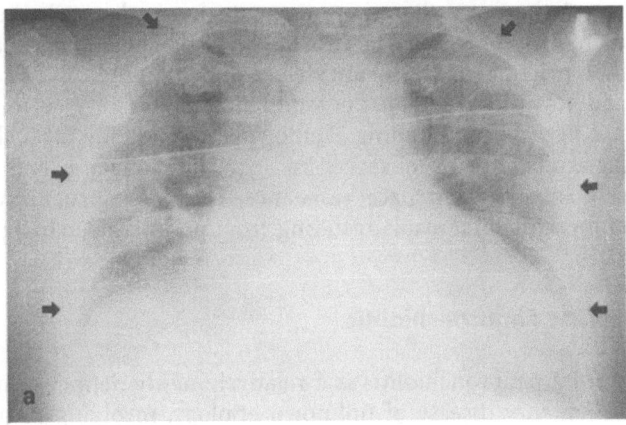

Fig. 5.36 a–c. The "hot center and cool periphery" sign in pulmonary edema in acute respiratory distress syndrome. **a** Anteroposteior chest radiograph shows blurred vascular markings and peripheral haze denoting lung congestion and edema (*arrows*). The heart is somewhat en-

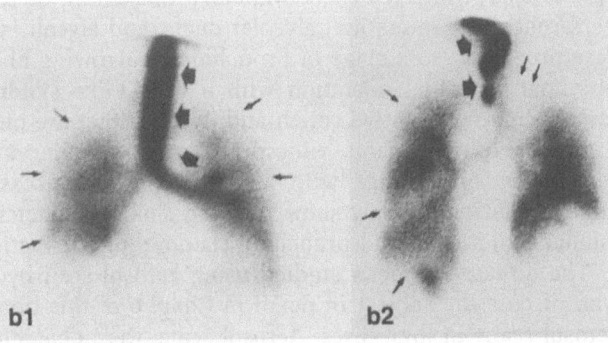

larged. **b1,2** Anterior and posterior aerosol scans reveal relatively increased tracer accumulation in the central lung surrounded by diminished peripheral deposition giving the "hot center and cool periphery" appearance (*small arrows*). The trachea is distended and shows intense tracer deposition (*large arrows*). Note rapid change in aerosol deposition pattern in the supine and prone views. **c** A follow-up scan reveals improved peripheral deposition with some residual defects (*arrows*). Basically, however, the pattern is the same as before, indicating that it is reproducible and characteristic of lung edema

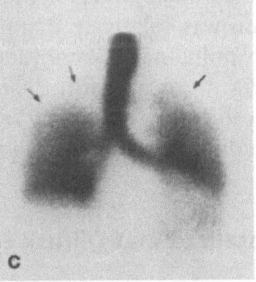

which were dilated (Figs. 5.35, 5.36). Scan alterations were far more prominent in respiratory distress syndrome than in chronic renal failure, and the difference was due to the cardiovascular change which was more severe in the former disease.

In this particular case, aerosol scans were made at two different occasions, one on admission and the other at 2-week follow-up after partial resolution of edema had occurred (Fig. 5.36). The follow-up scan showed much improved aeration but basically the same pattern that was characterized by "hot central lung and cool periphery," attesting to an excellent reproducibility of the scan alterations in acute lung edema. In both cases the aerosol scan showed cardiomegaly, helping to diagnose pulmonary edema of the cardiac origin. The perfusion defect in acute pulmonary edema seemed smaller and less distinct than the ventilation defect reverse mismatch, probably denoting alveolar flooding. Pathogenetically it was speculated that the intense airway deposition observed in acute pulmonary edema was related to diffusely increased airspace resistance, lowered mucociliary transport function, and excess of aerosols resulting from grossly disturbed penetration.

Diffuse Panbronchiolitis

Diffuse panbronchiolitis is a relatively newly defined, chronic, nonspecific inflammatory disease of unknown etiology, involving primarily the respiratory bronchioles in the "transitional zone" of lung [55, 56]. Pathologically the disease is characterized by inflammatory thickening of respiratory bronchioles, peribronchiolar interstitia, alveolar ducts, and alveoli [55]. Frequently the disease progresses to a stage of bronchiolar narrowing and stenosis resulting in proximal bronchial dilatation with a COPD-like syndrome [57]. The symptoms include productive cough and dyspnea that are often fatal.

Radiography presents widespread small nodular and reticular densities throughout both lungs with air trapping and occasional cor pulmonale. High-resolution CT may show the ring shadows, ductal shadows, and centrilobular punctiform and branching shadows of attenuation (Fig. 5.37) [56].

The disease has been studied using aerosol scan by Narita and Imai [58], who discuss the subject in detail in Chap. 6 of this book. We also performed aerosol scans in four cases. Aerosol scans were characterized by an irregular mixture of patchy airway depositions and airspace defects in the middle and transitional zones of the lung (Fig. 5.37). Generally the central airway deposition was relatively inconspicuous. At a glance, scan findings simulated those of pulmonary emphysema (Fig. 5.8C), simple bronchial asthma in attack (Fig. 5.16), and diffuse cystic bronchiectasis (Fig. 5.25). However the typical localization of patchy airway deposition and airspace defect in the intermediate zones were helpful [58, 59].

Localized and Diffuse Pulmonary Fibrosis

Pulmonary fibrosis or scarring is fibrous tissue formation in the lung at the site of healed tissue disruption caused by a variety of physical, chemical, and biological insults. Instances of unknown etiology are referred to as idiopathic. The common causes of localized fibrosis are necrotizing pneumonia, tuberculosis, parasitic infestation, mycosis, and irradiation and diffuse fibrosis may be seen in diffuse idiopathic pulmonary fibrosis, cystic fibrosis, sarcoidosis, asbestosis, and silicosis. Fibrosis may be minimal, moderate, or marked and either focal or diffuse. For a fibrosis to be clinically and scintigraphically significant it must be more than minimal in extent. Most of cases

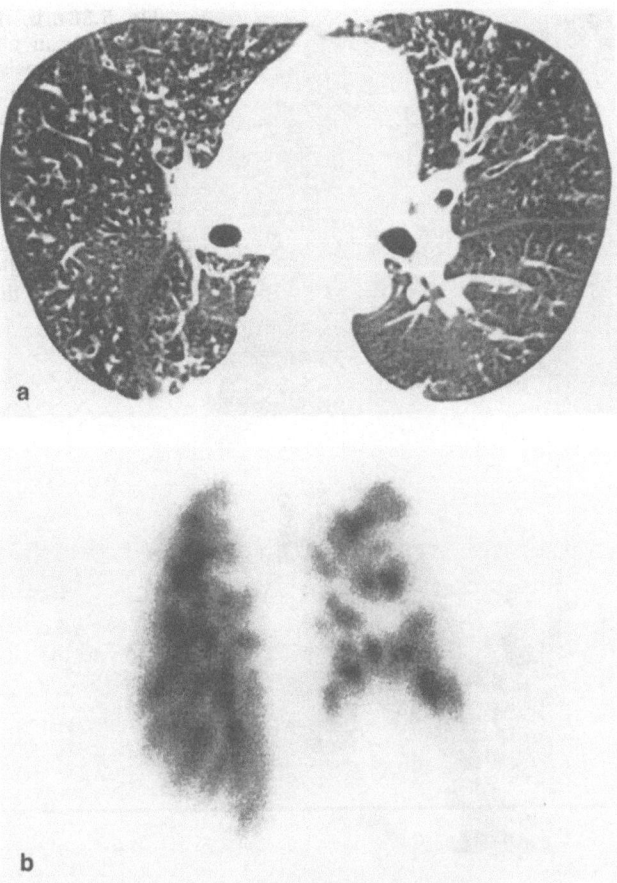

Fig. 5.37 a, b. Aerosol deposition in the transitional zone in diffuse panbronchiolitis. **a** Transaxial CT through the midlung shows the diffusely scattered ring and ductal shadows and centrilobular branching shadows of attenuation. **b** Anterior aerosol scan reveals irregular blotchy airway deposition mixed with airspace defects in the transitional and central zones of the lung. The central airway deposition is not conspicuous

in this series were minimal to moderate in extent and tuberculous in origin. Two cases were diffuse idiopathic pulmonary fibrosis.

Radiographically pulmonary fibrosis is characterized by linear, reticular, nodular, interstitial shadows with the obliteration of vascular shadows. The radiographic alterations are obvious when fibrosis is diffuse (Fig. 5.38), but it is not always easy to observe fibrosis when the change is minimal. For example, focal fibrosis involving a lung that is smaller in size than a segment may not be recognized as such (Fig. 5.34). Pulmonary hypertension with prominent central vasculature and cor pulmonale with a large heart are common end-stage complications of diffuse idiopathic pulmonary fibrosis.

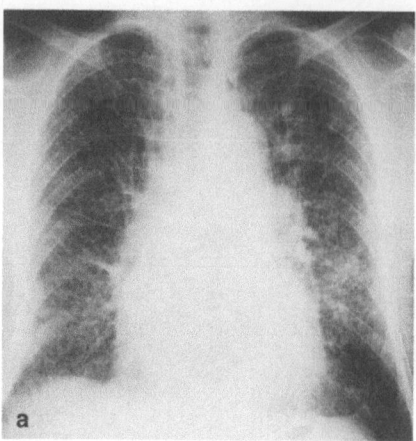

Fig. 5.38 a, b. Relatively inconspicuous aerosol scan alterations in diffuse pulmonary fibrosis. **a** Posteroanterior chest radiograph shows generalized pulmonary fibrosis in both lungs with linear nodular reticular shadows. The heart is somewhat enlarged with prominent hilar vasculature. **b** Anterior (*left*) and posterior (*right*) aerosol scans reveal multiple nonsegmental airspace defects in both lungs and cardiomegaly. Note that characteristically there is little airway deposition

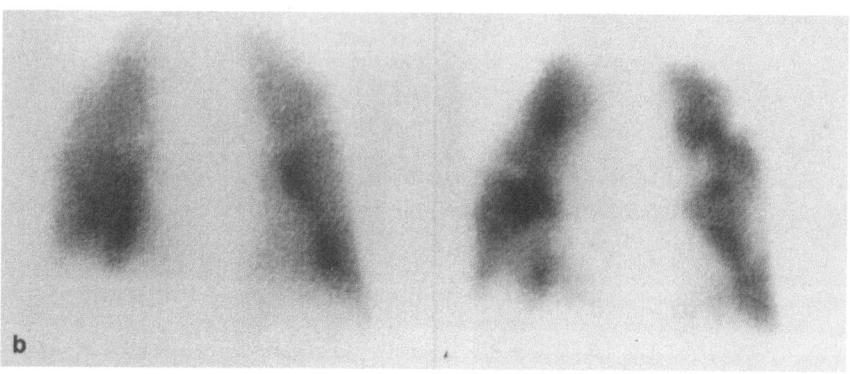

Scintigraphy can be used for the diagnosis of pulmonary fibrosis, both local and diffuse. Niden et al. [60] imaged a number of interstitial pulmonary diseases using ^{67}Ga, and more recently Siemsen et al. [50] documented the ^{67}Ga scan findings of diffuse interstitial pulmonary fibrosis and other lung diseases. Loken et al. [61] applied ^{99m}Tc-DTPA scan in a clinical study of cystic fibrosis, concluding that the test is very sensitive in showing airway alteration. The aerosol scan does not seem to have been used previously in systematic way for clinical evaluation of local and diffuse pulmonary fibrosis. We performed aerosol scans in patients with minimal focal tuberculous fibrosis and diffuse idiopathic fibrosis and confirmed the high sensitivity and value. Trivial fibrosis seen on radiogram frequently presented disproportionately prominent scan defect that was diagnostically meaningful (Fig. 5.34). The discrepancy was due to radiographically unrecognizable paracicatricial microatelectasis that attends fibrosis like a shadow.

It is to be noted that positive airway deposition is characteristic of tuberculous fibrosis, denoting bronchial involvement (Fig. 5.34). On the other hand, aerosol scan alterations in diffuse idiopathic pulmonary fibrosis are in-

deed mild compared to the prominent radiographic alterations (Fig. 5.38). Interestingly there was no airway deposition in this disease. Instead, partial
ventilation-perfusion mismatch was observed (Fig. 5.38). All these findings
were typical of the disease, the main pathology of which involves the interstitia, basically sparing the airspace and airway. In this connection it was of interest to note that, unlike diffuse idiopathic pulmonary fibrosis, cystic fibrosis manifests airway deposition due to bronchiectasis [61] which is a common complication of disease [62]. The aerosol scans in the long-standing diffuse idiopathic pulmonary fibrosis showed cardiomegaly and hilar scan defect, denoting cor pulmonale (Fig. 5.38).

Bronchogenic Carcinoma

Sociomedically bronchogenic carcinoma is one of the most important malignant tumors. There is a worldwide increase of epidemic proportions in this
tumor in both men and women, attributable to environmental factors and
life-style, notably air pollution and cigarette smoking [63]. The carcinoma
may arise from the central and peripheral bronchial mucosa. Generally the
peripheral variants do not produce respiratory symptoms unless well advanced, forming a bulky mass with the invasion of the neighboring ribs and
other tissues. In contrast, the central form tends to invade a large bronchus
and mediastinal structures in a relatively early stage, producing alarming
clinical signs and lung dysfunction.

Radiographic features are either tumefaction or infiltration in the central
or peripheral lung with emphysema or lung collapse (Figs. 5.39–5.41). More
often than not, carcinomas that incompletely occlude a bronchus cause a
check-valve causing emphysema (Fig. 5.39). Sooner or later such an occlusion
becomes complete, resulting in pulmonary collapse with the creation of the
well-known "S" or "inverted S" sign (Fig. 5.40).

Scintigraphically there are two different approaches to the nuclear imaging diagnosis of bronchogenic carcinomas, oncological and ventilation-perfusion scans. ^{67}Ga-citrate is one of the most widely explored tumor scan
agents. The ^{67}Ga scan is very sensitive but unfortunately nonspecific [50, 64].
As discussed in greater detail elsewhere in this textbook (see Chap. 8), the
tumor scans that use ^{201}Tl, ^{99m}Tc-methoxyisobutylisonitrile (MIBI), and pentavalent ^{99m}Tc-dimercaptosuccinic acid [(V)DMSA] offer the definite advantage of directly visualizing tumor tissues. However ventilation and perfusion
scans are indispensable for assessing aeration and blood flow in tumor and
the remaining lung (Figs. 5.39–5.41). For example, the paired lung scan is
useful for providing information on the bronchial patency in a tumor-in-
vaded lung by showing aerosol deposition in the nonperfused area of tumor,
a mismatch (Fig. 5.41).

Fazio et al. [65] have described their experience using the ventilation-perfusion scan to assess the therapeutic effect to carcinoma of irradiation or
chemotherapy. On the other hand, ^{131}I-labeled MAA perfusion scans have
been used for the screening of central lung cancer [66]. The aerosol scans in

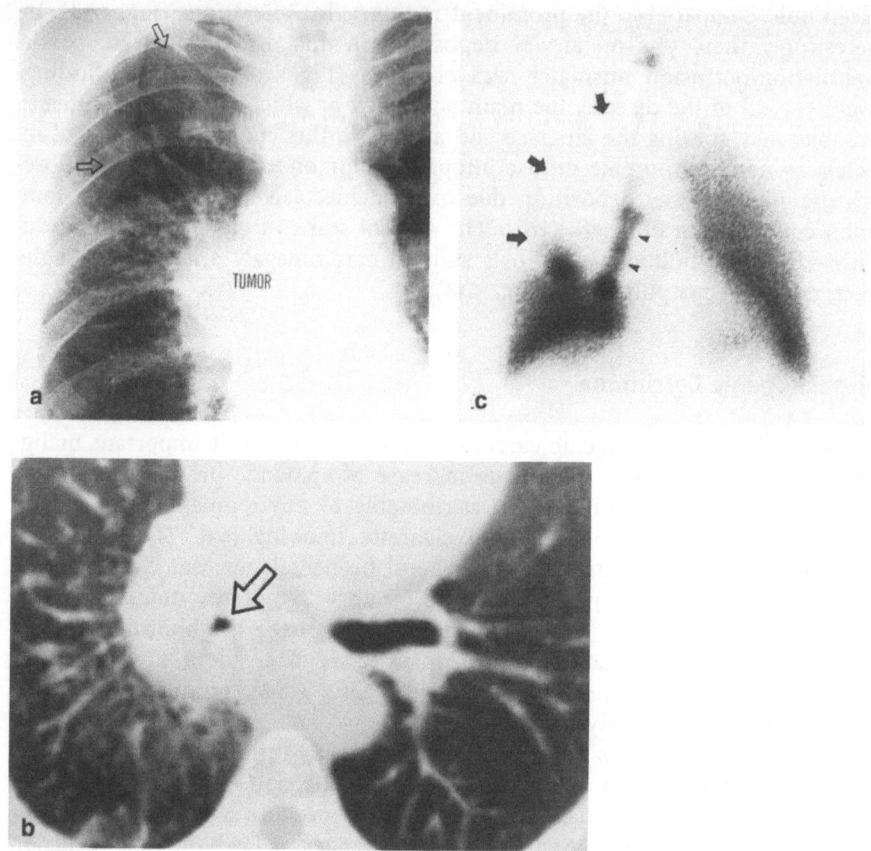

Fig. 5.39 a–c. Central bronchogenic carcinoma with focal emphysema. **a** Posteroanterior chest radiograph shows an ill-defined mass in the right hilum (*TUMOR*) with increased lucency in the ipsilateral upper lobe (*arrows*). **b** Transaxial CT through the right middle hilum reveals marked narrowing of the right hilar bronchus (*open arrow*). **c** Anterior aerosol scan portrays a large airspace defect in both the right upper and middle lobes, denoting obstructive emphysema (*arrows*). The bronchial narrowing is indicated by the prestenotic aerosol deposition in the mainstem and intermediate bronchi (*arrowheads*)

the present series demonstrated that peripheral carcinomas measuring a few centimeters or more can be portrayed as discrete scan defects (Fig. 5.41). Central carcinomas with peripheral lung collapse manifested a defect larger than tumor because of the addition of emphysema or collapse (Figs. 5.39, 5.40). The prestenotic bronchial deposition sign was useful in diagnosing bronchial obstruction that was difficult to detect radiographically [44] (Figs. 5.39, 5.40). Fazio et al. [65] described scan mismatch in two cases with upper lobe carcinoma. One of our two cases with upper left lobe carcinoma and typical "S" sign showed marked mismatch in the lower left lobe that was well ventilated in the presence of a complete perfusion defect (Fig. 5.40). It is

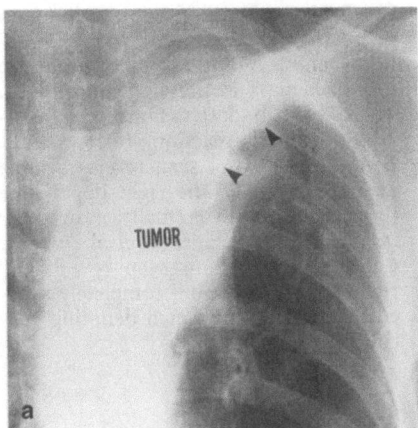

Fig. 5.40 a–c. Bronchogenic carcinoma and local lung collapse with the "S" sign. **a** Posteroanterior chest radiograph shows a tumor mass in the cranially shifted left hilar region (*TUMOR*) and a large collapsed lung opacity with concave border (*arrowheads*), creating the "S" sign. **b** Anterior aerosol scan reveals a large airspace defect in the left upper lobe (*arrowheads*) with the prestenotic aerosol deposition sign (*arrow*). **c** Anterior perfusion scan reveals complete defect in the whole left lung suggesting arterial invasion by tumor

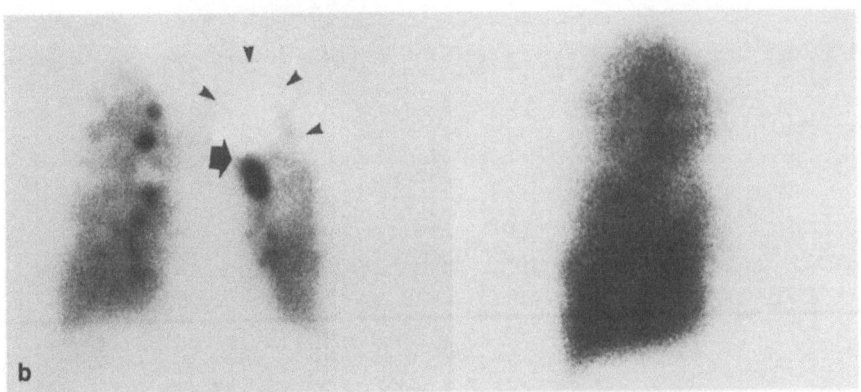

likely that the pulmonary artery had already been invaded by tumor while the airway was spared. The mismatch in the second case was focal and slight (Fig. 5.41). In general, the ventilation defects in lung cancer tended to be larger than radiographic lesion, as Ernst et al. [66] pointed out.

Metastatic Pulmonary Cancer

The types of pulmonary metastasis are hematogenous, lymphatic, and contiguous. Tumors that commonly metastasize to the lung include hepatocellular carcinoma, renal cell carcinoma, lung carcinoma, breast cancer, trophoblastic tumor, mediastinal malignancies, and bone sarcomas. Pulmonary metastases present either as a discrete or infiltrative solitary mass, multiple nodules, or "cannon balls" (Fig. 5.42) or lymphangitis. Of these, solitary metastasis often entails diagnostic problems [67].

CT-assisted radiography is the standard diagnostic approach to pulmonary metastasis. The lesion(s) may be either discrete or infiltrative mass,

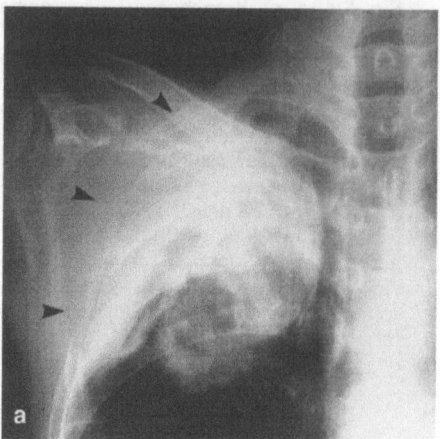

Fig. 5.41a–c. Ventilation-perfusion scan mismatch in carcinoma. **a** Posteroanterior chest radiograph shows a large roundish mass in the right upper lobe. There are rib destructions with associated pleural reaction (*arrowheads*). **b** Anterior aerosol scan revelas a large airspace defect in the right upper lobe (*arrowheads*) with a small aerated lung in the medial aspect (*open arrow*). **c** Anterior perfusion scan reveals the right upper lobe to be completely avascular, a partial mismatch denoting vascular invasion

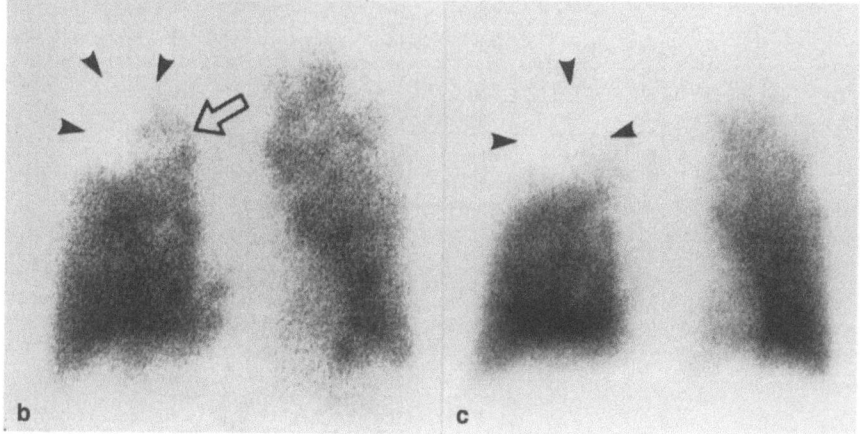

miliary nodules, "cannon balls" (Fig. 5.42), or irregular linear shadows with Kerley's A or B lines. Pleuropericardial involvement may supervene in advanced cases.

As with primary tumors, metastatic tumors of the lung can also be imaged using tumor scan agents such as ^{67}Ga-citrate [64]. In addition, the ventilation scan may be used to assess ventilatory state (Fig. 5.42). A successful scan delineation requires that the metastasis be larger than a few centimeters. A typical situation is that of "cannon ball" metastases from hepatoma, which create a number of well-defined rounded airspace scan defects (Fig. 5.42). Interestingly, there is a diffuse increase in aerosol deposition in the uninvolved lung. This is due to the relative excess of aerosols available for airspaces after the obliteration of a large volume of lung by multiple tumors (Fig. 5.42). The scan defects of "cannon ball" metastases resemble those of status asthmaticus (Fig. 5.19), diffuse cystic bronchiectasis (Fig. 5.25), and diffuse panbronchiolitis (Fig. 5.37). However, the sharp deli-

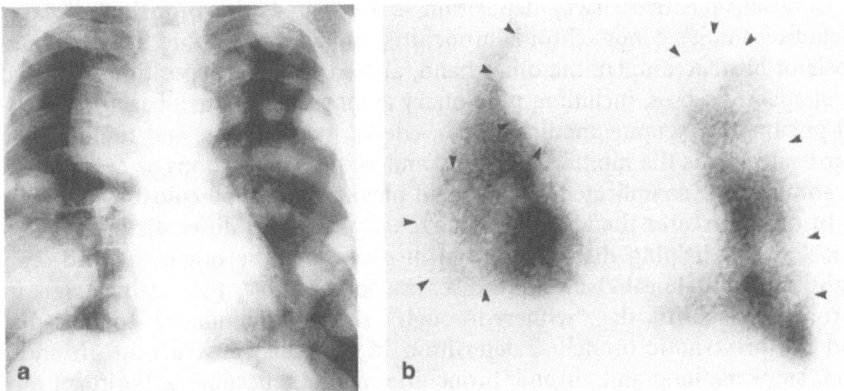

Fig. 5.42 a, b. Scan defects in metastastatic cancinomas of the lung. **a** Posteroanterior chest radiograph shows many well-defined mass shadows of metastatic hepatocecullular carcinomas in both lungs. **b** Anterior aerosol scan reveals many scan defects that compare well with radiographic lesions. Some are well-defined and some are not. Note that aerosol deposition is increased in uninvolved lungs due to relative excess of aerosols

neation and peripheral localization of metastases help to distinguish them from other diseases. Understandably the ventilation-perfusion scan is not suitable for lymphangitic or miliary metastases because these lesions are too small and fine. It must be remembered that lung miliary metastases from thyroid carcinoma can be imaged as diffuse mottled and patchy "hot" areas using ^{131}I especially when the tumor is well differentiated [68].

Summary and Conclusions

This study of the systematic application of the ^{99m}Tc-phytate aerosol inhalation scan to the diagnosis of COPD and other lung diseases shows that it is useful, economical, analytical, and practicable. When performed using a sufficient acquisition time and proper techniques, it can be elaborated into a state-of-the-art imaging modality that can provide many important and specific information in regard to the anatomy, pathology, patency, and aeration state of the airways and alveolar airspaces in normal and diseased conditions.

Basically aerosol scans can portray the alterations that occur in the conduit system of the airways and the gas-exchange system of the airspace. In general, the airway alteration is indicated simply by an increase in aerosol deposition. However the airspace aerosol depositions are either defective, decreased, or increased. The aerosol deposition patterns in the airways and airspaces can be assessed in terms of size, shape, location, and texture, and some patterns can be categorized into those that are common to a group of diseases and those that are specific to a disease.

Clinically positive airway deposition is associated with bronchial diseases including smoker's lung, chronic bronchitis, bronchiectasis, and bronchial stenosis or obstruction. On the other hand, altered airspace deposition is related to airspace diseases, including pulmonary emphysema, acute lobar or segmental pneumonia, synpneumonic abscess, edema, tuberculosis, and tumors. The third category is the mixture of airway and airspace alterations as exemplified in emphysema, complicated asthma, and pleomorphic tuberculosis.

In many diseases the airway and airspace alterations differ distinctly or to some extent, helping distinguish one disease from the other. Specific scan signs can be delineated in some diseases; for example, the "stripe" sign in chronic bronchitis, the "withered-bough" sign in pulmonary emphysema, and the prestenotic bronchial deposition in bronchial obstruction. In addition, smoker's lung and chronic bronchitis manifest peculiar arboriform airway deposition. It is of interest that pulmonary emphysemas manifest three different airway diversion patterns, distinguishing the panacinar, centriacinar, and increased-marking types of disease. In uncomplicated asthma, nonsegmental airspace defects appear diffusely in the entire lung with little airway deposition. Bronchiectasis is characterized by irregular eccentric airway deposition, typically in the lower lungs. Aerosol scan is of particular value in detecting the bronchiectasis hidden behind the heart.

Focal pulmonary fibrosis is indicated by localized airspace defect with little airway deposition. Generally the scan defect is much more prominent than radiographic alterations. The aerosol scan demonstrates typical prestenotic aerosol deposition in bronchial obstruction. The sign is useful in confirming bronchial patency in tuberculosis and carcinoma. Compensatory lung overinflation is characterized by a generalized increase in airspace deposition when change is more than moderate. Typically the airway deposition is also absent in this condition. Aerosol scans are useful for documenting disease stages and therapeutic response in bronchial asthma, bronchitis, smoker's lung, and tuberculosis. Ventilation-perfusion scans show mismatch in pulmonary carcinoma and reverse mismatch in acute pneumonia and pulmonary edema.

In conclusion, with improved image quality and a piecemeal analysis scheme, the ^{99m}Tc-phytate aerosol scan can be used as an important tool for both clinical and research studies of COPD and a large variety of other nonembolic bronchopulmonary diseases including infections, fibrosis, edema, and tumor.

References

1. Knipping HAW, Bolt W, Venerate LAM et al (1955) Eine neue Methode zur Prüfung der Herz- und Lungenfunktion. Die Funktionsanalyse in der Lungen- und Herzklinik mit Hilfe des radioaktiven Edelgases Xenon 133 (Isotopen-Thorakographie). Dtsch Med Wochenschr 80:1146–1147
2. Loken MK, Medina JR, Lillehei JP et al (1969) Regional pulmonary function evaluation using xenon-133, a scintillation camera and computer. Radiology 93:1261–1266

3. Kim EE, Hayine TP (1987) Pulmonary imaging. In: Kim EE, Haynie TP (eds) Nuclear diagnostic imaging – practical clinical applications. Macmillan, New York, pp 347–379

4. Treves ST, Packard AB (1995) Lungs. In: Treves ST (ed) Pediatric nuclear medicine, 2nd edn. Springer, Berlin Heidelberg New York, pp 159–197

5. Bahk YW, Chung SK (1994) Radioaerosol lung scanning in chronic obstructive pulmonary disease and related disorders. In: Bahk YW, Isawa T (eds) Radioaerosol imaging of the lung. IAEA, Vienna, pp 88–135

6. Isawa T (1995) General discussion. In: Isawa T (ed) Pulmonary nuclear medicine (in Japanese). Kinkodo, Sendai, pp 3–61

7. Dyson NA, Hugh-Jones P, Newbery GR et al (1960) Studies on regional lung function using radioactive oxygen. BMJ 1:231–238

8. West JB, Dollery CT (1960) Distribution of blood flow and ventilation-perfusion ratio in the lung measured with radioactive CO_2. J Appl Physiol 15:405–410

9. Clark JC, Mathews CME, Silvester DJ et al (1967) Using cyclotron-produced isotopes at Hammersmith Hospital. Nucleonics 25:54–62

10. Taplin GV, Poe ND, Greenberg A (1966) Lung scanning following radioaerosol inhalation. J Nucl Med 7:77–87

11. Pircher FJ, Temple JR, Kirsch WJ et al (1965) Distribution of pulmonary ventilation determined by radioisotope scanning. A preliminary report. Am J Roentgenol 94:807–814

12. Taplin GV, Isawa T (1968) Regional alveolar liquid diffusibility by lung scintigraphy. UCLA Rep (Biol Med) UC-48:4–48

13. Kotrappa P, Raghunath B, Subramanyam PSS et al (1977) Scintiphotography of lungs with dry aerosol-generation and delivery system. J Nucl Med 18:1082–1085

14. Burch WM, Sullivan PJ, McLaren CJ (1986) Technegas – a new ventilation agent for lung scanning. Nucl Med Commun 7:865–871

15. Anazawa Y, Isawa T, Teshima T et al (1990) Measurement of size of aerosols produced by different generators and effect of physical factors on aerosol size. Jpn J Thorac Dis 26:863–867

16. Isawa T, Teshima T, Anazawa Y et al (1991) Technegas for inhalation lung imaging. Nucl Med Commun 12:47–55

17. Taplin GV (1969) Scintiscanning in the assessment of regional pulmonary function. In: Gordon BL, Carleton RA, Faber LP (eds) Clinical cardiopulmonary physiology. Grune and Stratton, New York, pp 437–464

18. Taplin GV, Johnson DE, Dore EK et al (1964) Lung photoscans with macroaggregates of human serum radioalbumin. Experimental basis and initial clinical trials. Health Phys 10:1219–1227

19. Wagner HN Jr, Sabiston DC Jr, McAfee JG et al (1964) Diagnosis of massive pulmonary embolism in man by radioisotope scanning. N Engl J Med 271:377–384

20. Rhodes BA, Stem HS, Buchanan TW (1971) Lung scanning with 99m-technetium microspheres. Radiology 99:613–621

21. Isawa T, Teshima T, Anazawa Y et al (1994) Comparison of aerosol inhalation lung images using BARC and other nebulizers. In: Bahk YW, Isawa T (eds) Radioaerosol imaging of the lung. IAEA, Vienna, pp 49–63

22. Barter SJ, Cunningham DA, Lavender JP et al (1985) Abnormal ventilation scans in middle aged smokers. Am Rev Respir Dis 132:148–151

23. Alderson PO, Secker-Walker RH, Forrest JV (1974) Detection of obstructive pulmonary disease. Radiology 111:643–648

24. Fazio F, Lavender PJ, Steiner RE (1978) [81m]Krypton ventilation and ^{99m}Tc perfusion scans in chest disease: comparison with standard radiographs. Am J Roentgenol 130:421–428

25. Snider GL, Kleinerman J, Thurlbeck WM et al (1985) The definition of emphysema. Am Rev Respir Dis 132:182–185

26. Heitzman ER (1984) Chronic obstructive pulmonary disease. In: Heitzman ER (ed) The lung: radiologic-pathology correlation, 2nd edn. Mosby, St Louis, pp 422–456

27. Thurlbeck WM, Simon G (1978) Radiographic appearance of the chest in emphysema. Am J Roentgenol 130:429–440
28. West JB (1971) Distribution of mechanical stress in the lung, a possible factor in localisation of pulmonary disease. Lancet 1:839–841
29. Lavender JP, Finn JP (1987) V/Q patterns in nonthromboembolic lung diseases. In: Loken MK (ed) Pulmonary nuclear medicine. Appleton and Lange, Norwalk, pp 101–131
30. Isawa T, Wasserman K, Taplin GV (1970) Lung scintigraphic and pulmonary function studies in obstructive airway disease. Am Rev Respir Dis 102:161–172
31. Cunningham DA, Lavender JP (1981) Krypton 81m ventilation scanning in chronic obstructive airways disease. Br J Radiol 54:110–116
32. Dunnill MS (1988) Relationship of chronic bronchitis to emphysema. In: Dunnill MS (ed) Pulmonary pathology, 2nd edn. Churchill Livingstone, Edinburgh, pp 124–125
33. Ciba Guest Symposium (1959) Terminology, definition and classification of chronic pulmonary emphysema and related conditions. Thorax 14:286–299
34. Reid L (1968) Pathology of chronic bronchitis. Lancet 1:275–278
35. American Thoracic Society (1962) Chronic bronchitis, asthma, and pulmonary emphysema. A statement by the Committee on Diagnostic Standards for Nontuberculous Respiratory Disease: definitions and classification of chronic bronchitis, asthma, and pulmonary emphysema. Am Rev Repir Dis 85:762–768
36. Burrows B (1982) Simple chronic bronchitis and asthmatic bronchitis. In: Wyngaarden JB, Smith LH (eds) Cecil textbook of medicine, 16th edn. Saunders, Philadelphia, pp 365–367
37. Dunnill MS (1988) Asthma. In: Dunnill MS (ed) Pulmonary pathology, 2nd edn. Churchill Livingstone, Edinburgh, pp 61–79
38. Dunnill MS (1960) The pathology of asthma, with special references to changes in the bronchial mucosa. J Clin Pathol 13:27–33
39. Kim BS, Park YH, Park JM et al (1991) Radioaerosol inhalation imaging in bronchial asthma. Korean J Nucl Med 25:46–52
40. Dunnill MS (1988) Bronchiectasis. In: Dunnill MS (ed) Pulmonary pathology, 2nd edn. Churchill Livingstone, Edinburgh, pp 81–95
41. Lavender JP, Finn JP (1987) Bronchiectasis. In: Loken MK (ed) Pulmonary nuclear medicine. Appleton and Lange, Norwalk, p 123
42. Vandevivere J, Spehl M, Dab J et al (1980) Bronchiectasis in childhood: comparison of chest roentgenograms, bronchography and lung scintigraphy. Pediatr Radiol 9:193–198
43. Lavender JP, Finn JP (1987) Acute lung disease. In: Loken MK (ed) Pulmonary nuclear medicine. Appleton and Lange, Norwalk, pp 104–106
44. Chung SK, Kim HH, Bahk YW (1997) Prestenotic bronchial radioaerosol deposition: a new ventilation scan sign of bronchial obstruction. J Nucl Med 38:71–74
45. Dunnill MS (1988) Compensatory emphysema. In: Dunnill MS (ed) Pulmonary pathology, 2nd edn. Churchill Livingstone, Edinburgh, p 116
46. Dunnill MS (1988) Pulmonary pathology, 2nd edn. Churchill and Livingstone, Edinburgh
47. Heitzman ER (1984) The lung: radiologic-pathologic correlation, 2nd edn. Mosby, St Louis
48. Kjellman B (1967) Regional lung function studied with xenon-133 in children with pneumonia. Acta Paed Scand 56:467–476
49. Lavender JP, Irving H, Armstrong JD (1981) II: Krypton-81m ventilation scanning: acute respiratory disease. Am J Roentgenol 136:309–316
50. Siemsen JK, Grebe SI, Waxman AD (1987) The use of gallium-67 in pulmonary disorders. Semin Nucl Med 8:235–249
51. Pierce AK (1982) Pathophysiology of pulmonary edema. In: Guenter CA, Welch MH (eds) Pulmonary medicine, 2nd edn. Lippincott, Philadelphia, pp 262–264
52. Mack JF, Moss AJ, Harper WW et al (1965) The bronchial arteries in cystic fibrosis. Br J Radiol 38:422–429

53. Lavender JP, Finn JP (1987) Pulmonary edema. In: Loken MK (ed) Pulmonary nuclear medicine. Appleton and Lange, Norwalk, pp 114–116
54. Kim EE, Haynie TP (1987) Cardiovascular disease. In: Kim EE, Haynie TP (eds) Nuclear diagnostic imaging: practical clinical applications. MacMillan, New York, p 374
55. Honma H, Yamanaka A, Tanimoto S et al (1983) Diffuse panbronchiolitis – a disease of transient zone of the lung. Chest 83:63–69
56. Nishimura K, Kitaichi M, Izumi T et al (1992) Diffuse panbronchiolitis: correlation of high-resolution CT and pathologic findings. Radiology 184:779–785
57. Maeda M, Saiki S, Yamanaka A (1987) Serial section analysis of the lesion in diffuse panbronchiolitis. Acta Pathol Jpn 37:693–701
58. Watanabe H, Itoh S, Imai T et al (1991) Study on the Tc-99m aerosol deposition patterns of diffuse panbronchiolitis: the analysis of the hot spot formation mechanism by SPECT of the aerosol inhalation scintigraphy and the chest CT. Jpn J Clin Radiol 36:43–50
59. Kim HH, Choi BG, Bahk YW et al (1994) Radioaerosol scan manifestations of diffuse panbronchiolitis. Korean J Nucl Med 28:192–199
60. Niden AH, Mishkin FS, Khurana MM (1976) Gallium-67 citrate lung scans in interstitial lung disease. Chest 69:2266–2268
61. Loken MK, Sirr SA, Boudreau RJ et al (1987) Quantitative measurements of regional ventilation in patients with cystic fibrosis. In: Loken MK (ed) Pulmonary nuclear medicine. Appleton and Lange, Norwalk, pp 155–174
62. Heitzman ER (1984) Cystic fibrosis. In: Heitzman ER (ed) The lung: radiologic-pathologic correlation, 2nd edn. Mosby, St Louis, pp 449–453
63. Dunnill MS (1988) Carcinoma of the bronchus and lung. In: Dunnill MS (ed) Pulmonary pathology, 2nd edn. Churchill and Livingston, Edinburgh, pp 333–401
64. Kinoshita F, Ushino T, Maekawa A et al (1974) Scintiscanning of pulmonary diseases with ^{67}Ga-citrate. J Nucl Med 15:227–233
65. Fazio F, Pratt TA, McKenzie CG et al (1979) Improvement in regional ventilation and perfusion after radiotherapy for unresectable carcinoma of the bronchus. Am J Roentgenol 133:191–200
66. Ernst H, Krüger J, Vessal K (1969) Lung scanning as a screening method for cancer of the lung. Cancer 23:508–512
67. Dunnill MS (1988) Secondary tumours in the lung. In: Dunnill MS (ed) Pulmonary pathology, 2nd edn. Churchill Livingston, Edinburgh, p 437
68. Blahd WH, Nordyke RA, Bauer FK (1960) Radioactive iodine (I131) in the postoperative treatment of thyroid cancer. Cancer 13:745–756

6 Diffuse Panbronchiolitis and Related Diseases

T. Imai and N. Narita

Diffuse panbronchiolitis (DPB) is a disease entity first proposed by Yamanaka et al. [1] and Honma et al. [2]. Chronic inflammation of the respiratory bronchioles is the major lesion associated with this disease [1–3]. The disease is peculiar to Japanese, and involvement of genetic or constitutional factors in its onset has been suggested [4]. DPB shows diverse pathophysiological features, such as exertional dyspnea with stridor, repeated infection of the lower airways, and marked obstructive disturbances of ventilation. A differential diagnosis of DPB is essential because the symptoms and pathophysiological features of DPB largely overlap with those of bronchial asthma, chronic bronchitis, bronchiectasis, and chronic pulmonary emphysema.

DPB is frequently complicated by chronic sinusitis. DPB, chronic bronchitis, and bronchiectasis complicated by chronic sinusitis are collectively referred to sinobronchial syndrome (SBS) [5, 6]. This chapter describes DPB, then SBS, and finally bronchial asthma.

Diffuse Panbronchiolitis

Coughing, sputum, and exertional dyspnea are the major clinical symptoms of DPB. This disease can be viewed as inflammation of the respiratory bronchioles and the peribronchial area. Infiltration of lymphocytes and plasma cells is detected in the respiratory bronchioles, causing stenosis or obstruction of these bronchioles [1, 7]. Emphysematous changes begin to appear as this disease advances. In cases of advanced DPB cylindrical bronchiectasis is often caused by repeated infection in the relatively thick small bronchi and in the subsegmental bronchi. These lesions are usually distributed diffusely in both lungs and tend to be more marked in the middle to lower lung fields and in the dorsal area [8].

These morphological features are reflected in diagnostic images and pulmonary function. In the early stages of DPB additional air is trapped in the lungs due to bronchiolar stenosis, and this is noted on chest X-rays. Airway stenosis or obstruction gradually increases, leading to hyperinflation. A characteristic small nodular shadow up to 2 mm in diameter with unclear margin appears on X-rays as a result of the spread of inflammation to the area around the respiratory bronchioles [9] (Fig. 6.1). In advanced stages emphy-

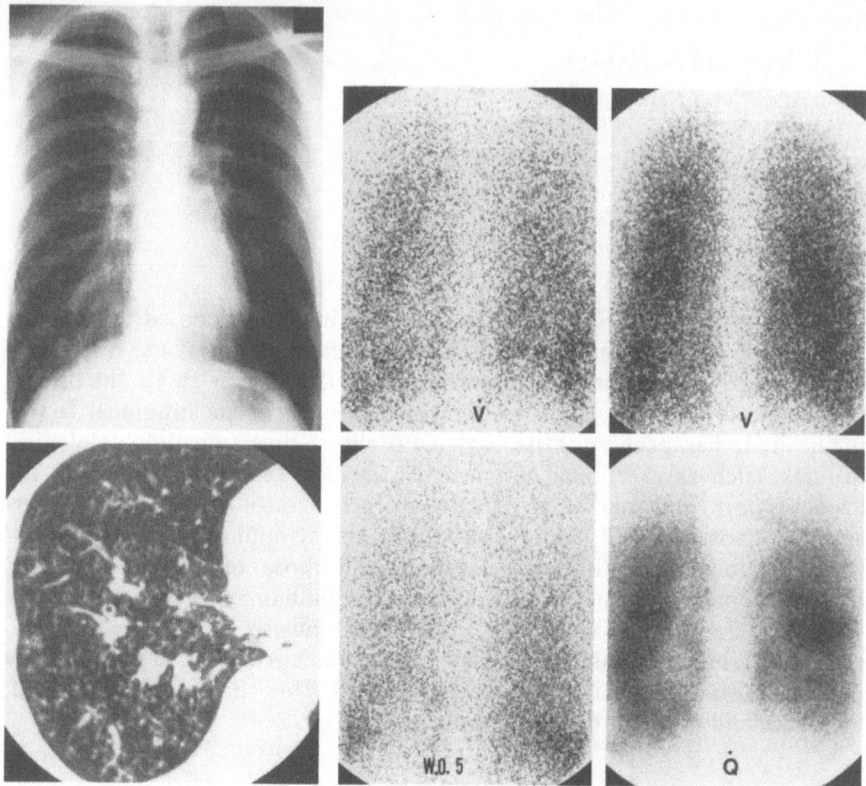

Fig. 6.1. Diffuse panbronchiolitis. Chest X-ray reveals hyperinflation in both lungs and small nodular shadowed in both lower lung fields. CT shows diffuse centrilobular region with small rounded areas of high attenuation around the ends of the broncho-vascular branches. Posterior ventilation image from ^{133}Xe gas scintigraphy shows inhomogeneous distributions in both lungs, and washout 5 min image shows delayed washout in the peripheral lower field of both lungs. Lung perfusion posterior image (^{99m}Tc-MAA) shows inhomogeneous distribution especially in the lower lung field

sematous lesions are more apparent. These lesions become more evident as the duration of illness lengthens. Repeated infection can cause thickening of the walls of proximal segments of the nonrespiratory bronchioles and spread to the thick bronchi. This change and pool of secretions sometimes lead to the appearance of tramlines, peribronchial thickening, reticular shadows, or linear shadows. Cylindrical bronchiectasis is sometimes seen [10] (Fig. 6.2). On chest CT images there are small rounded areas of high attenuation distributed centrilobularly along the peripheral bronchioles and the branches of the pulmonary artery (Fig. 6.1). Dilated bronchioles and bronchi and thick walls are often visible. As the disease advances, dilation and wall thickening spreads to the proximal segments of the bronchi [11, 12] (Fig. 6.2).

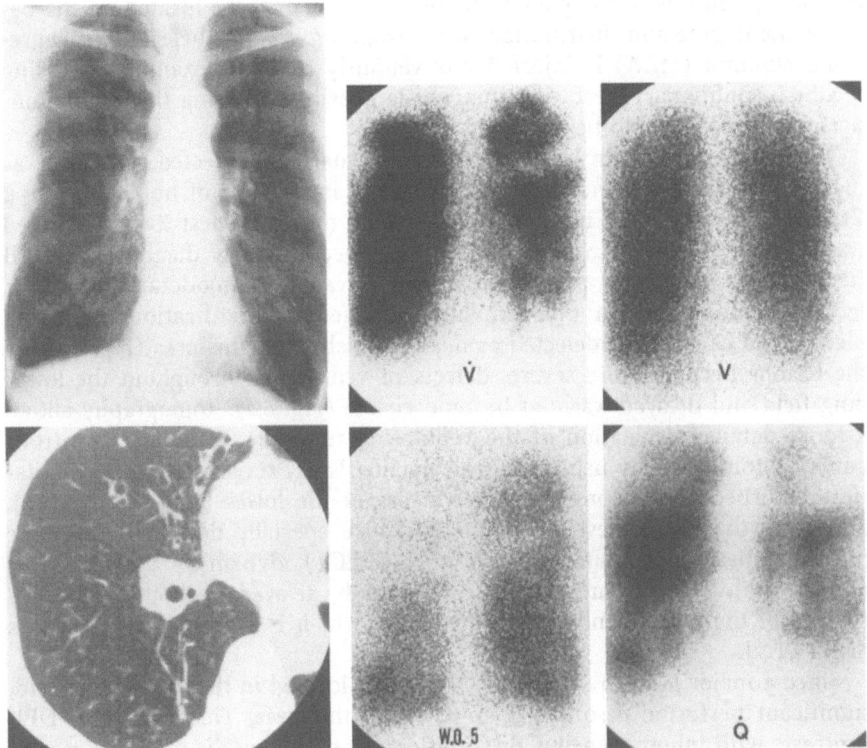

Fig. 6.2. Diffuse panbronchiolitis. Chest X-ray reveals flattened diaphragm, hyperinflation of both lungs, diffuse small nodular shadows throughout both lungs, and tramlines in the lower field of both lungs and in the upper lung field of right lung. CT shows diffuse small rounded areas of high attenuation, thickening of bronchial walls and bronchiectasis. Posterior ventilation images from ^{133}Xe gas scintigraphy shows a high degree of inhomogeneous distribution in the bilateral lungs, especially in the right lung. In segments, lobe-related ventilatory insufficiency was noted. Delayed washout of ^{133}Xe gas is observed in the entire right lung and the left middle and lower lung fields washout 5-min image. Posterior perfusion image reveals decreased blood flow consistent with the area showing delayed washout

Ventilation-Perfusion Scintigraphy

Changes often observed in respiratory function in the presence of DPB include severe obstructive dysfunction of ventilation and an accompanying decrease in $FEV_{0.01}$. As the disease advances, the residual volume and the residual rate increase, and the vital capacity decreases, often leading to a condition called "mixed ventilatory disturbance of restrictive and obstructive disorder" [2]. Nuclear medicine provides a useful means for evaluating regional pulmonary function.

A ventilation test using ^{133}Xe gas allows imaging of three distinct phases: ventilation imaging, equilibrium wash-in imaging, and equilibrium wash-out imaging. With this technique obstructive disorders can be located on the basis of the degree and distribution of air trapping. ^{99m}Tc-labeled macroaggregated albumin (MAA) is injected intravenously after the examination using ^{133}Xe gas; pulmonary perfusion imaging is possible, allowing the ventilation-perfusion imbalance to be evaluated.

Obstructive lesions in cases of DPB can usually be detected sensitively as markedly delayed washout of ^{133}Xe gas in the lower field of both lungs [13]. Even in stages at which little change is visible on plain chest X-rays, delayed washout of ^{133}Xe gas is visible and can be used for early diagnosis of DPB [14]. As the severity of peripheral lesions advances to moderate levels, defects become visible in the ventilation images as stratification along the pleura, and can also be detected as delayed washout in this area (Fig. 6.1). As the lesions become more severe, defects of ventilation throughout the lower lung field and delayed washout become visible (Fig. 6.2). Tomography allows a more detailed evaluation of the ventilating function. Transverse positron-emission tomogragphy using positron nuclide N2-13 reveals stratified ventilation-disturbed areas along the outer layers of the lower lung field [15, 16]. Following the recent development of a device specially designed for single photon emission computed tomography (SPECT), dynamic ^{133}Xe SPECT is now possible. This technique reveals markedly delayed washout in the periphery of the middle and lower lung fields, which is a characteristic of this disease [17].

Since a major lesion responsible for DPB is located in the lower lung field, significant perfusion disorder is apparent in this area. This feature of DPB contrasts with inhomogeneous distributions of perfusion disorder in cases of chronic pulmonary emphysema. Pulmonary perfusion scintigraphy reveals multiple perfusion defects in various segments of the lungs. In cases of advanced DPB, segmental perfusion defects are sometimes visible due to dilatation of the relatively thick small bronchi and subsegmental bronchi [18]. Comparison of a pulmonary perfusion scintigraphy with an ^{133}Xe gas ventilation scintigraphy indicates reduced blood flow in the area showing delayed washout. Quantitative evaluation on the basis of the V/Q ratio indicates that ventilation is more severely impaired than perfusion in the lower lung field [14] (Fig. 6.2).

^{99m}Tc-Technegas

^{99m}Tc-Technegas is ultrafine particles of carbon (0.005 μm or less in diameter) labeled with ^{99m}Tc [19–21]. Inhaled Technegas is deposited in alveoli and allows imaging of regional pulmonary function. This can be used in combination with MAA for the evaluation of pulmonary perfusion. Technegas is distributed approximately homogeneously in normal lungs, without showing increased deposition (so-called "hot spots") in the trachea or bronchi. In diseased lungs it shows various patterns of inhomogeneous distribution. Technegas posterior images taken immediately after inhalation by patients with

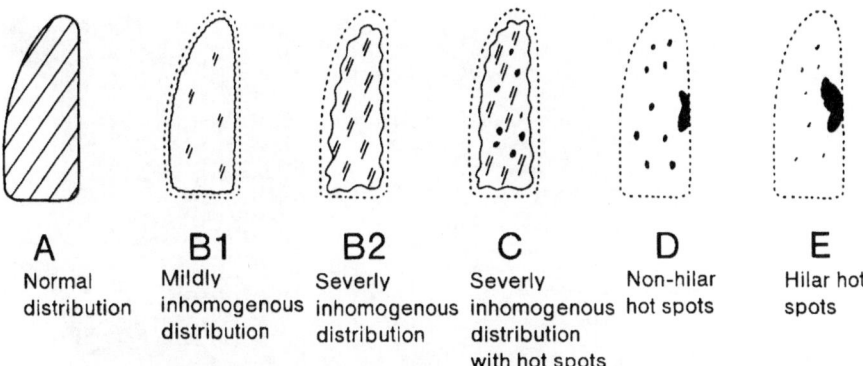

| A | B1 | B2 | C | D | E |
| Normal distribution | Mildly inhomogenous distribution | Severly inhomogenous distribution | Severly inhomogenous distribution with hot spots | Non-hilar hot spots | Hilar hot spots |

Fig. 6.3. Classification of posterior Technegas images. The degree of inhomogeneous distribution is classified into six types by the deposition pattern on AICS

Table 6.1. Relationship between lung deposition patterns of Technegas and respiratory diseases (updated with new cases; from [22])

Diseases	Deposition pattern					
	A	B1	B2	C	D	E
Healthy controls	8	–	–	–	–	–
Obstructive pulmonary disease						
Chronic pulmonary emphysema	–	–	2	2	3	–
Diffuse panbronchiolitis	–	–	1	2	2	–
Chronic bronchitis	–	–	1	2	–	–
Bronchiectasis	–	–	–	2	–	–
Interstitial pulmonary disease						
Idiopathic interstitial pneumonia	–	6	–	–	–	–
Asbestosis	1	8	2	1	–	–
Collagen vascular disease	–	4	–	–	–	–
Sarcoidosis	–	1	–	–	–	–
Total	9	19	6	9	5	0

various lung diseases were classified into six patterns (Fig. 6.3). In cases of interstitial pulmonary disease, Technegas distribution in lungs is slightly inhomogeneous. In cases of obstructive pulmonary disease, it is often very inhomogeneous. In cases in which chronic pulmonary emphysema or DPB are complicated by severe obstructive pulmonary dysfunction, hot spots can be easily seen [22] (Table 6.1). Technegas can also be used for multiple direction planar imaging and SPECT (Fig. 6.4).

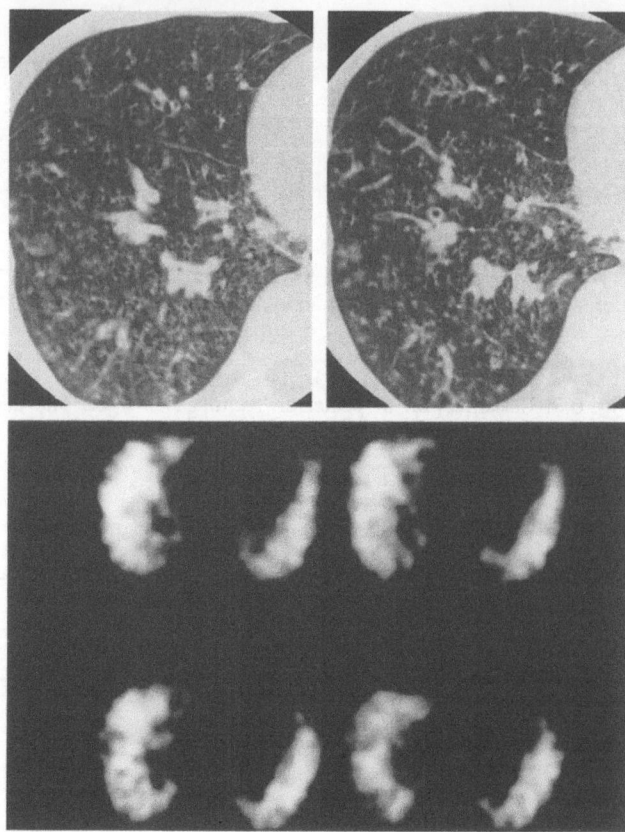

Fig. 6.4. Diffuse panbronchiolitis (CT and Technegas SPECT images). Images show diffuse centrilobular region with small rounded areas of high attenuation in the lower lung field. Technegas transverse SPECT images show inhomogeneous distribution of Technegas in the lower lung fields, especially in the outer zone

Aerosol Inhalation Scintigraphy

If a liquid radioisotope-labeled substance is inhaled repeatedly in the form of an aerosol produced by a nebulizer, it is deposited in the airway and alveoli after impaction, sedimentation, and diffusion. The optimum particle size of this aerosol for deposition in small bronchi and alveoli is about 2 μm. Aerosols with particles larger than 5 μm tend to be deposited in the large airways and the pharynx. Aerosols show various deposition patterns depending on the condition of the airways [23–27]. Aerosol deposition patterns reveal airway resistance levels and indicate areas of impaired regional ventilation. Low ventilation is shown by a reduced deposition, while airway stenosis or obstruction is visible as hot spots or absence of deposition [28, 29]. Because of these features, aerosol inhalation scintigraphy (AIS) is useful in the diagnosis

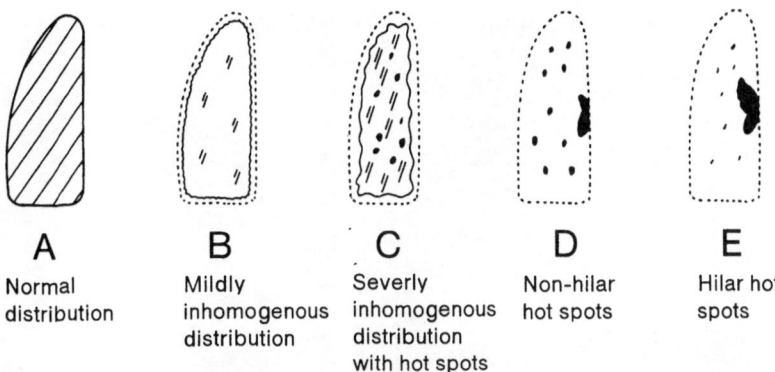

Fig. 6.5. Classification of posterior aerosol inhalation scintigrams. The degree of inhomogeneous distribution is classified into five types based on that in healthy controls

Table 6.2. Relationship between lung deposition patterns of radioactive aerosol and chronic obstructive pulmonary diseases (from [33])

Diseases	Deposition patterns				
	A	B	C	D	E
Chronic pulmonary emphysema ($n=19$)	–	2	5	5	7
Diffuse panbronchiolitis ($n=27$)	–	3	9	10	5
Chronic bronchitis ($n=18$)	6	5	4	2	1
Total ($n=64$)	6	10	18	17	13

of chronic obstructive pulmonary disease and has often been used for this purpose since its first report in 1965 by Taplin [23]. We classified aerosol deposition in lungs into 5 patterns (Fig. 6.5). The deposition pattern in cases of DPB differs clearly from that in cases of chronic bronchitis or chronic pulmonary emphysema. In cases of chronic pulmonary emphysema, the hilar pattern is often noted, while in cases of DPB the peripheral pattern is predominant [30] (Table 6.2, Fig. 6.6).

In patients with DPB cinebronchography indicates marked narrowing of the lumens of the trunchus ii:.ermedius, the lower lobe bronchus, and the segmental bronchus [31]. In bronchoscopic findings, redness, swelling, and pooled secretion are seen diffusely in the mucosa of the central to subsegmental bronchi [32]. Hot spot formation is due to the stenosis and obstruction of these bronchial segments. Comparing transverse SPECT images with X-ray CT images, we assessed the distribution of aerosol deposition in the inner zone and the outer zone. Aerosol deposition showing homogeneous distribution is rated as the normal type, that showing inhomogeneous distribution as the inhomogeneous type, that without deposition as the defect type, and that with hot spots as the hot spot type. According to this classification, in DPB the hot spot type is usually seen in the inner zone, while the

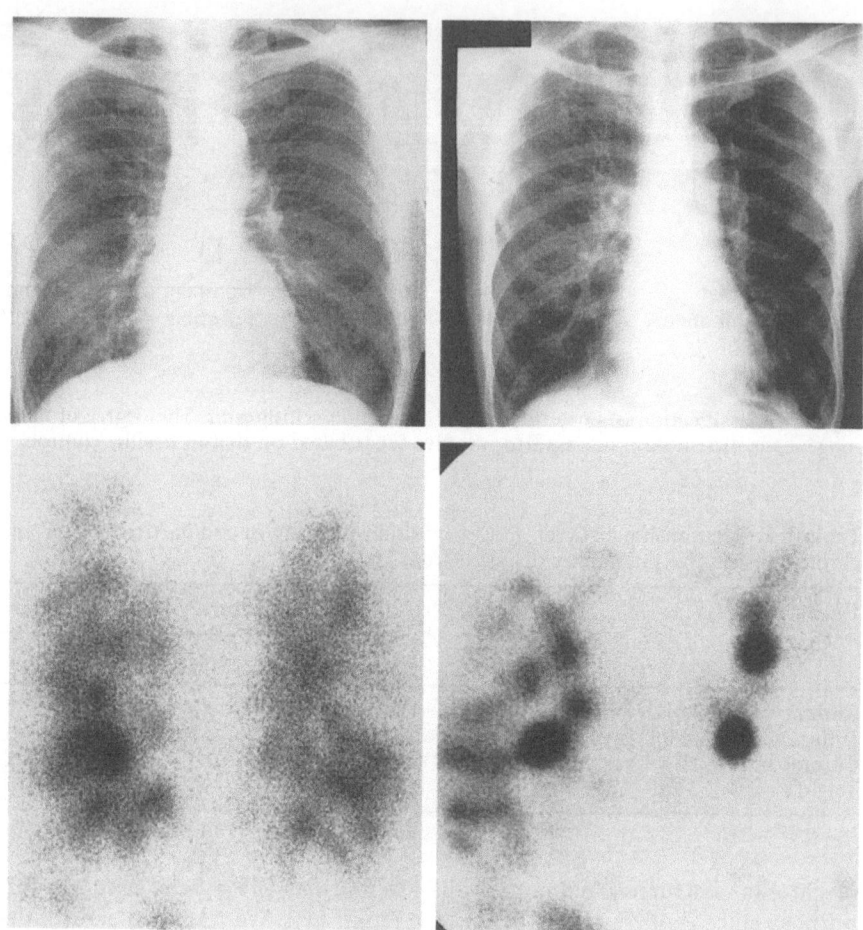

Fig. 6.6. Aerosol inhalation scintigram in chronic obstructive pulmonary diseases. Severe inhomogeneous distribution is revealed in both cases. AIS shows peripheral pattern DPB (*left*) and hilar pattern in chronic pulmonary emphysema (*right*)

Table 6.3. Bronchial morphological abnormalities and hot spots (from [33])

	Inner zone	Outer zone
Number of bronchial morphological abnormalities (A)	37	743
Number of hot spots (B)	54	30
Number of agreement of bronchial morphological abnormalities and hot spots (C)	31	4
Matching rate of bronchial morphological abnormalities to hot spots (C/A)	83.8%	0.5%
Matching rate of hot spots to bronchial morphological abnormalities (C/B)	57.4%	13.3%

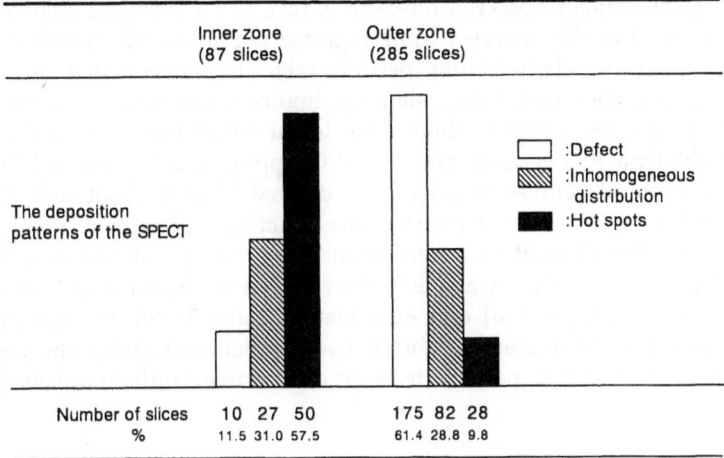

Fig. 6.7. The deposition patterns of the SPECT images of AIS. Transverse SPECT images 11 mm-thick from the middle lung field involving six slices below the carina, the area one-third proximal is regarded as the proximal area and the one-third distal the distal area. The regions of the apex and base of the lung are regarded as the distal area. (From [33])

defect type is usually seen in the outer zone [33] (Fig. 6.7). When hot spots are compared with morphological abnormalities of the airway on composite X-ray CT-SPECT images, the location of hot spots often agrees with that of morphological abnormalities of the airway in the inner zone, suggesting that abnormal airway morphology is a major factor responsible for hot spot formation in the central airway (Table 6.3).

Evaluation of the Response of DPB to Erythromycin

In the past DPB was viewed as a disease with poor prognosis. However, following the development of long-term erythromycin (EM) therapy [34], its prognosis has been improved markedly. EM does not directly kill or eradicate the pathogen. Instead, it modifies the airway environment associated with colonization and proliferation of bacteria, for example, by suppressing excessive mucus secretion in cases of chronic airway infection. Earlier studies on the mechanism of its action suggested the augmentation of the defense mechanism in a host by suppressing the development of infection (through inhibition of bacterial attachment), by inhibiting the production of elastase and protease, by elevating the activity of natural killer cells, or by increasing the production of various cytokines [35–37].

As the pulmonary function is improved by long-term EM therapy, CT images of the lungs of patients with DPB show a decrease in mucus plugging and in the number and size of centrilobular and branched linear areas of attenuation, while dilative changes of the airway continue to be seen. Morphological changes observed on chest X-rays or CT decrease relatively soon after the start of this therapy, while regional pulmonary dysfunction continues to be seen for relatively long periods even after a reduction in morphological abnormalities [38]. Cases showing improvement have been examined using ^{133}Xe gas; the mean washout time in the lower lung field and the total lung field tend to decrease, and the V/Q approaches the normal level [13]. Reduced local ventilation (visible as delayed ^{133}Xe washout in both lower lung fields) is seen even after respiratory function and arterial blood gas level improve. Therefore, if an examination using ^{133}Xe gas is repeated, it is useful to determine the time when EM therapy can be discontinued. Aerosol inhalation scintigraphy [39] and examination using Technegas also provide sensitive means for evaluating obstructive ventilation disorder and are very useful in evaluating therapeutic effects on obstructive ventilation disorder.

Mucociliary Clearance

The mucociliary transport (MCT) system is one of the major components of the airway defense mechanism. A number of methods are available for its evaluation [40–43]. Aerosol inhalation lung cinescintigraphy, developed in 1981 by Isawa et al. [44, 45], takes a series of pictures of the radioisotope deposited in the airway after inhalation in the form of aerosols and reproduces them as dynamic images. This method allows the MCT to be evaluated visually under physiological conditions. We have used this technique (aerosol inhalation cine-scintigraphy, AICS; Fig. 6.8) to classify the patterns of the transfer of the bolus movement of radioactive aerosol from the main

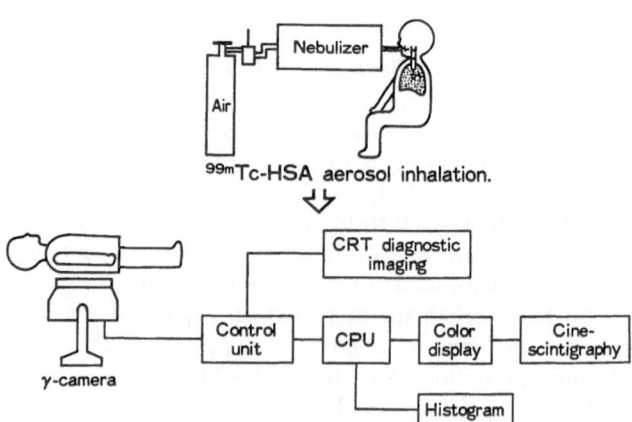

Fig. 6.8. Aerosol inhalation cine-scintigraphy. Subjects inhaled ^{99m}Tc-labeled human serum albumin aerosols generated from a nebulizer. Then they assumed a supine position on the table, and posterior view images were obtained dynamically at 20s/frame for over 2 h with a gamma-camera. The 20-s stored serial frames were edited into a cinematographic presentation at 200ms/frame

Fig. 6.9. Classification of the bolus movement of radioactive aerosol (BRA) from the main bronchi to the trachea. The patterns of BRA were classified into four types using the movement in healthy control subjects (type I). Types II–IV represent increasing degrees of impaired mucociliary transport function

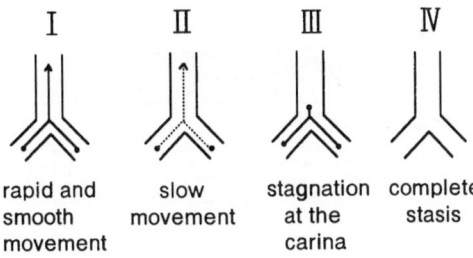

bronchus to the trachea, for the purpose of evaluating the MCT (Fig. 6.9). Since DPB is a disease specific to Japanese, no foreign investigators have published a study of the MCT in patients with DPB. Our studies reveal that the MCT shows various abnormalities in cases of chronic lower airway diseases such as bronchiectasis, chronic bronchitis, and DPB, and that the abnormalities of the MCT are most severe in cases of DPB [46–48] (Fig. 6.10). Various factors suppressing ciliary beats, such as abnormalities of the cilia themselves and persistent infection of the lower airways, are visible in patients with DPB [48–50]. Furthermore, an increase in airway mucus has been reported in cases of DPB. These findings suggest that the MCT is impaired by abnormalities of both mucus and cilia.

Erythromycin Therapy and Mucociliary Clearance

Disturbances of MCT can be reduced by EM therapy. Our long-term study, using AICS, reveals that the MCT shows improvements in patients responding to EM therapy, and that it returns to normal in some cases. Normalization of the MCT is sometimes seen in parallel to a reduction in clinical symptoms (Figs. 6.11, 6.12). In some cases, however, the MCT remains disturbed even after a reduction in clinical symptoms, and it improves only after treatment is prolonged. These findings suggest that evaluation of the MCT using AICS is important for objective evaluation of the responses of DPB to EM therapy and is useful for determining the timing of ending treatment and following up patients after the end of treatment [39, 51].

Sinobronchial Syndrome

SBS is a disease entity first proposed in 1969 by Huzly [52]. This concept includes both upper airway lesions (especially chronic sinusitis) and nonspecific chronic infected lesions of the lower airways. In Japan 85% of DPB cases are complicated by chronic sinusitis, and Mikami et al. [6] have therefore proposed including DPB as an aditional disease of SBS along with chronic bronchitis and bronchiectasis. This syndrome is thought to be caused by disturbances of the respiratory defense system due to genetic or constitutional

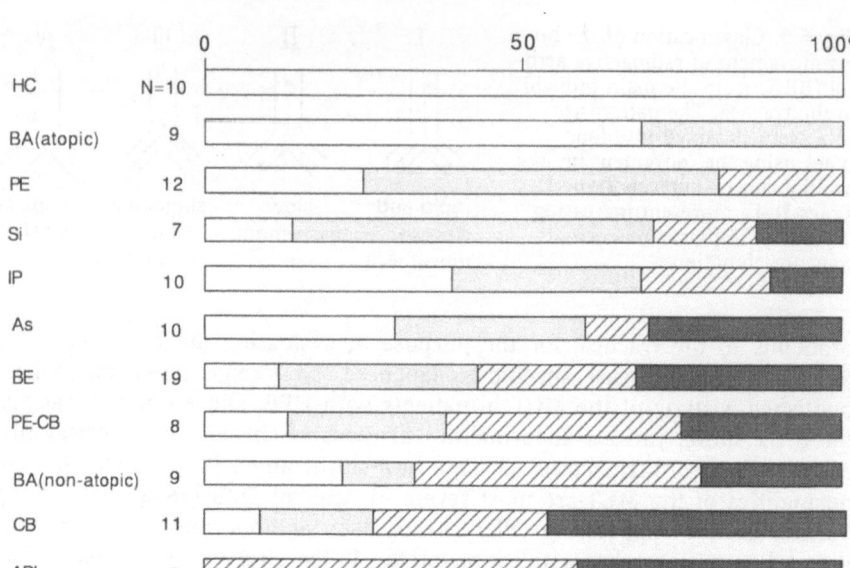

Fig. 6.10. Relationship between the type of the BRA and respiratory diseases. The proportion of patients showing type III+IV was high among patients with BE, CB, BA, or DPB. In particular, type IV was noted in 94.1% of patients with DPB, and MCT was severely impaired in DPB. *HC*, healthy control; *BA*, bronchial asthma; *PE*, pulmonary emphysema; *Si*, silicocis; *IP* interstitial pneumonitis; *As*, asbestosis; *BE*, bronchiectasis; *PE-CB*, pulmonary emphysema with chronic bronchitis; *CB*, chronic bronchitis; *API*, acute pulmonary infection; *DPB*, diffuse panbronchiolitis. (From [46])

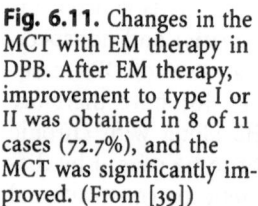

Fig. 6.11. Changes in the MCT with EM therapy in DPB. After EM therapy, improvement to type I or II was obtained in 8 of 11 cases (72.7%), and the MCT was significantly improved. (From [39])

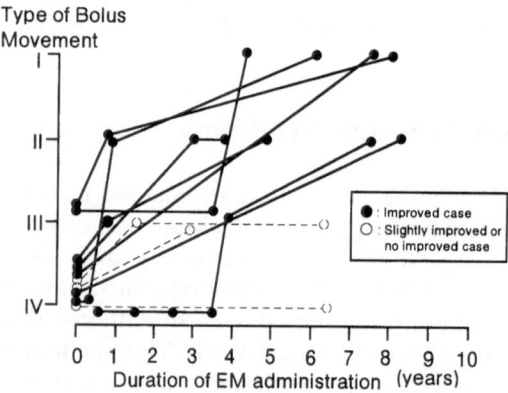

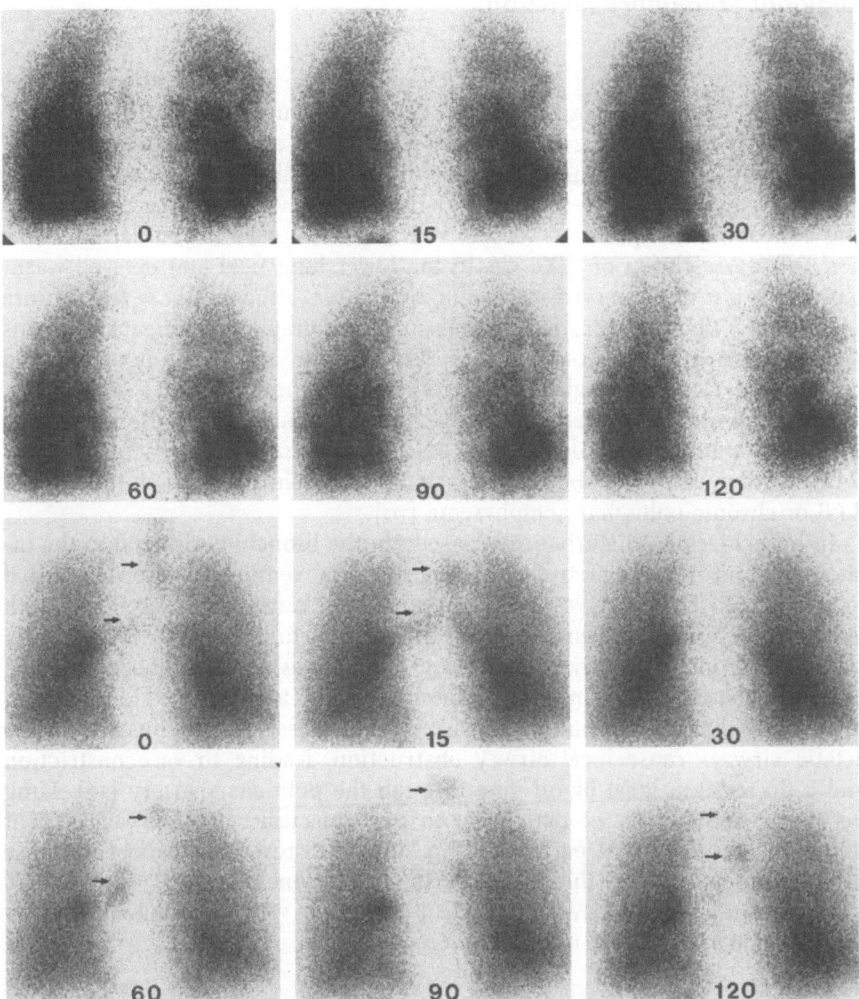

Fig. 6.12. AICS before and after EM therapy in a case of DPB. Before EM therapy the bolus movement of radioactive aerosol ascended only slightly from the main bronchi to the carina in 2 h (type III), suggesting advanced impairment of the MCT. After therapy, immediately after inhalation the BRA rapidly ascended from the bilateral main bronchi to the trachea (type I). The MCT was significantly improved

factors common to both the upper and lower airways. Chronic sinusitis and chronic inflammation of the lower airways are features common to the conditions constituting this syndrome. In cases of SBS without accompanying airway destruction, sinusitis is predominant. In such cases persistent infections by bacteria cause the release of elastase from infiltrated inflammatory cells, leading to weakening of the airway walls and bronchiectasis [9].

Regional Pulmonary Function

Chronic bronchitis is a disease characterized by excessive secretion from the bronchi. Fletcher's criteria [53, 54] are used to diagnose this disease. The impaired ventilation and perfusion noted in cases of chronic bronchitis are attributable primarily to ventilation disorder due to airway stenosis (caused by infection, hyperplasia of secretory glands, excessive mucus secretion, etc.) and concomitant hypoxemic vasoconstriction secondary to ventilation disorder. Diffuse retention of ^{133}Xe gas in the lower lung field and delayed washout of this gas are observed in chronic bronchitis, although these features are less marked than in DPB. Lung perfusion scintigraphy of patients with this disease often reveals spot-shaped perfusion-poor areas and nonsegmental perfusion defects, although these signs are often not very clear. AIS reveals diffuse inhomogeneous aerosol distribution predominantly in the lower lung field. Hot spots are also detected in cases of very severe obstructive ventilation disorder, although they are less marked in chronic bronchitis than in DPB or chronic pulmonary emphysema [30].

In bronchiectasis disturbances are seen in the bronchi peripheral to the dilated site and in alveolar tissue, accompanied by ventilation disorder caused by puriform secretions retained in the dilated parts of the bronchi [55]. Furthermore, persistent inflammation of the bronchi and ventilation disorder cause the bronchial artery to dilate and sometimes to anastomoze with the pulmonary artery thus making a shunt, leading to a marked decrease in blood flow through the pulmonary artery, and massive secretions within the ectatic airways cause local airway obstruction, leading to vasoconstriction and a decrease in local blood flow through the pulmonary artery [56]. Lung perfusion scintigraphy of patients with bronchiectasis often reveals evident nonsegmental defects of perfusion (Fig. 6.13). AIS reveals a marked decrease in aerosol deposition in the dilated parts of the bronchi [57, 58].

If Technegas and MAA SPECT are performed, ventilation and perfusion can be evaluated in more detail (Fig. 6.14).

Mucociliary Clearance

In cases of SBS persistent infection of the lower airway by bacteria normally indigenous of the upper airways (e.g., Hemophilus influenzae) is seen in the lower airway. Disturbances of MCT are revealed by AICS, suggesting that these disturbances are related to the progression of SBS [59] (Figs. 6.15, 6.16).

MCT of patients with bronchiectasis was evaluated by ^{99m}Tc-labeled human serum albumin aerosol inhalation scintigraphy. Impaired MCT was seen at the dilated parts of the bronchi in 95%, suggesting that infection and bleeding is promoted by this impairment [60]. Abnormal ultrastructure of the cilia was also seen in cases of bronchiectasis, suggesting its importance in the pathogenesis [61, 62].

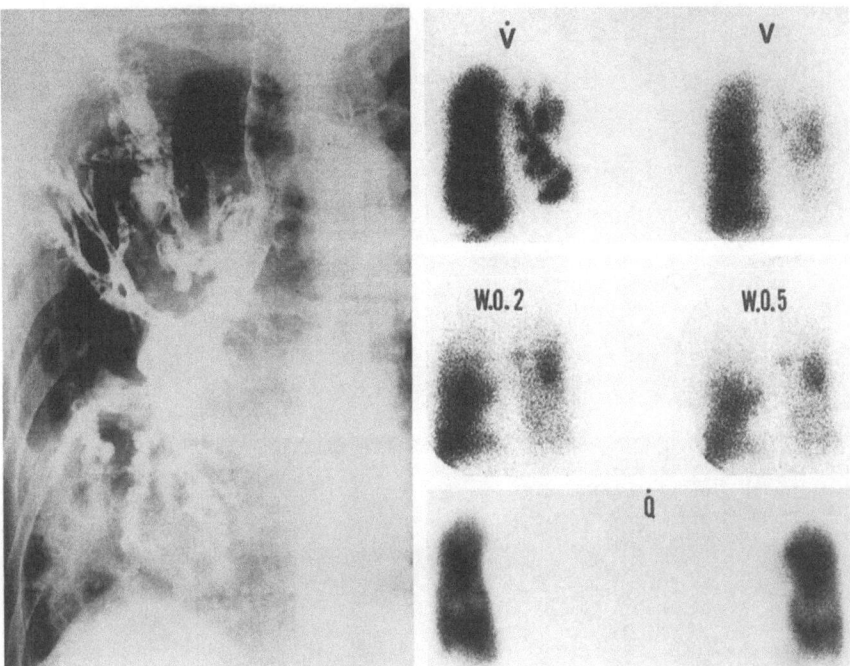

Fig. 6.13. Sino-bronchiectasis (^{133}Xe and ^{99m}Tc-MAA scintigraphy). Bronchography revealed cystic bronchodilatation in the middle and lower fields. ^{133}Xe gas ventilation imaging revealed nonsegmental defects in the middle and lower fields, and washout imaging showed delayed washout. Perfusion scintigraphy (^{99m}Tc-MAA) revealed defects throughout the entire left lung, and perfusion disorder was more severe

Evaluation of Responses of SBS to Treatment

It has recently been reported that EM is effective not only in DPB but also in chronic bronchitis and bronchiectasis. EM therefore seems to be effective by reducing the amount of sputum and improving MCT in SBS, as in the treatment of DPB. SBS is usually progressive, but its progression is sometimes suppressed by EM therapy [63]. In addition to EM, 14-membered ring macrolide antibiotics have also been shown to be effective in treating SBS. The mechanism of the action of macrolide antibiotics resembles that of EM [64]. Our study also revealed improvement of the MCT following EM therapy in some cases (Fig. 6.15).

Bronchial Asthma

In the past bronchial asthma was defined from functional aspects. In recent years bronchial asthma has been viewed as chronic inflammatory airway disturbances. According to this view, attacks of asthma in predisposed indivi-

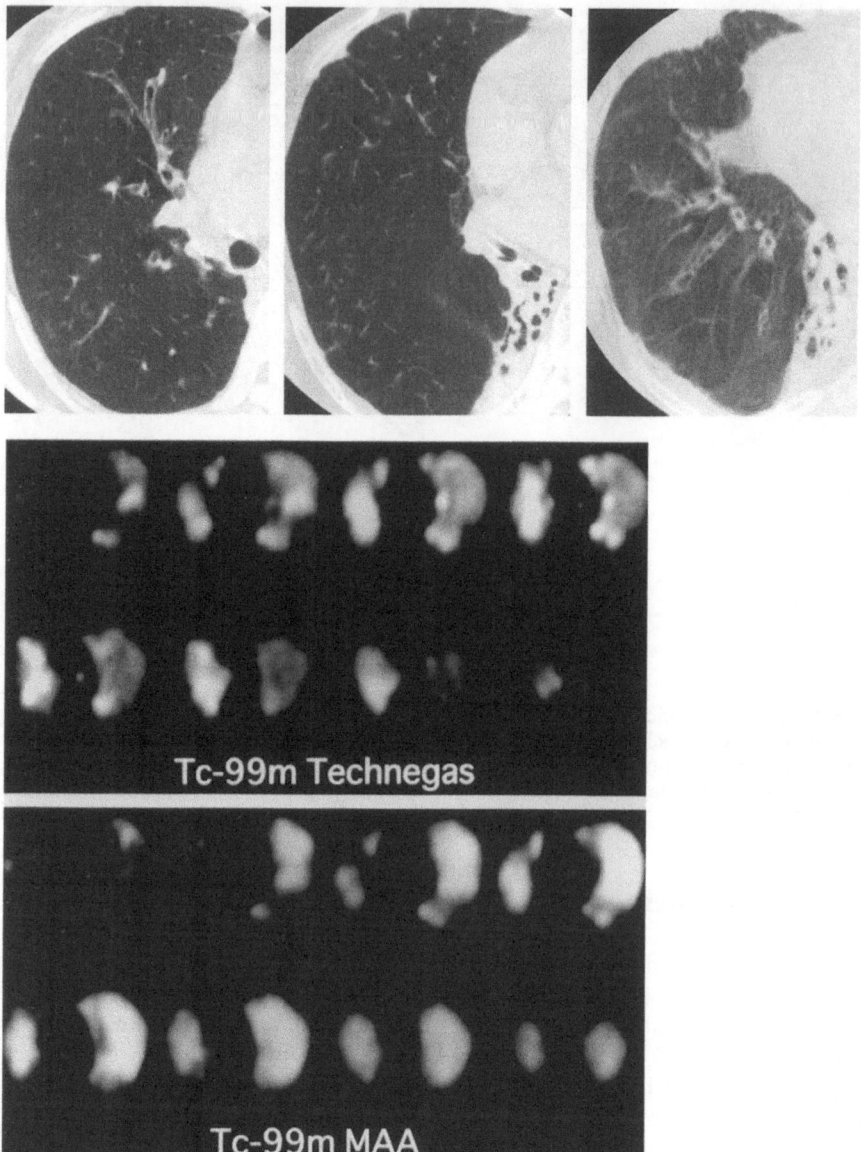

Fig. 6.14. Sino-bronchiectasis (CT and Technegas SPECT images). CT revealed thickening of bronchial walls and bronchiectasis in upper and lower right lung fields and also in the left lung. Technegas and perfusion SPECT transverse images (lower to upper slices) showed multiple defects in both lungs. Perfusion defects were more widespread than Technegas deposition, so perfusion was impaired more severely than ventilation in the areas of bronchiectasis

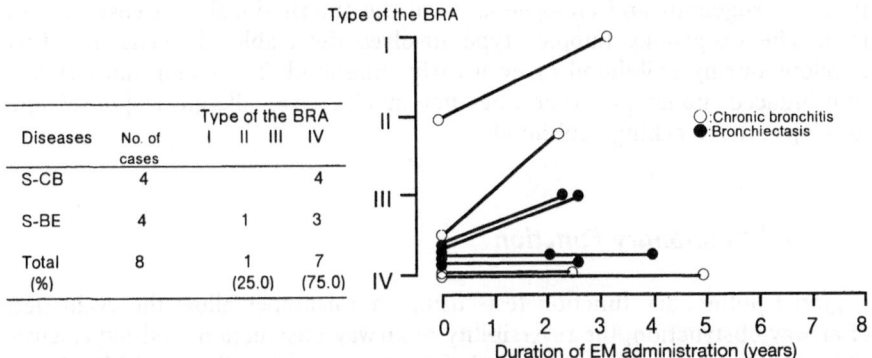

Type of the BRA

Diseases	No. of cases	Type of the BRA			
		I	II	III	IV
S-CB	4				4
S-BE	4			1	3
Total	8			1	7
(%)				(25.0)	(75.0)

○:Chronic bronchitis
●:Bronchiectasis

Duration of EM administration (years)

Fig. 6.15. AICS and changes in the MCT with EM therapy in cases with SBS. Concerning the pattern of BRA from main bronchi to the trachea, 93.8% of cases were classified as type III+IV. Severely impaired MCT was noted. Erythromycin therapy improved MCT in some cases of SBS. *S-CB*, chronic bronchitis with sinusitis; *S-BE*, bronchiectasis with chronic sinusitis; *BRA*, bolus movement of radioactive aerosol; *EM*, erythromycin

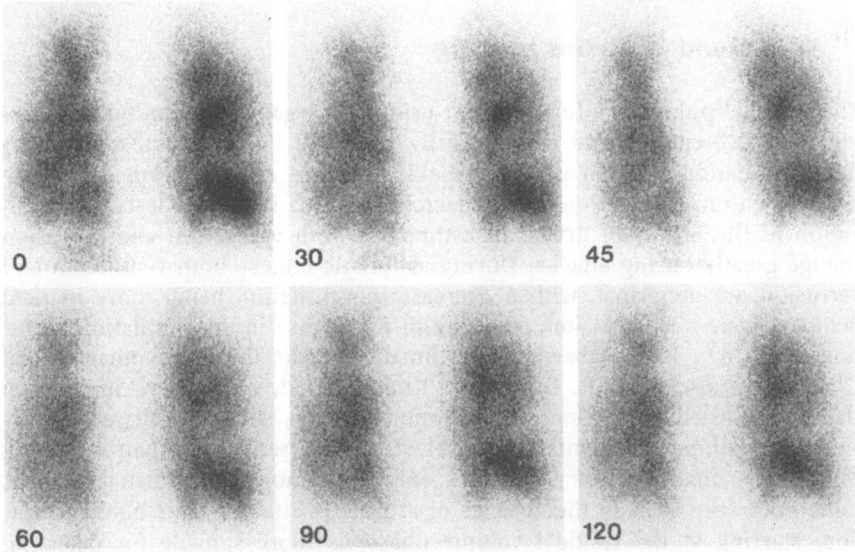

Fig. 6.16. AICS in a case of sino-bronchiectasis. Serial changes in posterior images were noted. There was no BRA from the main bronchi to the trachea within 2 h of aerosol inhalation. Severely impaired MCT was noted

duals are triggered by inflammation. These individuals show reversible air flow restrictions which are extensive but variable, and airway inflammation can cause airway hypersensitivity to various stimuli [65]. Clinical classifications of bronchial asthma now available include those proposed by Rackemann [90] and Swineford et al. [91] Bronchial asthma is divided into two types – exogenous and endogenous – in the International Consensus report [66]. The exogenous (atopic) type involves detectable allergens and first develops during childhood or even early childhood. The endogenous (infection-induced, nonatopic) type does not involve clear allergic responses and develops after reaching adulthood.

Regional Pulmonary Function

Regional pulmonary function tests using radioisotopes allow the evaluation of airway obstruction, the reversibility of airway obstruction, and hypersensitivity of the airways. They provide information useful in distinguishing bronchial asthma from other chronic obstructive lung diseases (COPD), assessing the severity of asthma, and evaluating the response to treatment. Since bronchial asthma is often complicated by COPD, it is essential to determine whether bronchial asthma or COPD is responsible for obstructive ventilation disorder which persists after treatment.

^{81m}Kr Gas and ^{133}Xe Gas Imaging

The regional pulmonary function test using ^{81m}Kr gas can be performed during natural breathing and can be easily repeated. Because of these features the examination is often used for making images of ventilation during attacks of asthma, evaluation during exercise, asthma induction tests, and evaluation of the effects of drugs. In asthmatics both ventilation and perfusion change greatly during attacks. During asthmatic attacks both ventilation and perfusion are abnormal, with a decrease in ventilation being more marked than a decrease of perfusion, resulting in a decrease in the ventilation/perfusion ratio [67]. In the absence of asthmatic attacks the bolus inhalation of ^{81m}Kr gas is also possible. If bolus ^{81m}Kr is inhaled, ventilatory kinetics can also be revealed in its local distribution pattern, allowing airway disturbances of asthmatic patients to be evaluated more sensitively than in resting continuous inhalation of ^{81m}Kr gas [68]. Inhomogeneous distribution is sometimes seen even in the absence of asthmatic attacks. Thus bolus inhalation, starting at the residual volume phase, is more suitable for detecting mild abnormalities associated with bronchial asthma [69].

The evaluation of the washout of ^{133}Xe during scintigraphy is useful in examining the presence or absence of pulmonary emphysema which makes asthma severe and intractable. Late-onset asthma, which develops after the age of 40 years is often more severe and intractable than early-onset asthma, which is the atopic type in most cases. Irreversible lesions during the absence of late-onset asthma attacks have been examined using ^{133}Xe and ^{99m}Tc-MAA, patients with late-onset intractable asthma often have disturbances of ventilation and perfusion even in the absence of attacks, and these disturbances tend to be more severe as the duration of sickness lengthens, suggesting the involvement of organic changes of the lungs in the intractable course of asthma [70].

Ventilation and Perfusion During Drug Load

The principal characteristic of bronchial asthma is elevated sensitivity of the airway in response to various nonspecific stimuli. Airway sensitivity to a drug is evaluated by measuring the $FEV_{1.0}$ and airway resistance following inhalation of the drug which causes contraction of the bronchial smooth muscle. In Japan directwriting recording of the dose-response curves of the airway to methacholine is often used, which determines the threshold level for the response to methacholine while monitoring respiratory resistance [71].

^{81m}Kr gas is useful in examining the regional ventilatory distribution following induction of asthmatic attacks. The ventilatory distribution changes sharply some time following a methacholine; the decrease in ventilation is not homogeneous but differs from area to area, and the lobar to segmental ventilation defects are visible [72]. The decrease in ventilation occurs in both lower lung fields soon after methacholine inhalation, and the decrease in these fields tends to be greater than that in the upper lung fields [73, 74] (Fig. 6.17). This may be related to some extent to enhanced airway sensitivity but seems to be more closely related to enhanced absorption of the drug because of higher ventilation in the bilateral lower lung field due to gravity.

β_2-Adrenoreceptor agonists are very useful in treating acute attacks of bronchial asthma. However, several reports showing a decrease in PaO_2 following inhalation of β_2-stimulants have been published. A study using ^{81m}Kr suggests that the decrease in PaO_2 following the administration of bronchodilators is due to deterioration in the V/Q ratio and an increase in the shunt-like effect caused by the strong vasodilative action of these agents.

Aerosol Inhalation Scintigraphy

Changes caused by asthmatic attacks have been shown by AIS to be reversible. Uneven distribution, defects, and excessive deposition of aerosols in the lungs are seen during asthmatic attacks. These changes are seen in the airway segments peripheral to the segmental or subsegmental bronchi. The areas showing hot spots are approximately identical to the areas showing asthma-associated lesions [75-77]. Aerosol distribution in the lungs tends to remain somewhat abnormal even in the absence of attacks [78]. The irregular distribution in the periphery, which can be seen for some time after the administration of bronchodilators, indicates lesions of the peripheral airways. Regarding the aerosol distribution in lungs in the absence of asthmatic attacks and the type of asthma, we have found that severely uneven distribution is more frequent in cases of nonatopic asthma (Table 6.4). This techni-

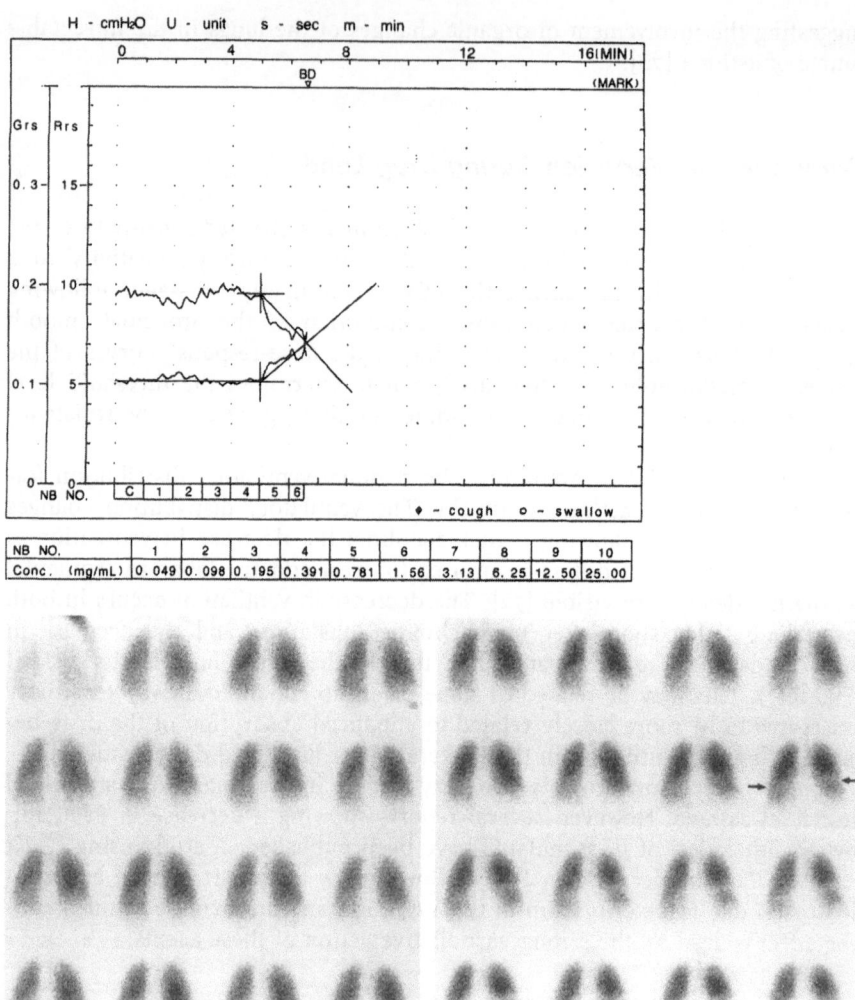

Fig. 6.17. Directwriting recording of the dose-response curves of the airway to methacholine combined with ^{81m}Kr gas ventilation imaging. With inhalation of incrementally increased dosage of methacholin, respiratory resistance (Rrs; cmH$_2$O l^{-1} s^{-1}) increase and calculated respiratory conductance (Grs; l s^{-1} cmH$_2$O^{-1}) from Rrs decrease. ^{81m}Kr gas ventilation imaging was performed at 10 s/frame to obtain serial posterior images. The ^{81m}Kr gas ventilation images show reduced ventilation in the bilateral lower lung fields with increases in airway resistance during inhalation of methacholine

Table 6.4. Aerosol inhalation scintigraphy in cases with asthma

	Deposition patterns of radioactive aerosol				
	A	B	C	D	E
Atopic type					
During remission	2	9	3	–	–
During attack	–	2	2	1	3
Nonatopic type					
During remission	–	4	9	4	3
During attack	–	–	1	1	1

Table 6.5. Aerosol inhalation cine-scintigraphy in cases with asthma: bolus movement of radioactive aerosol (BRA) from the main bronchi to the trachea

	Type of BRA			
	I	II	III	IV
Atopic type				
During remission	7	7	–	–
During attack	1	2	3	2
Nonatopic type				
During remission	1	9	6	4
During attack	–	–	2	1

que is useful in assessing the responses to treatment and following up the course of asthma in individual cases.

Mucociliary Clearance

Transbronchial biopsy and bronchoalveolar lavage reveals that injury of the airway epithelium such as detachment of the ciliated epithelial cells occurs even during remission of mild asthma [79]. It has been reported that failure in mucociliary function is seen in bronchial asthma, and that the resultant mucus plugging of the peripheral airway is often responsible for the death of asthmatic patients [80, 81]. Examinations using X-rays and radioactive aerosols [82–84] reveal that the incidence of impaired mucociliary clearance in the central and peripheral segments of the airway is higher in asthmatics than in healthy controls [85–87]. Our study demonstrated a correlation between the type of asthma and the mucociliary transport function; the disturbance was more severe in nonatopic than in atopic asthma (Table 6.5).

Factors probably responsible for disturbances of the MCT include chemical mediators released by allergic responses and viscoelasticity of mucus [83, 87, 88]. The severe disturbances of the MCT observed during remission of nonatopic asthma are noteworthy in the factors responsible for the onset of

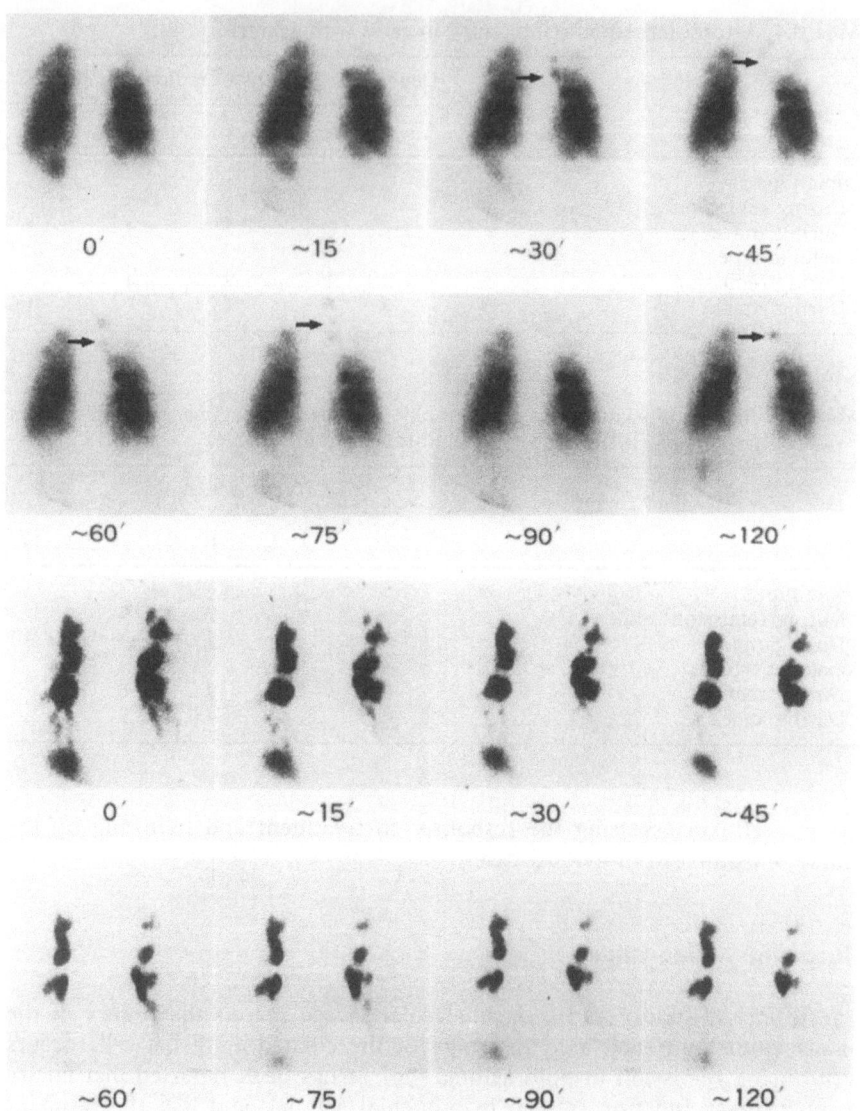

Fig. 6.18. AICS in a case with bronchial asthma. Serial posterior AICS images during remission and during mild attacks in a patient with atopic asthma are shown. The BRA was observed during remission, while there was no BRA during mild attacks

this type of asthma. Reduced mucociliary transport during attacks of bronchial asthma has been shown in canine models of asthma [88] and in humans [82]. Postmortem examination of patients who died of asthma reveals extensive mucus plugging of the airways. This suggests that mucociliary transport decreases during asthmatic attacks. Our evaluation of humans in vivo using AICS also shows severely disturbed MCT during asthmatic attacks (Table 6.5, Fig. 6.18). This suggests that disturbances of the MCT are also reversible, as in airway constriction. Normalization of the MCT is one of the most important goals of treatment of bronchial asthma [89]. The evaluation of MCT by means of AICS is useful in evaluating the response of bronchial asthma to treatment.

References

1. Yamanaka A, Saiki S, Tamura S et al (1969) Problems in chronic obstructive pulmonary disease, with special reference to diffuse panbronchiolitis. Naika 23:442–451
2. Honma H, Yamanaka A, Tanimoto S et al (1983) Diffuse panbronchiolitis: a disease of the transitional zone of the lung. Chest 83:63–69
3. Fraser RG, Paré JA, Paré PD et al (1990) Diagnosis and diseases of the chest, 3rd edn. Saunders, Philadelphia, pp 2224–2229
4. Sugiyama Y, Kudoh S, Maeda H et al (1990) Analysis of HLA antigens in patients with diffuse panbronchiolitis. Am Rev Respir Dis 141:1459–1462
5. ACCP-ATS Joint Committee (1975) Pulmonary terms and symbols. Chest 67:583–593
6. Mikami R (1975) Relationship between upper and lower respiratory tract in the pathogenesis of chronic respiratory infection. Approach for common factor in pathogenesis of sino-bronchial syndrome. J Jpn Bronchoesophagol Soc 26:74–81
7. Maeda M, Saiki S, Yamanaka A et al (1987) Serial section analysis of the lesions in diffuse panbronchiolitis. Acta Pathol Jpn 37:693–704
8. Saiki S (1987) Bronchial changes of diffuse pan-bronchiolitis. J Jpn Bronchoesophagol Soc 38:176–180
9. Nakata K, Tanimoto H (1981) Diffuse panbronchiolitis. Jpn J Clin Radiol 26:1133–1142
10. Sugiyama Y (1993) Diffuse panbronchiolitis. Clin Chest Med 14:765–772
11. Akira M, Kitani F, Yong-Sik L et al (1988) Diffuse panbronchiolitis: evaluation with high-resolution CT. Radiology 168:433–438
12. Nishimura K, Kitaichi M, Izumi T et al (1992) Diffuse panbronchiolitis: correlation of high-resolution CT and pathologic findings. Radiology 184:779–785
13. Fukuda K, Hasegawa S (1992) Analysis of chronic obstructive pulmonary diseases by long-term evaluation with Xe-133 functional imaging. Jpn J Med Imaging 12:138–146
14. Komatuzaki K (1995) Utility of Xe-133 ventilation scintigraphy in evaluation airflow limitation in diffuse panbronchiolitis. Jikeikai Med J 110:103–109
15. Senda M, Murata K, Itoh H, et al (1986) Quantitative evaluation of regional pulmonary ventilation using PET and nitrogen-13 gas. J Nucl Med 27:268–273
16. Murata K, Itoh H, Senda M et al (1989) Stratified impairement of pulmonary ventilation in "diffuse panbronchiolitis" PET and CT studies. J Comput Assist Tomogr 13:48–53
17. Suga K, Nishigauchi K, Matsumoto T et al (1994) Regional pulmonary xenon-133 washout study using dynamic SPECT images obtained by a triple-headed SPECT system. Nippon Acta Radiol 54:1424–1426
18. Tomioka H, Tanaka E, Amitani R et al (1988) Lung perfusion scintigraphy with Tc-99m MAA in 46 patients with chronic airway disease. Jpn J Thorac Dis 26:975–982
19. Burch WM, Sullivan PJ, McLaren CJ et al (1986) Technegas – a new ventilation agent for lung scanning. Nucl Med Commun 7:865–871
20. Sullivan PJ, Burke WM, Burch WM et al (1988) A clinical comparison of technegas and xenon-133 in 50 patients with suspected pulmonary embolus. Chest 94:300–304

21. Isawa T, Teshima T, Anazawa M et al (1991) Technegas for inhalation lung imaging. Nucl Med Commun 12:47–55
22. Sasaki Y, Imai T, Kasuga H et al (1991) Clinical evaluation of Tc-99m technegas. Jpn J Respir 10:821–829
23. Taplin GV, Poe ND (1965) A dual lung scanning technic for evaluation of pulmonary function. Radiology 85:365–368
24. Newman SP, Agnew JE, Pavia D et al (1982) Inhaled aersols: lung deposition and clinical applications. Clin Phys Physiol Meas 3:1–20
25. Goldberg IS, Lourenco RV (1973) Deposition of aerosols in pulmonary disease. Arch Intern Med 131:88–91
26. Morrow PE (1974) Conference on the scientific basis of respiratory therapy. Aerosol therapy. Aerosol characterization and deposition. Am Rev Respir Dis 110:88–99
27. Heyder J (1981) Mechanism of aersosl particle deposition. Chest 80:820–823
28. Taplin GV, Poe ND, Dore EK et al (1967) Bronchial patency and aerated space assessment by scintiscanning. Lahey Clin Found Bull 16:297–312
29. Hayes M, Taplin GV (1980) Lung imaging with radioaerosols for the assessment of airway disease. Semin Nucl Med 10:243–251
30. Watanabe H (1989) Study of the deposition patterns of aerosol inhalation scintigraphy. I. Comparison of the deposition patterns of aerosol inhalation scintigraphy with lung function tests in pulmonary diseases. J Nara Med Assoc 40:385–399
31. Frazer RG (1961) Measurement of the caliber of human bronchi in three phases of respiration by cinebronchography. J Can Assoc Radiol 12:102–112
32. Sugiyama Y, Izumi T, Kitamura S et al (1983) Bronchoscopic and histological appearances of the central airway in patients with diffuse panbronchiolitis. Jpn J Chest Dis 42:652–659
33. Watanabe H, Itoh S, Imai T et al (1991) Study on the Tc-99m aerosol deposition patterns of diffuse panbronchiolitis; the analysis of the hot spot formation mechanism by the SPECT of the aerosol inhalation scintigraphy and the chest CT. Jpn J Clin Radiol 36:43–50
34. Sawaki M, Mikami R, Mikasa K et al (1986) The long term chemotherapy with erythromycine in chronic lower respiratory tract infections. Second report; including cases with Pseudomonas infections. Kansenshogaku Zasshi 60:45–50
35. Kita W, Sawaki M, Oku D et al (1991) Suppression of virulence factors of Pseudomonas aeruginosa by erythromycin. J Antimicrob Chemother 27:273–284
36. Mikasa K, Kita E, Sawaki M et al (1992) The anti-inflammatory effect of erythromycin in zymosan-induced peritonitis mice. J Antimicrob Chemother 30:339–348
37. Tanakadate A, Sasaki K, Nemoto H et al (1991) Effect of long-term, low doses of erythromycine on diffuse panbronchiolitis (DPB). J Med Soc Toho Jpn 38:211–220
38. Kawakami K (1994) Use of radioisotopes to study the function and morphology of the lung. Jpn J Thorac Dis 32:223–230
39. Imai T, Sasaki Y, Ohishi H et al (1995) Clinical aerosol inhalation cine-scintigraphy to evaluate mucociliary transport system in diffuse panbronchiolitis. J Nucl Med 36:1355–1362
40. Sackner MA, Rosen MJ, Wanner A (1973) Estimation of tracheal mucous velocity by bronchofiberscopy. J Appl Physiol 34:495–499
41. Friedman M, Scott FD, Poole DO et al (1977) A new roentgenographic method for estimating mucous velocity in airways. Am Rev Respir Dis 115:67–74
42. Yeates DB, Aspin N, Levison H, Jones MT et al (1975) Mucociliary tracheal transport rates in man. J Appl Physiol 39:487–495
43. Morrow PE, Gibb FR, Gazioglu KM (1967) A study of particulate clearance from the human lungs. Am Rev Respir Dis 96:1209–1221
44. Isawa T, Teshima T, Hirano T et al (1981) Radioaerosol inhalation lung cine-scintigraphy; a preliminary report. Tohoku J Exp Med 134:245–255
45. Isawa T, Teshima T, Hirano T et al (1984) Mucociliary clearance mechanism in smoking and nonsmoking normal subjects. J Nucl Med 25:352–359

46. Itoh S, Mikami R, Ryujin Y et al (1984) Applications of aerosol inhalation cine-scintigraphy for clinical investigation of mucociliary transport. Jpn J Thorac Dis 22:961–969
47. Ryujin Y, Itoh S, Kasuga H et al (1984) Mucociliary clearance in diffuse pan-bronchiolitis, pulmonary emphysema and chronic bronchitis estimated by aerosol inhalation cine-scintigraphy. Jpn J Thorac Dis 22:479–485
48. Ninomiya H, Ichikawa Y, Koga H et al (1991) Elastase activity in broncho alveolar lavage fluid from patients with diffuse panbronchiolitis. Kansenshogaku Zasshi 65:672–680
49. Tegner H, Ohlsson K, Toremalm NG et al (1979) Effect of human leukocyte en-zyme on tracheal mucosa and its mucociliary activity. Rhinology 17:199–206
50. Smallmann LA, Hill SL, Stockley RA et al (1984) Reduction of ciliary beat fre-quency in vitro by sputum from patients with bronchiectasis: a serine proteinase effect. Thorax 39:663–667
51. Imai T, Ohishi H, Katada H et al (1990) Bronchoscopic findings and aerosol inha-lation cine-scintigraphy in cases with diffuse panbronchiolitis treated effectively by erythromycine. J Jpn Soc Bronchol 12:382–390
52. Huzly A (1969) Sinobronchiales Syndrome. Beitr Klin Tuberk 136:265–280
53. American Thoracic Society (1962) Chronic bronchitis, asthma and pulmonary em-physema: a statement by the committee on diagnostic standards for non-tubercu-lous respiratory diseases. Am Rev Respir Dis 85:762–769
54. Medical Research Council (1965) Definition and classification of chronic bronchi-tis for clinical and epidemiological purpose. Lancet i:775–779
55. Bass H, Henderson JAM, Hecksher T et al (1968) Regional structure and function in bronchiectasis. A correlative study using bronchography and Xe-133. Am Rev Respir Dis 97:598–609
56. Isawa T, Shiraishi K, Yasuda T et al (1967) Effect of oxygen concentration in in-spired gas upon pulmonary arterial blood flow. Am Rev Respir Dis 96:1199–1208
57. Lorrenco RV, Loddenkemper R, Carton RW et al (1972) Patterns of distribution and clearance of aerosols in patients with bronchiectasis. Am Rev Respir Dis 106:857–866
58. Ashford NS, Buxton-Thomas MS, Flower CDR et al (1988) Aerosol lung scintigra-phy in the detection of bronchiectasis. Clin Radiol 39:29–32
59. Narita N, Mikami R, Sawaki M et al (1987) Symposium II: sinobronchial syn-drome and it's related subjects. II. Mechanism of the defence of airway. J Jpn Bronchoesophagol Soc 38:163–170
60. Isawa T, Teshima T, Hirano T et al (1990) Mucociliary clearance and transport in bronchiectasis: global and regional assessment. J Nucl Med 31:543–548
61. Corbeel L, Cornillie F, Lauweryns J et al (1981) Ultrastructural abnormalities of bronchial cilia in children with recurrent airway infections and bronchiectasis. Arch Dis Child 56:929–933
62. Waite DA, Wakefield SJ, Mackay JB et al (1981) Mucociliary transport and ultra-structural abnormalities in polynesian bronchiectasis. Chest 80:896–898
63. Nishi K, Myou S, Fujimura M et al (1993) Effect of erythromycin on mucociliary transport and clinical symptoms in patients with sinobronchial syndrome. Jpn J Thorac Dis 31:1367–1376
64. Takeda H, Miura H, Kawahira M et al (1989) Long-term administration study on TE-031 (A-56268) in the treatment of diffuse panbronchiolitis. Kansenshogaku Zasshi 63:71–78
65. National Institutes of Health, National Heart Lung and Blood Institute (1995) Global Initiative for Asthma (Global stategy for asthma management and preven-tion. NHLBI/WHO work shop report). Publication, no 95-3659
66. US Department of Health and Human Services (1992) International consensus report on diagnosis and management of asthma. Publication no 92-3091 Bethes-da. Eur Respir J 5:601–641
67. Wilson AF, Surprenant EL, Beall GN et al (1970) The significance of regional pul-monary function changes in bronchial asthma. Am J Med 48:416–423

68. Kawakami K, Katsuyama N, Fukuda Y et al (1981) A Kr-81m inhalation method for detection of absence of uniform ventilation in asthma. Clin Nucl Med 6:463–467

69. Kawakami K, Kastuyama N, Anno I et al (1978) An application of Kr-81m gas for chronic obstructive pulmonary disease. A comparison of various inhalation techniques. Nippon Act Radiol 38:1044–1053

70. Ishihama H (1994) Analysis of the dynamic states of pulmonary ventilation and perfusion in bronchial asthmatics using Xe- 133 gas ventilation scintigraphy and Tc-99m MAA lung perfusion scntigraphy. Acta Med Okayama 106:415–428

71. Takishima T, Hida W, Sasaki H et al (1981) Direct-writing recorder of the dose-response curves of the airway to methacholine. Chest 80:600–606

72. Fazio F, Palla A, Santrolicandro A et al (1979) Studies of regional ventilation in asthma using 81m Kr. Lung 156:185–194

73. Kitada O, Sugita M, Kawasaki M et al (1986) Studies on a comparison between continuous changes in respiratory impedance and in regional ventilatory distribution, and on the sites of airway obstruction induced by the methacholine provocation test. Arerugi 35:1011–1021

74. Itoh S (1981) Regional pulmonary ventilation and perfusion studies with 81mKr after acetylcholine inhalation in bronchial asthma. J Nara Med Assoc 32:387–401

75. Woolock AJ, Macklem PT, Hogg JC et al (1969) Effect of vagal stimulation on central and peripheral airway in dogs. J Appl Physiol 26:806–813

76. Chan-Yeung M, Abboud R, Tsao MS et al (1976) Effect of helium on maximal expiratory flow in patients with asthma before and during induced bronchoconstriction. Am Rev Respir Dis 113:433–443

77. MacFadden ER Jr, Lyons HA (1969) Serial studies of factors influencing airway dynamics during recovery from acute asthma attacks. J Appl Physiol 27:452–459

78. Suzuki T (1981) Evaluation of the regional lung function revealed in radioaerosol scintigram of chronic obstructive pulmonary disease. Nippon Acta Radiol 40:156–167

79. Holgate ST, Wilson JR, Howarth PH et al (1992) New insights into airway inflammation by endobronchial biopsy. Am Rev Respir Dis 145:S2–S6

80. Dunnill MS (1960) The pathology of asthma, with special reference to changes in the bronchial mucosa. J Clin Pathol 13:27–33

81. Hilding AC (1943) The relation of ciliary insufficiency to death from asthma and other respiratory diseases. Ann Otol Rhinol Laryngol 52:5–19

82. Mezey RJ, Cohn MA, Fernandez RH et al (1978) Mucociliary transport in allergic patients with antigen-induced bronchospasm. Am Rev Respir Dis 118:677–684

83. Ahmed T, Greenblatt DW, Birch S et al (1981) abnormal mucociliary transport in allergic patients with antigen induced bronchospasm: role of alow reacting substance of anaphylaxis. Am Rev Respir Dis 124:110–114

84. Bateman JRM, Pavia D, Sheahan NF et al (1983) Impaired tracheobronchial clearance in patients with mild stable asthma. Thorax 38:463–467

85. Pavia D, Bateman JRM, Sheahan NF et al (1985) Tracheal mucociliary clearance in asthma: impairment during remission. Thorax 40:171–175

86. Agnew JE, Bateman JRM, Pavia D et al (1984) A model for assessing bronchial mucus transport. J Mucl Med 25:170–176

87. Dulfano MJ, Luk CK (1982) Sputum and ciliary inhibition in asthma. Thorax 37:646–651

88. Wanner A, Zarzecki S, Hirsch J et al (1975) Tracheal mucus transport in experimental canine asthma. J Appl Physiol 39:950–957

89. Matthys H (1991) Management of bronchial asthma. Respiration 58:34–36

90. Rackemann FM (1947) A working classification of asthma. Am J Med 3:601–606

91. Swineford O Jr (1954) Asthma: classification of causes. A recommended classification and a critical review. J Allergy 25:151–167

7 Pneumoconiosis

H. Shida, K. Chiyotani, and K. Honma

Introduction

Recent advances in radiological technology have led to increased diagnostic efficacy and accuracy in detecting pulmonary parenchymal changes and pleural abnormalities due to occupational dust exposure:

- Exclusively small rounded opacities on conventional posteroanterior (PA) radiographs: silicosis, caused by inhalation of a high concentration of free silicon dioxide dusts
- Small opacities mixed with rounded and irregular shapes (rounded/irregular): mixed dust fibrosis (MDF) or atypical silicosis, caused by inhalation of less free silicon dioxide dusts or asbestos fiber
- Exclusively small irregular opacities on PA chest radiographs: MDP or asbestosis and silicatosis

In developed countries, with the decreasing prevalence of silicosis and asbestosis and the development of modern diagnostic instruments, the rounded/irregular opacities representing MDF have been recognized as more common than exclusively small, rounded/irregular opacities. Comparative studies are essential between the actual features of such PA findings of exclusively rounded, rounded/irregular, occasionally large opacities and irregular opacities, computed radiography (CR), computed tomography (CT), scintigraphy (SG), and autopsy specimens. Small irregular opacities on PA/CR in MDF/atypical silicosis and asbestosis often represent reticular or honeycomb patterns on CT, which are histologically composed of silicotic nodules (SN), pigmented macules including birefringent dust particles exposed to the polarized light, interstitial fibrosis (IF) accompanied by honeycombing and emphysematous change, and rounded atelectasis.

Large opacities on PA/CR sometimes show consolidated/conglomerated SN in silicosis, and necrotic massive fibrosis in MDP, tuberculous lesions, and rounded atelectasis in non-asbestos pneumoconiosis and MDF through CR, CT, SG and pathological specimens. The above changes are illustrated using seven cases with various changes induced by free silica/mixed dusts and asbestos fibers, such as small rounded and rounded/irregular opacities, large opacities, and irregular opacities on PA/CR; nodular and irregular patterns combined with conglomeration, tuberculous cavity, and rounded atelectasis on CT; and SN plus MDF and IF in pathological specimens.

Table 7.1. Summary of findings in seven cases of pneumoconiosis

Case	PA	CT	Pathology	MAA	^{67}Ga
1	1/1, q/q, ca	N+ca	SN=MDF+ca	+	+++
2	A, 2/2 r/r, es	N+C+hi	MDF+SN+PMF	++	–
3	3/3, r/r, ax, bu, em, es	N+ax+bu+em+es	SN>MDF+bu+em	+++	None
4	2/2 r/r, ca, ef	N+Ra+ef	MDF>SN+RA	None	+ ++
5	1/1, r/r, cv, pt	N+C+cv	MDF+PMF+pt	+++	++
6	3/3 s/s, ho	I+ho+em+pq	IF+asbestosis+pq	+++	None
7	3/3 t/t	I+ho	IF+MDF+anthoracosis	+++	None

N, Nodular patterns; I, irregular patterns (including reticular, reticulolinear, strand, bandlike, and bundle); C, conglomeration; RA, rounded atelectasis; bu, bulla(e) or bleb(s); ca, cancer; cn, calcified nodules; cv, cavitary lesion(s); em, emphysema; es, egg shell calcification of hilum and mediastinum; ho, honeycomb lung; pq, pqc; calcified plaques, pleural plaques; pt; diffuse pleural thickening. MAA: +, mild decrease in perfusion; ++, moderate decrease in perfusion; +++, severe decrease in perfusion. ^{67}Ga-citrate: –, no significant uptake; ++, moderate increased uptake; +++, marked increased uptake. SN, silicate nodules; MDF, mixed dust fibrosis; IF, interstitial fibrosis

Methods

Almost all cases of pneumoconiosis visiting Rosai Hospital for Silicosis routinely undergo CR, CT, SG; autopsy is performed in cases of death. The subjects in the present study were seven patients whose respective data are summarized in Table 7.1. The range of chest radiographic findings were classified by 1980 International Labor Office (ILO) International Classification of Chest Radiographs on Pneumoconioses [1].

CT provides much more detailed information than PA radiography regarding nodular and reticular changes, pulmonary emphysema, conglomeration involving bronchial trees, and pleural effusion. SG using ^{99m}Tc-labeled macroaggregated albumin (MAA) demonstrates the distribution of pulmonary arterial perfusion, and ^{67}Ga-citrate shows high concentrations of radioactive nuclide in the areas of cellular activity in cancerous mass, progressive massive fibrosis, rounded atelectatic area, inflammation, and fibrotic regions.

We compared the following changes on radiographic images with autopsy findings; pulmonary fibrotic change, emphysematous change, architectural parenchymal disorder or damaged pulmonary vasculature, and pleural abnormalities caused by inhalation of dusts.

Posteroanterior Radiography

The ILO [1] classification provides a means of quantitatively coding the radiographic findings of all pneumoconioses, including silicosis, coal worker's pneumoconiosis, and asbestosis. Small opacities, the basic pattern for pneumoconiosis, are classified according to shape/size, profusion, and localization. Small rounded opacities characteristic of silicosis are classified into three shape/size groups based on the approximate diameter of the predominant nodules: p for opacities up to 5 mm in diameter, q for 1.5–3 mm opacities, and r for 3–10 mm opacities. The small irregular opacities characteristic of asbestosis are graded according to width: fine as s, medium as t, coarse or blotchy as u, with the similar cutting points to p, q, and r definitions.

Profusion, or density, of small opacities is divided into four major categories: 0 for normal or nearly normal, 1 for slight, 2 for moderate, and 3 for advanced. The intermediate grading of these 4 profusion scales uses a dual notation; for example, 2/2 means profusion is definitely moderate, and 2/3 that the major category is 2 but with category 3 being seriously considered as an alternative.

Large opacities indicate PMF [2]. These are divided into three categories: A, an opacity having a greatest diameter over 10 mm and up to including about 50 mm, or several opacities each larger than about 10 mm, the sum of whose greatest diameter does not about 50 mm; B, one or more opacities larger or more numerous than those in category A, whose combined area does not exceed the equivalent of the upper right zone; C, one or more opacities whose combined area exceeds the equivalent of the upper right zone.

Computed Radiography

We use CR because the imaging plate improves the quality of images and provides much more diagnostic information. CR proves satisfactory, however, only when the radiographic quality is reasonable for diagnosis of pneumoconiosis. CR images are highly compatible with human vision and permit more diagnostic information by use of tonal conversion. Fine, small rounded, or irregular opacities can be clarified by spatial frequency modification to eliminate contrast deficiencies and blurring.

Life-sized CR images have recently become widely available. In our study CR was performed by a TCR 201 unit (Toshiba Medical, Tokyo, Japan.). Magnified views were obtained by using an optical filling disk and contrast enhancement; this permits very fine, small, rounded opacities or irregular opacities to be imaged much more clearly than with conventional PA chest radiographs. We compared CR images and conventional radiographs. On the former it was sometimes difficult to discern the p-sized, small, rounded opacities on the reduced-size CR film; in such cases the magnified views of CR were used.

Computed Tomography

CT was performed with a helical CT scanner (TCT-900S Helical; Toshiba Medical) equipped with 2304 solid detectors of an 0.35 mm spatial resolution, and specially designed filter functions of FC3 or FC4 for imaging pulmonary parenchyma and FC1 for imaging soft tissues, and with the super resolution mode. The imaging parameters included 120 kVp, 200–250 mA, and 0.6- to 1.0-s scan times. Soft-tissue images were produced with window widths of 200–1000, window levels of 0–600, and filter function FC1. Scans of the parenchyma were obtained with window widths of 800–1500, window levels of 500–850, and filter function FC3 or FC4. Section thicknesses of 5–10 mm were used.

SG was performed with a GCA-90 B system (Toshiba Medical) and obtained in supine position. ^{99m}Tc-MAA was injected in supine position, with an activity of 185 MBq. ^{99m}Tc-MAA SG planner images reflects the distribution of pulmonary perfusion. ^{67}Ga-citrate was also injected, with an activity of 185 MBq. ^{67}Ga-citrate studies may reflect cellular activity within areas of immature fibrosis or neoplasms; it is impossible to differentiate between lung cancer and PMF. We assessed reduction in pulmonary perfusion on planner SG by the naked eye. Emission CT was not performed for the quantitative evaluation of pulmonary perfusion because of several difficulties in comparison with CT images. ^{133}Xe perfusion and ventilation studies were not performed because of poor accuracy and less effectiveness of estimation of pulmonary function tests for pneumoconioses.

Autopsy

We investigated macro- and microsections, cut surface of the lungs, namely the Gough-Wentworth (G-W) [3] whole-lung section, and histopathological sections.

Case Presentations

In the following case descriptions the relationship between SN and mixed dust fibrosis (MDF) is presented as: SN>MDF, silicosis is dominant; MDF>SN, mixed dust fibrosis is dominant; or SN=MDF, equal findings.

Case 1 (SN=MDF)

The patient was a 74-year-old man who had worked in a metal mine for 30 years. He was a former smoker and eventually died of lung cancer.

PA chest radiographic findings showed opacity type q/q, profusion category 1/1, and lung cancer.

CR revealed small rounded opacities 1.5–2.0 mm in diameter scattered in both upper lungs, showing low profusion. A tumorlike protrusion was noted in the right hilar region associated with diaphragmatic elevation (Fig. 7.1).

CT demonstrated a few parenchymal nodules in both upper lungs and a tumorlike bulge in the right upper hilar and mediastinal regions with nar-

Fig. 7.1. Case 1. Posteroanterior CR image reveals of the chest reveals a small number of small rounded opacities scattered in both upper lungs. A tumorlike protrusion is noted in the right hilum

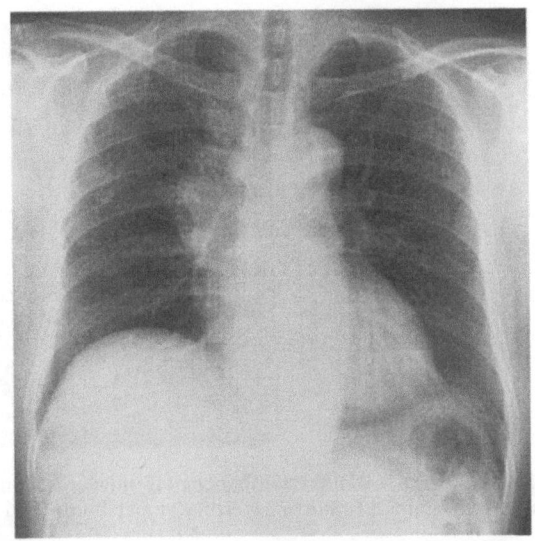

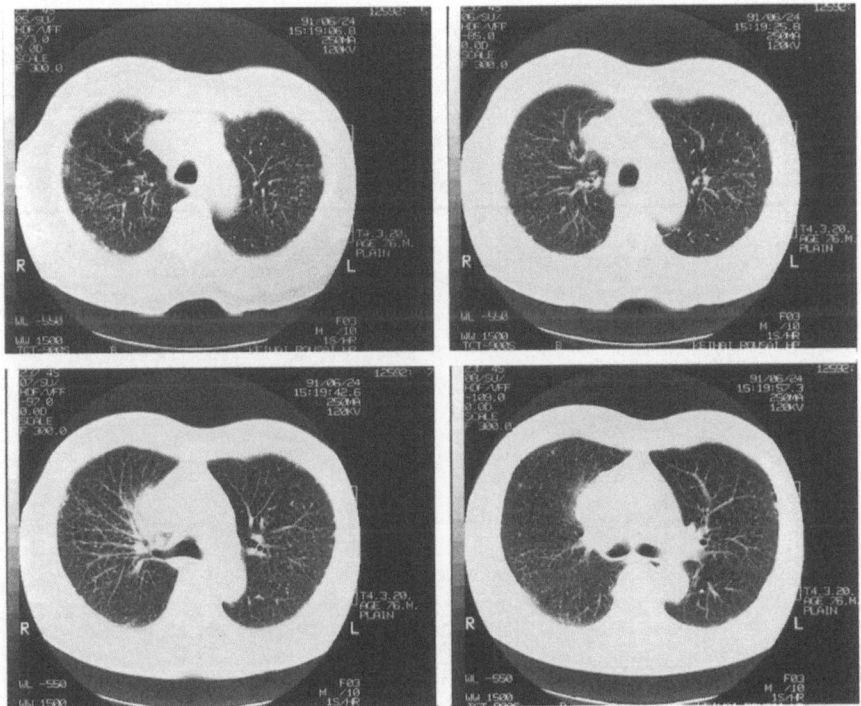

Fig. 7.2. Case 1. CT images (1-s scan time, 10-mm collimation, window width of 1500, window level of 500, FC3 filter) of the upper lung demonstrate a small number of parenchimal nodules in both upper lungs. A tumorlike bulge in the upper right hilar and mediastinal regions with narrowing of the upper anterior bronchial trees

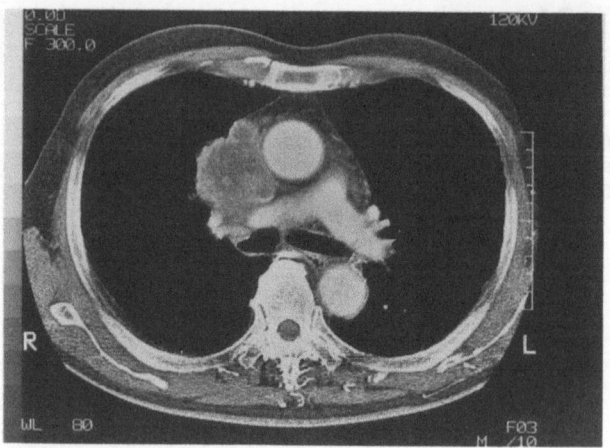

Fig. 7.3. Case 1. Contrast-enhanced CT image demonstrates irregularly contoured and unevenly stained tumor mass in the upper hilum and metastatic lymph nodes

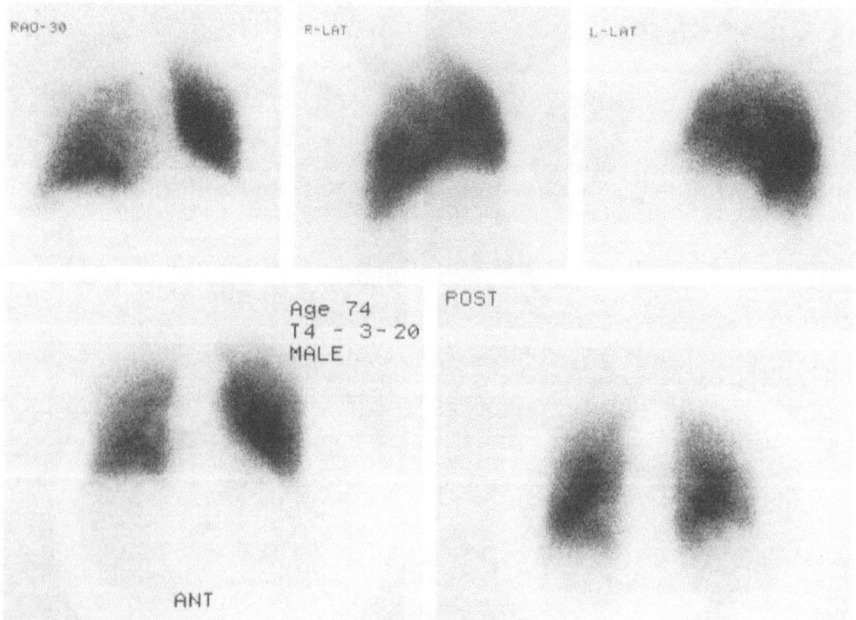

Fig. 7.4. Case 1. ^{99m}Tc-MAA SG images show mildly decreased deposition of radionuclide in both upper and middle lungs. *ANT,* Anterior; *L-LAT,* left lateral; *RO-30°,* right oblique at 30°; *R-LAT,* right lateral; *POST,* posterior

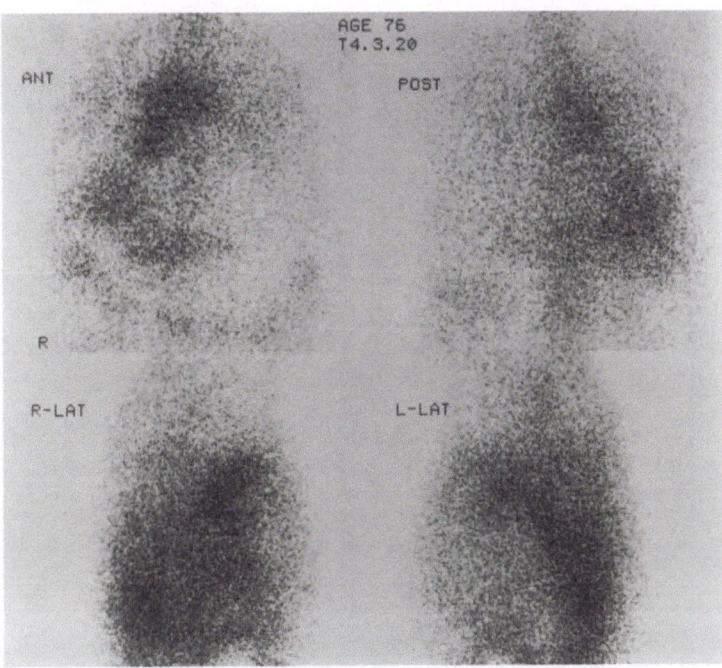

Fig. 7.5. Case 1. ^{67}Ga-citrate SG reveals marked uptake of radionuclide in the tumor mass in the upper hilum and mediastinal regions

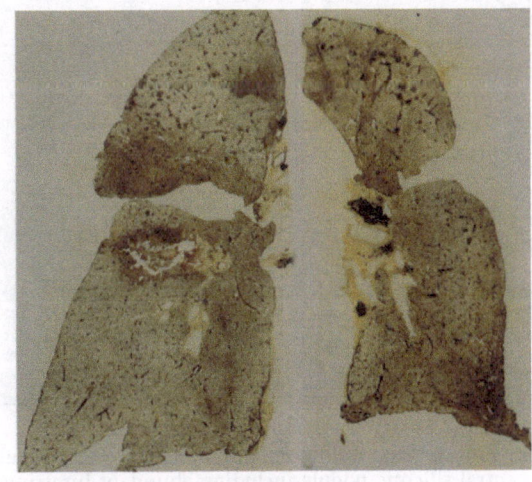

Fig. 7.6. Case 1. Whole lung section (G-W fixative) demonstrates sparse and pigmented nodular lesions in the upper lobes and a necrotic tumor mass involving the mediastinal portion of the right lower lobe

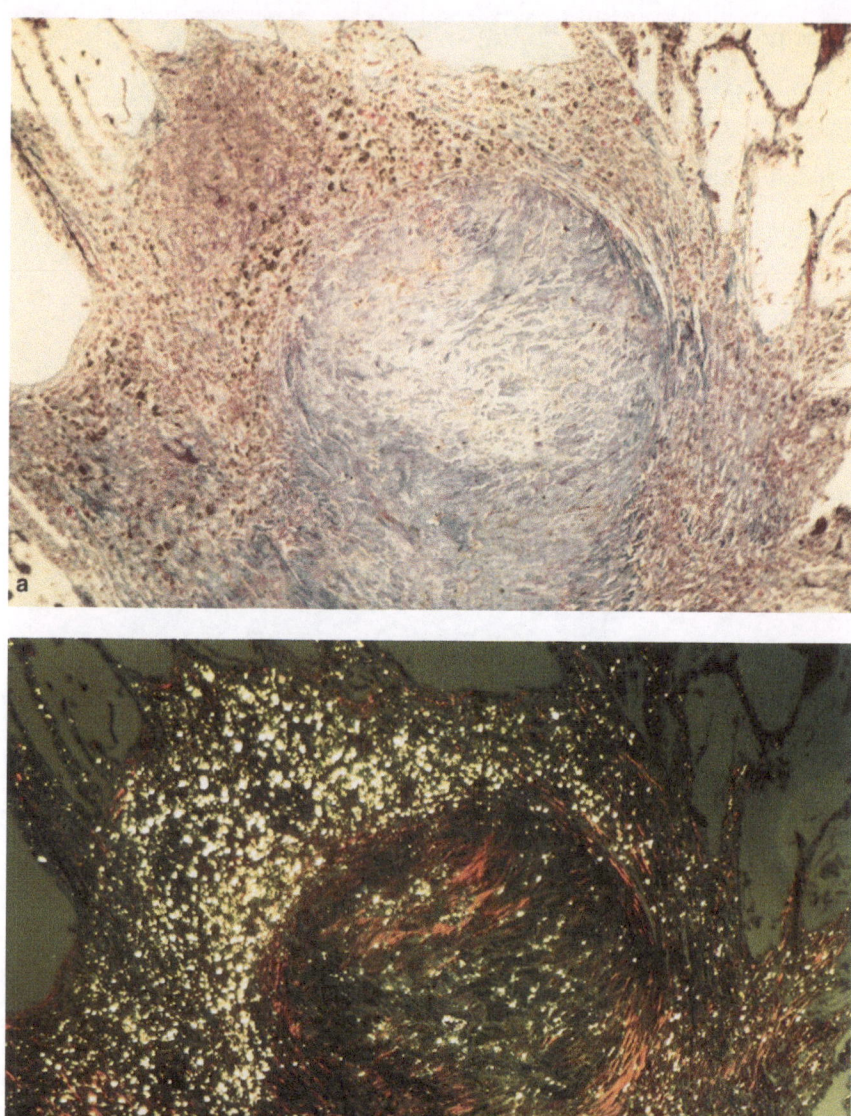

Fig. 7.7 a, b. Case 1. Photomicrographs show an irregularly contoured MDF lesion with a central silicotic nodule including abundant birefringent dust particles visualized under the polarized light, suggesting of MDF lesion (SN=MDF). Original magnification, 40×, Elastica Masson stain

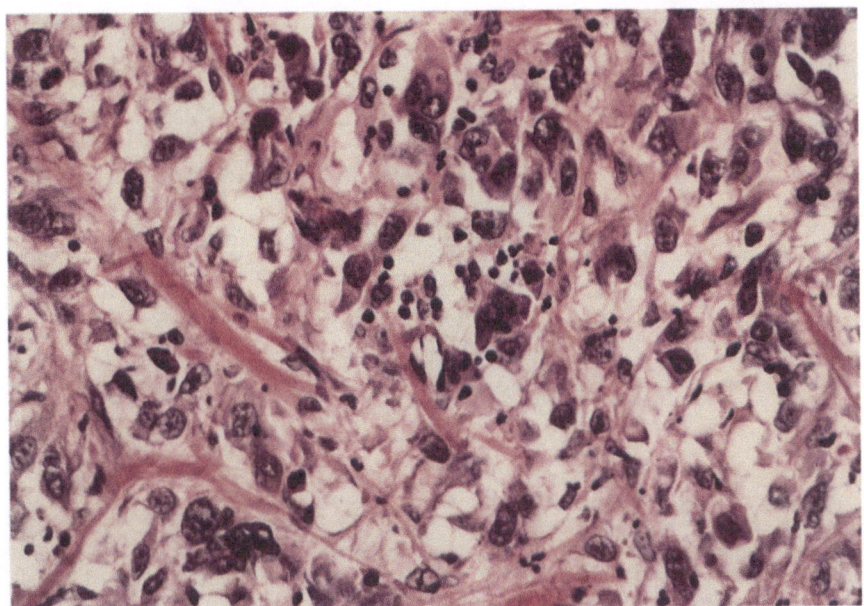

Fig. 7.8. Case 1. Histological section confirms pleomorphic large cell carcinoma

rowing of the upper bronchial trees (Fig. 7.2). Contrast enhancement CT demonstrated irregularly contoured and unevenly stained tumor mass in the right hilum and metastatic lymph nodes (Fig. 7.3).

^{99m}Tc-MAA SG showed mildly decreased deposition of radioactive tracer in the upper right lung (Fig. 7.4).

^{67}Ga-citrate SG revealed marked uptake of radionuclide in the tumor mass in the upper right hilum and mediastinal regions, suggesting of lung cancer accompanied with metastatic lymph nodes (Fig. 7.5).

G-W whole-lung section revealed sparse dissemination of SN in both upper lobes, suggesting changes of a mild silicosis, and a necrotic tumor measuring 8×3 cm involving the medial portion of the upper right lobe and extending into the anterior main bronchus of the right pulmonary artery. There were carcinoma metastases to lymph nodes in the cervical, supraclavicular, paratracheal, and pulmonary hilar regions (Fig. 7.6).

Histological findings included irregularly contoured, fibrotic lesions including abundant birefringent dust particles exposed to polarized light, suggesting MDF and early SN in the center (Fig. 7.7). Histological study confirmed large-cell carcinoma (Fig. 7.8).

Case 2 (SN=MDF)

The patient was a 79-year-old man who had worked in a metal mine for 24 years. He was a former smoker and eventually died of respiratory failure.

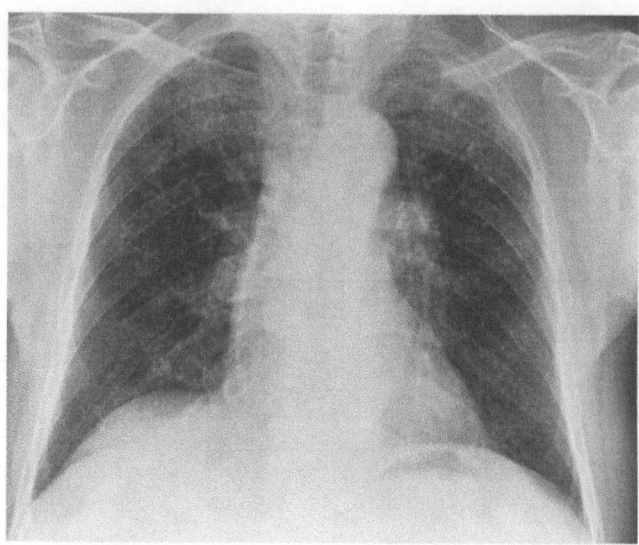

Fig. 7.9. Case 2. Posteroanterior chest CR image reveals well-circumscribed, small, rounded opacities in both upper and middle lungs. An ill-defined large opacity 5 cm in diameter is presented in the upper lung

PA showed exclusively small rounded opacities and a large opacity of category A. Chest radiographic findings were opacity type r/r, profusion 2/2, A, eggshell calcification.

CR image revealed fairly well-circumscribed, small rounded opacities 3–5 mm in diameter of low profusion in both middle and upper lungs. An ill-defined large opacity 5 cm in diameter was presented in the upper right lung. These findings were classified as r/r in shape/size and 1/1 in profusion with a grade A large opacity. Such large opacity usually indicates PMF. Lymphadenopathy with calcium deposition is noted in both hilar regions. There was also eggshell calcification (Fig. 7.9).

CT revealed numerous parenchymal nodules throughout the lungs and subpleural nodules in the upper left posterior zone. Two conglomerations in both upper lungs were also noted (Fig. 7.10).

^{99m}Tc-MAA SG showed a moderate decrease in distribution of radionuclide in both upper and lower posterior lungs (Fig. 7.11). This finding suggests decreased pulmonary perfusion caused by fibrotic changes.

^{67}Ga-citrate SG showed no significant uptake in large opacities.

G-W whole-lung section revealed confluent pigmented fibrous nodules in the both upper and middle lobes, associated with fibrous pleural adhesions. Two areas of PMF in both upper lobes were noted (Fig. 7.12).

Histological findings included SN surrounded by irregularly contoured MDF lesion. A small amount of birefringent dust particles under the polarized light were found within irregularly contoured fibrotic lesions (Fig. 7.13).

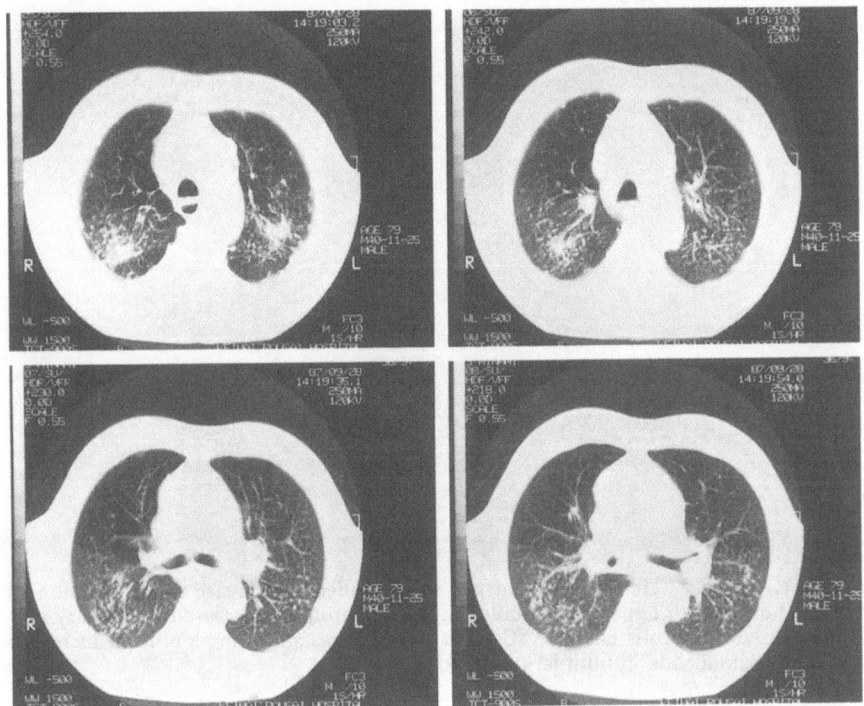

Fig. 7.10. Case 2. CT images (1-s scan time, 10-mm collimation, window width 1500, window level 500, FC3 filter) reveal nodules throughout the lungs and subpleural nodules in the upper left posterior zone. Two conglomerations in both upper lungs are also noted

Case 3 (SN>MDF)

The patient was a 79-year-old man who had worked in a copper mine for 17 years. He was a former smoker and died of retroperitoneal hemorrhage.

PA showed exclusively small rounded opacities of 3/3 r/r, coalescence of nodules, bullae, emphysema, and eggshell calcification. PA chest radiographic findings according were r/r in shape/size, category 3/3 in profusion; we also observed coalescence of nodules, bullae, em, and eggshell calcification in the right hilar region.

CR revealed fairly well-circumscribed, small rounded opacities, up to 5.0 mm in diameter widespread and densely disseminated throughout the lungs, and several small rounded opacities were confluented. Emphysematous hyperlucency in both lower lungs was accompanied with bullae (Fig. 7.14).

CT demonstrated numerous fairly well-circumscribed nodules evenly distributed throughout the lungs with confluent nodules, and strandlike pleural scarring in the lower left lung. Bullae in various size in the left middle anterior zone and emphysematous change in both lower lungs were noted. The pulmonary vasculature was obscured (Fig. 7.15).

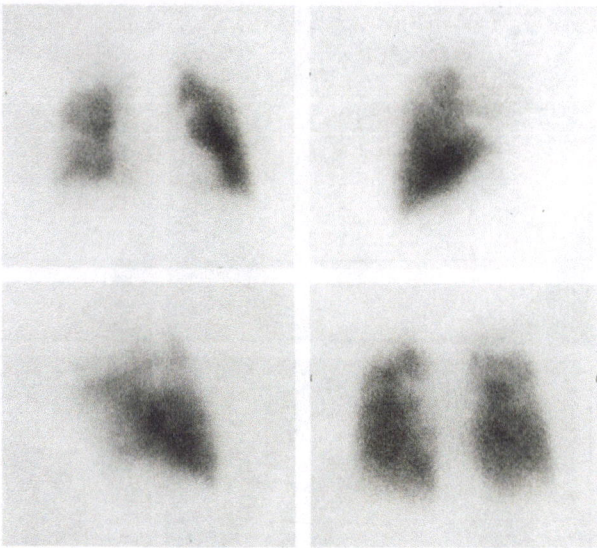

Fig. 7.11. Case 2. ^{99m}Tc-MAA SG images show moderate decrease in distribution of radionuclide in both upper and middle lungs, suggesting of decreased pulmonary perfusion caused by fibrotic change. ^{67}Ga-citrate SG images show no significant increased uptake of radionuclide in both large opacities

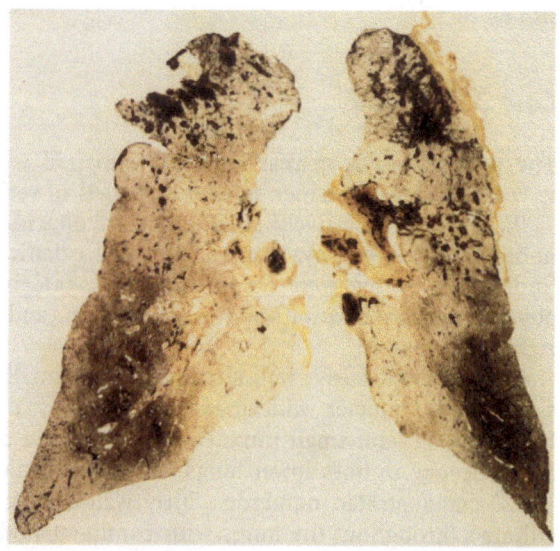

Fig. 7.12. Case 2. Whole lung section (G-W fixative) demonstrates confluent pigmented fibrous nodules in both upper lobes, associated with fibrous pleural adhesion. Two areas of PMF in both upper lobes are noted

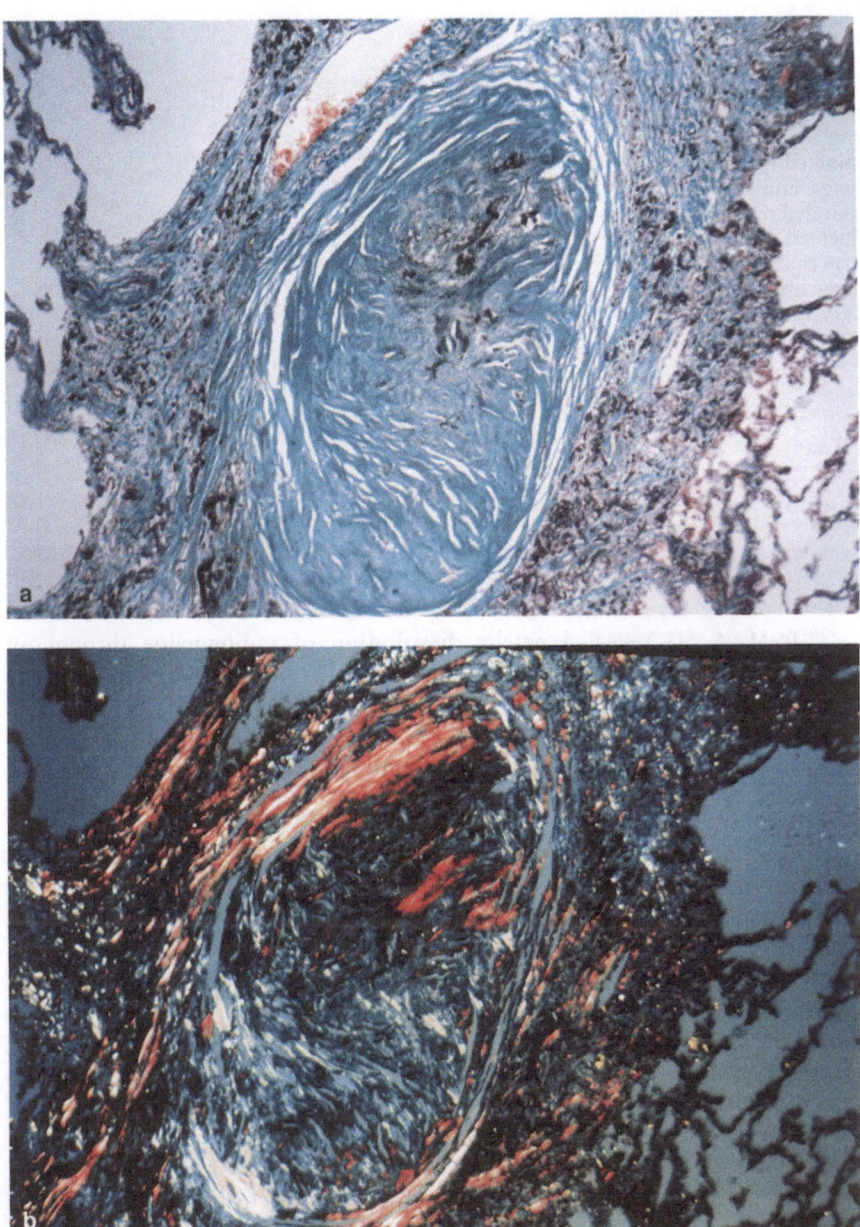

Fig. 7.13 a, b. Case 2. Photomicrographs demonstrate SN surrounded by an irregularly contoured MDF lesion. A small number of birefringent dust particles under polarized light are found within irregularly contoured fibrotic lesions (SN=MDF)

Fig. 7.14. Case 3. Posteroanterior CR chest image
reveals numerous fairly
well-circumscribed, small,
rounded opacities wide-
spread and densely disse-
minated throughout the
lungs, and several small
rounded opacities are confluented. Emphysematous
hyperlucency in both lower
lungs are noted. Pulmo-
nary vasculature is ob-
scured

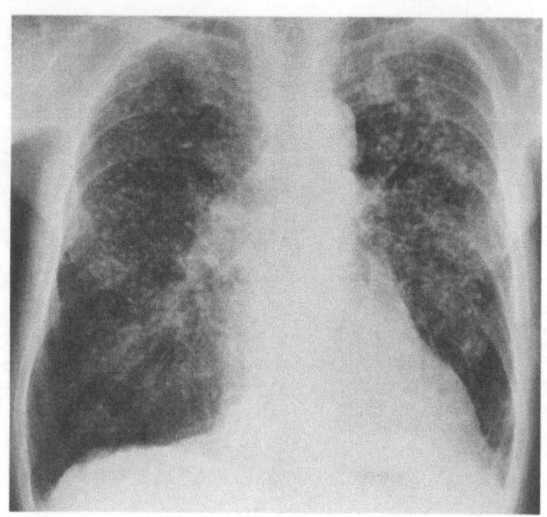

^{99m}Tc-MAA SG revealed patchy distribution of radionuclide throughout the lungs with considerably reduced deposition in both posterior lung zones due to emphysematous change (Fig. 7.16).

G-W whole-lung section revealed numerous pigmented nodules up to 5 mm in diameter throughout the lungs with confluence and emphysematous change. Pigmented induration of the hilar lymph nodes were noted (Fig. 7.17).

Histological findings revealed typical SN with varying degrees of conflu-ence (Fig. 7.18).

Case 4 (MDF>SN)

The patient was a 60-year-old man who had worked as a boilerman for 8 years and in a gravel-crushing factory for 33 years. He was a former smoker and died of gastric cancer.

PA showed small rounded opacities and a large opacity radiographs. Chest radiographic findings were r/r in shape/size and category 2/2 in profusion with suspicion of carcinoma and effusion in the right costophrenic angle.

➤

Fig. 7.15 a, b. Case 3. CT images (1-s scan time, 10-mm collimation, window width 1200, window level 600) demonstrate numerous fairly well-circumscribed nodules evenly disseminated throughout the lungs with confluent nodules and strandlike pleural scarring in the lower left lung. Bullae in various size in the left middle anterior zone and emphysematous change in both lower lungs are noted. Pulmonary vasculature obscured

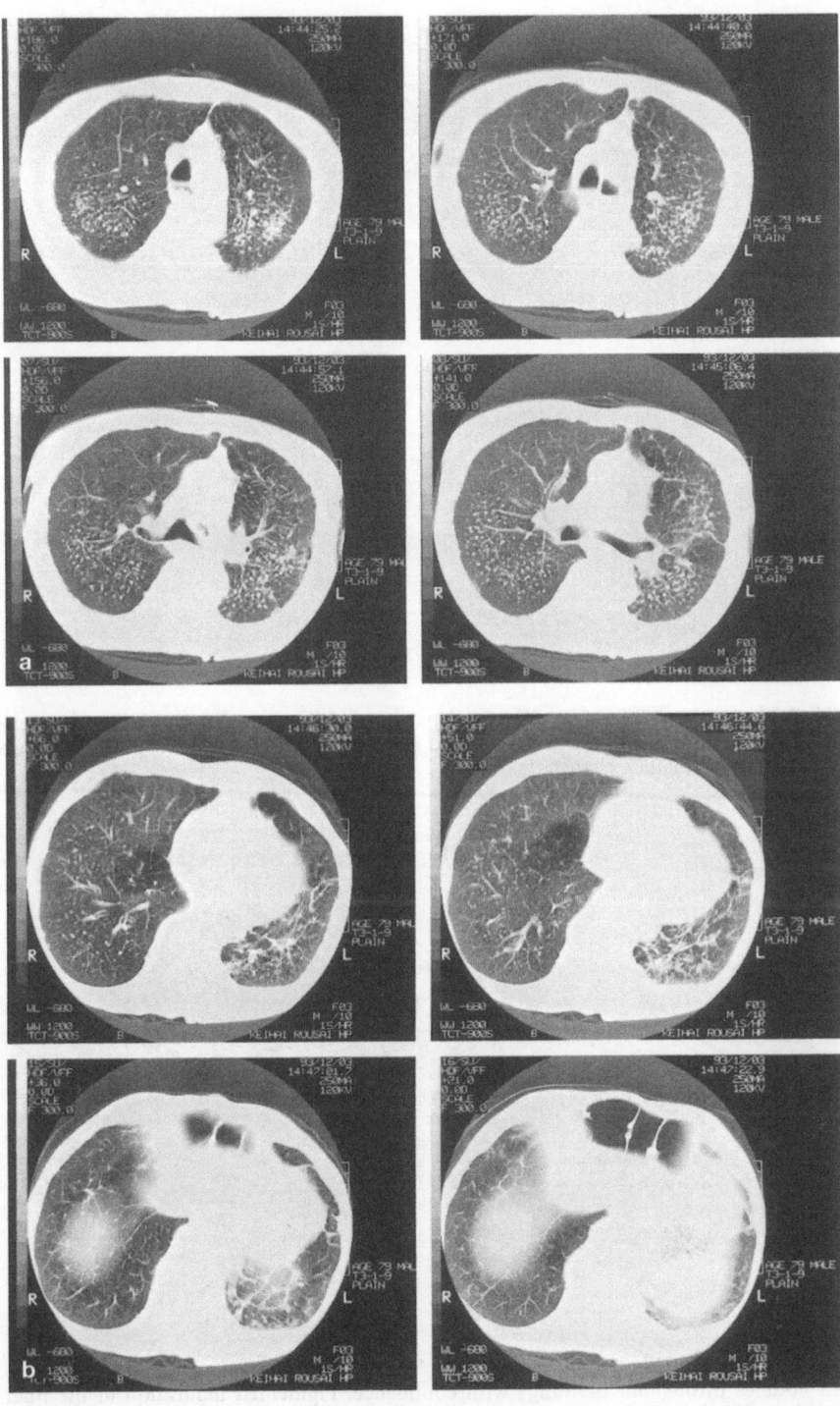

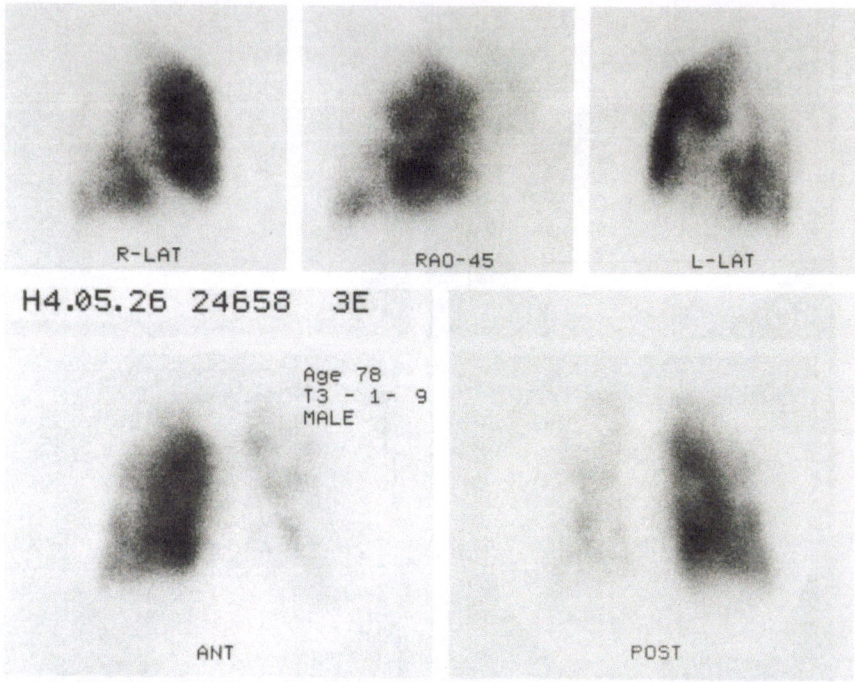

Fig. 7.16. Case 3. ^{99m}Tc-MAA SG reveal patchy distribution of radionuclide through-out the lung zones with markedly reduced deposition of MAA in both posterior lungs due to emphysematous change

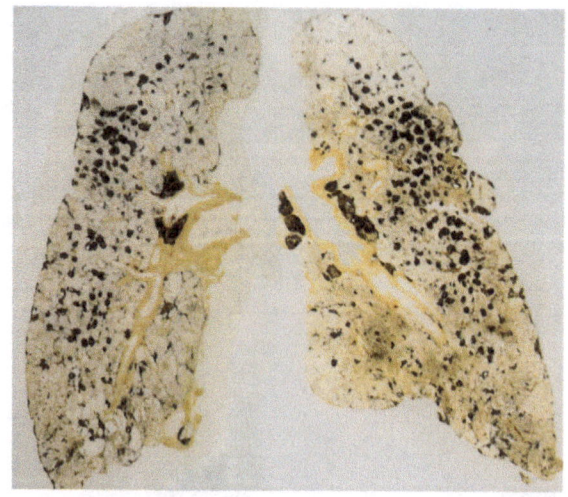

Fig. 7.17. Case 3. Whole lung section (G-W fixative) demonstrates numerous pigmen-ted nodules throughout the lungs with confluence. Pigmented induration of the hilar lymph nodes are noted

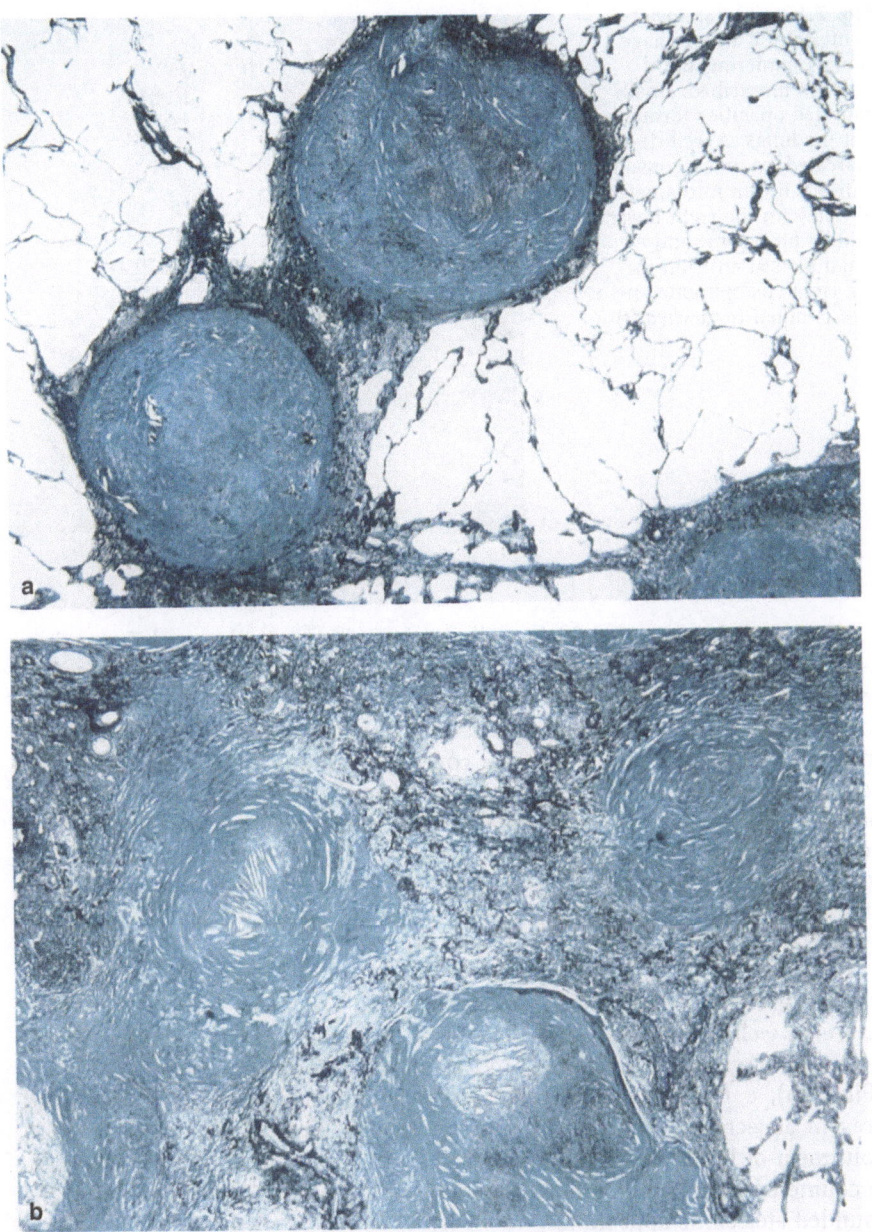

Fig. 7.18 a, b. Case 3. Histological findings revealed typical SN showing varying degrees of confluence

Fig. 7.19. Case 4. Poster-oanterior CR chest image reveals numerous fairly well-circumscribed, small, rounded opacities through-out the lungs. A well-de-marcated, rounded consoli-dation 3.0 mm in diameter is visible in the right lower middle lung zone, and a small pleural effusion in the right costophrenic an-gles is noted (*arrowheads*)

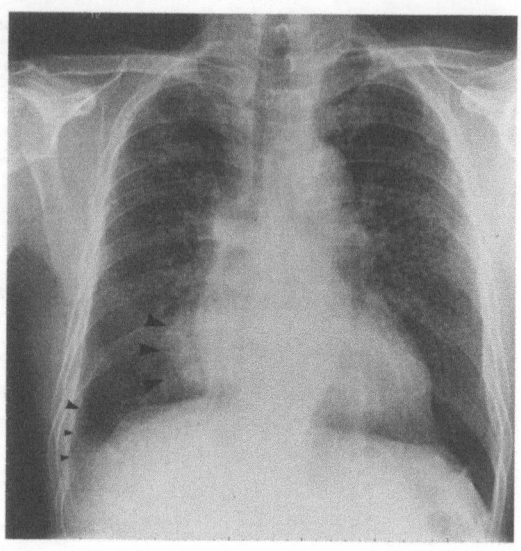

CR revealed numerous fairly well-circumscribed, small rounded opacities 3–5 mm in diameter scattered densely and diffusely throughout the lungs. A well-demarcated, rounded consolidation of 3.0 cm in diameter was visible in the lower right lung zone accompanied by a small amount of pleural effusion in the right costophrenic angle. The consolidation was thought to represent a carcinoma or rounded atlectasis. Large opacities seen in silicotic patients often represent PMF and are usually located in the upper lung zones, not accompanied by pleural effusion. The large opacity seen in this case was interpreted as a rounded area of rounded shrinkage of a lobe or rounded atelectasis, which is much more frequently associated with asbestos dust ex-posure and with pleural effusion (Fig. 7.19).

CT demonstrated numerous, well-circumscribed parenchymal nodules evenly distributed throughout the left lung and obscuring pulmonary vascu-lature. A well-demarcated, tumorlike mass was also seen in the lower right posterior region accompanied by a small amount of pleural effusion (Fig. 7.20), a finding suggestive of either a neoplastic lesion or a rounded area of atelectasis. The latter interpretation was more likely considering in-volvement of bronchial trees and a small amount of pleural effusion. We have encountered four other silicotic patients in whom CT demonstrated the rounded atelectatic appearance.

[67]Ga-citrate SG showed increased uptake of radionuclides in the tumorlike, rounded consolidation in the lower right lung and diffuse uptake in both lungs (Fig. 7.21). These findings were considered suggestive of fibrotic nod-ules since the uptake of ^{67}Ga-citrate indicates cellular activity in a fibrotic le-sion or neoplastic disease.

At pathological examination, numerous silicotic nodules up to 5 mm in di-ameter were seen scattered throughout the lungs on G-W whole-lung section

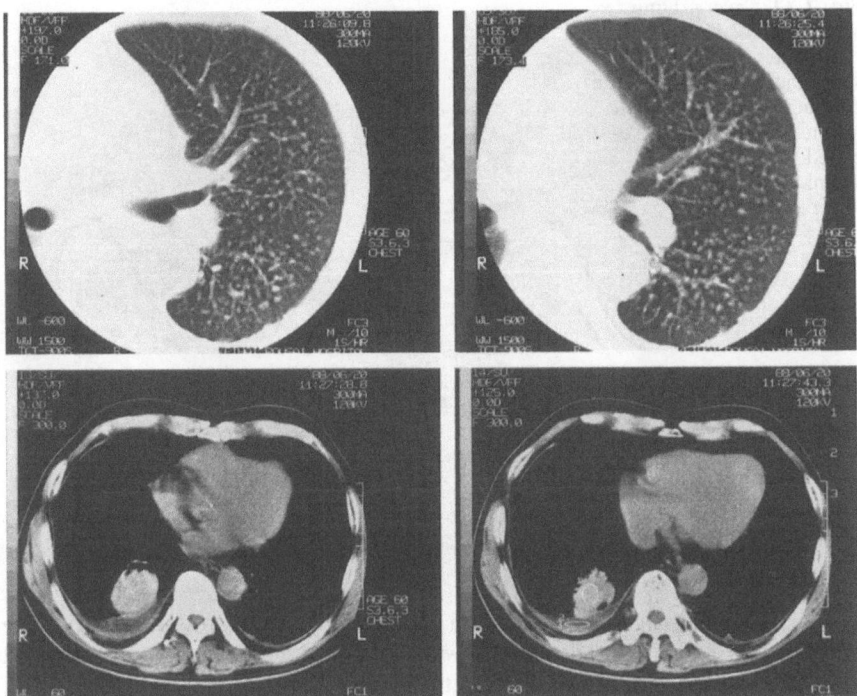

Fig. 7.20. Case 4. CT images (1-s scan time, 10-mm collimation, window width 1500, window level of 600, FC3 filter) demonstrate numerous, well-circumscribed nodules throughout the lungs, and obscuring pulmonary vasculature. At soft tissue algorithm (window width 200, window level 60, FC1 filter), a well-demarcated, tumorlike mass is also seen in the lower right posterior region and a small pleural effusion (*arrowheads*)

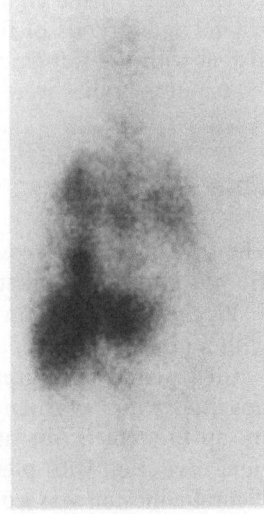

Fig. 7.21. Case 4. The ^{67}Ga-citrate SG shows increased uptake of radionuclide in the middle posterior region of the right lung and diffuse uptake in both lungs

Fig. 7.22. Case 4. Lung section (G-W fixative) demonstrates numerous SN throughout the lungs and a confluent massive fibrotic lesion (*arrowheads*) associated with a rounded shrinkage process in the lower right lobe

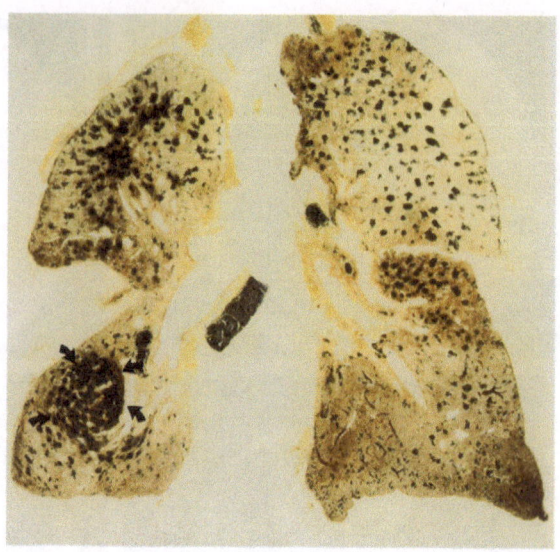

(Fig. 7.22). A massive fibrotic lesion, associated with a rounded shrinkage process, was present in the right lower lobe. Although the lesion resembled PMF, it consisted of numerous SN within a small area of lobar shrinkage and was considered as a feature of atelectasis. Because of coexistent pleural effusion the diagnosis of PMF was considered to be unlikely. No malignant tumor was found. Pleural adhesion and pigmented induration of the hilar lymph nodes were noted.

Photomicrography demonstrated well-developed SN. Abundant birefringent dust particles exposed to polarized light both within and outside the nodule were observed (Fig. 7.23).

The mass in the right lower lobe was composed of atelectatic lung parenchyma and strands of fibrotic pleura which invaginated into the former, consistent with the features of rounded atelectasis (Fig. 7.24).

Asbestos bodies were not found.

Case 5 (MDF)

The patient was a 76-year old man who had been a brickworker for 31 years. He was a former smoker and died of pneumonia.

PA chest radiographic findings were opacity type r/r, profusion category 1/1 with a grade B large opacity, with cavity.

CR-PA chest radiograph showed sparse, well-circumscribed, small rounded opacities 5 mm in diameter in the upper left lung. An ill-defined large opacity up to 5 cm in diameter was presented in the upper right lung. In addition, cavitation with pleural thickening in the upper left lung was visualized. Pleural adhesion was noted in the right costophrenic angle (Fig. 7.25).

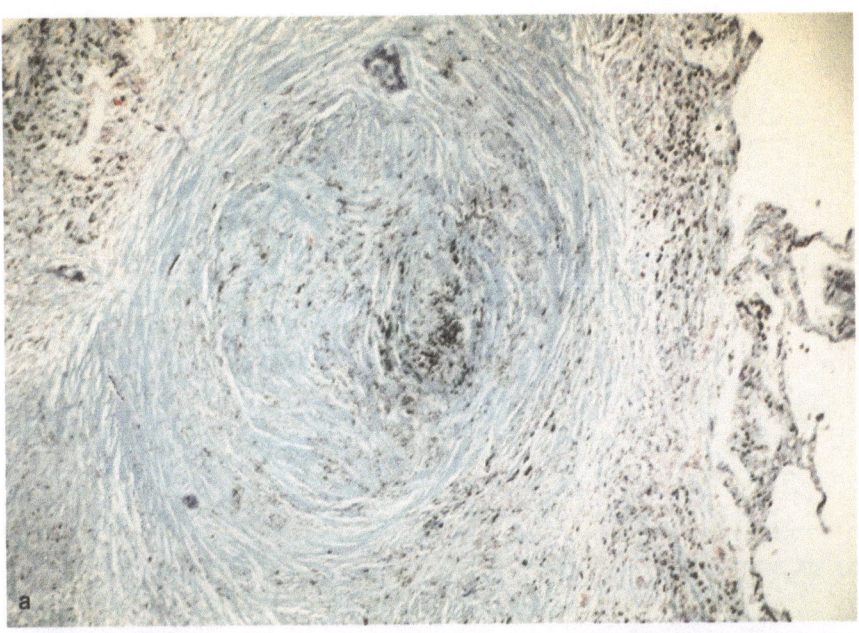

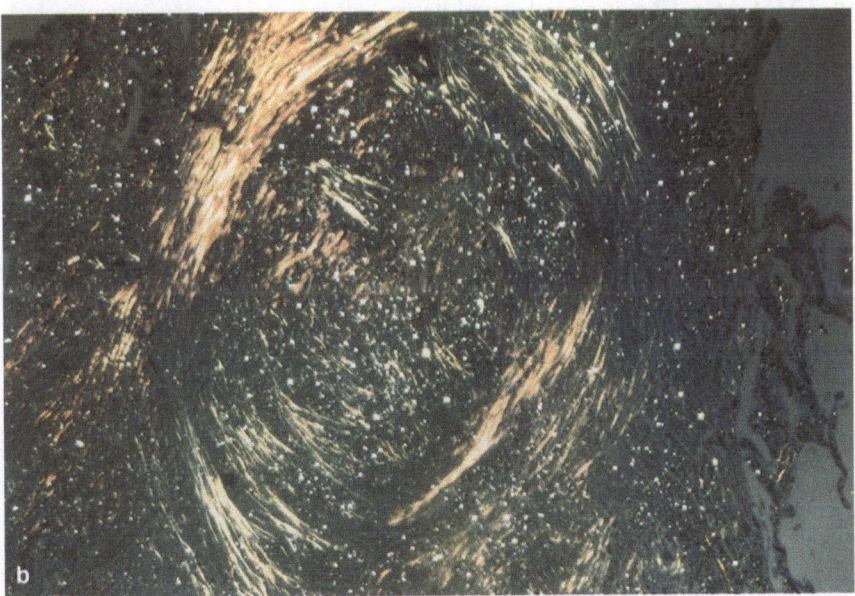

Fig. 7.23 a, b. Case 4. Photomicrographs demonstrate well-developed SN. Abundant birefringent dust particles both within and outside the nodules are observed under the polarized right. Original magnification, –40, Elastica Masson stain

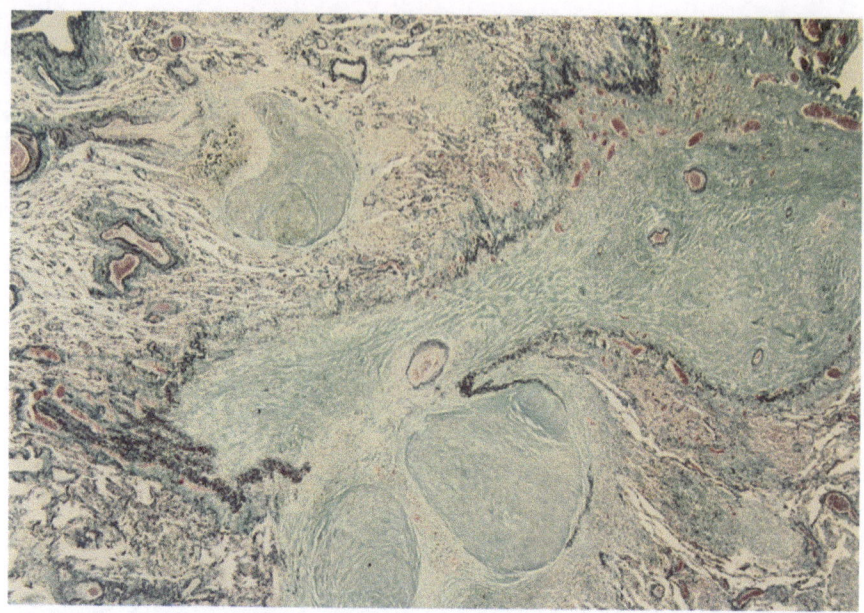

Fig. 7.24. Case 4. Fibrous pleural strand invaginates into the lung parenchyma which is atelectatic and consistent with the findings of rounded atelectasis

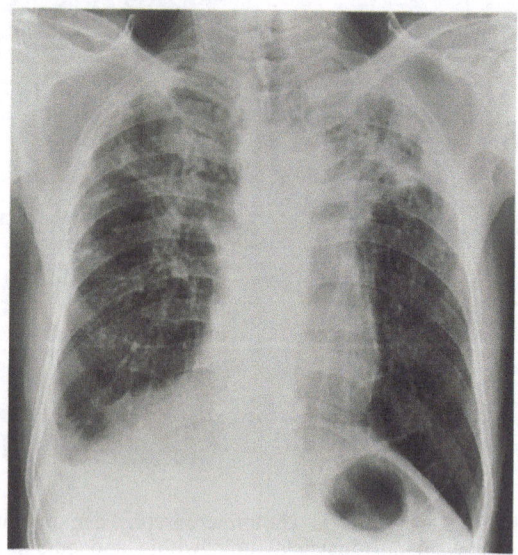

Fig. 7.25. Case 5. Posteroanterior CR chest image reveals sparse, well-circumscribed, small, rounded opacities in the upper left lung. An ill-defined large opacity is present in the upper right lung. In addition, cavitation with pleural thickening in the upper left lung and pleural adhesion are noted. The right costophrenic angle is obliterated

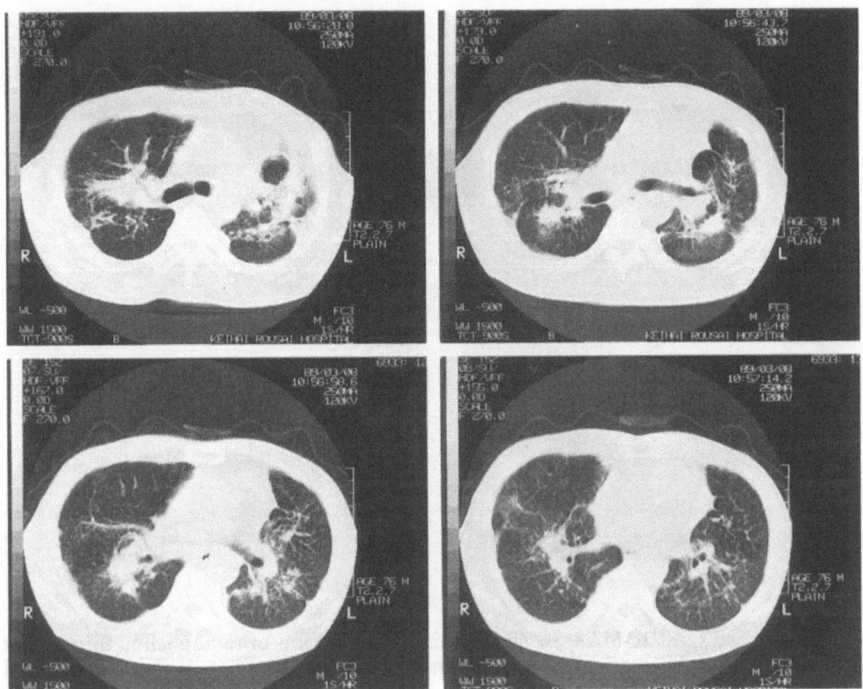

Fig. 7.26. Case 5. CT images (1-s scan time, 10-mm collimation, window width 1500, window level 500, FC3 filter) demonstrate conglomerations and cavitary lesion with thick wall in the upper left lung. Sparse, well-demarcated nodules are disseminated throughout the lungs. Pulmonary vasculature is severely damaged. Lymph nodes are involved in both hilar regions

CT demonstrated conglomerations and cavitary lesions with thick walls in the upper left lung. Sparse, well-demarcated, nodules were disseminated throughout the lungs. Pulmonary vasculature was severely damaged. Lymph nodes were enlarged in both hilar regions (Fig. 7.26).

^{99m}Tc-MAA SG revealed patchy distribution of radionuclide throughout the lungs, with markedly reduced distribution of MAA in both upper and middle regions, suggestive of considerable decrease in pulmonary perfusion (Fig. 7.27).

^{67}Ga-citrate SG revealed increased uptake of radionuclide in the large opacities at CR and CT images especially marked in the upper right lung zone. The increased uptake indicates persistent cellular activity in the areas of PMF (Fig. 7.28).

G-W whole-lung section demonstrated massive fibrotic lesions in the left upper lobe and in the hilar portion of the right lung, small numbers of individual pigmented fibrous nodules around the mass lesions, and pigmented fibrous induration of both hilar lymph nodes. Fibrous pleural adhesions were present. Tuberuculous cavitary lesion was not noted (Fig. 7.29).

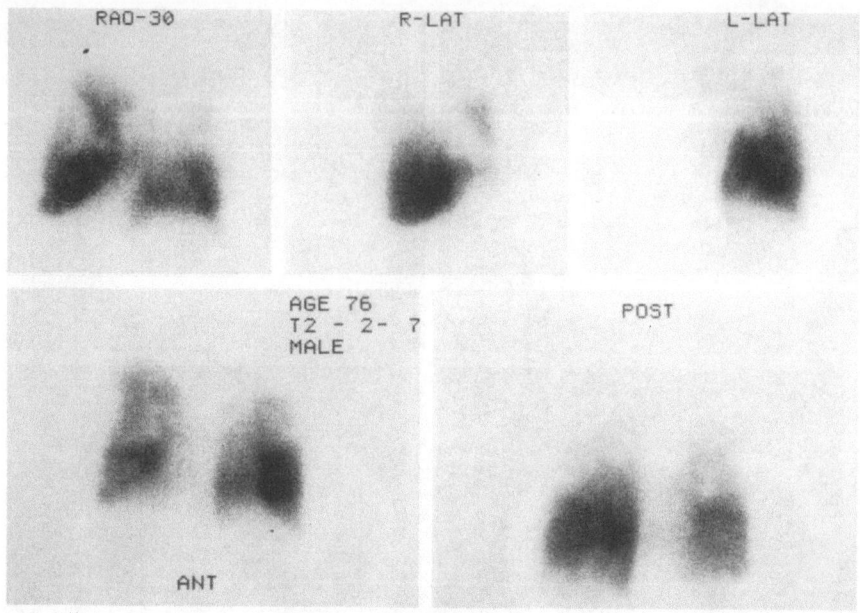

Fig. 7.27. Case 5. ^{99m}Tc-MAA SG show patchy distribution of radionuclide throughout the lungs, especially markedly reduced distribution of the MAA in both upper and middle regions

Histological findings revealed massive fibrosis showing early cavitary degenerative changes (Fig. 7.30).

An MDF nodule was seen in a part of a mixed dust fibrotic nodule, showing irregular-contoured fibrous tissue (stellate nodule) containing pigment-laden macrophages. A small amount of birefringent dust particles in the nodule exposed to the polarized light was observed and MDF nodules connected with the adjacent ones by fibrous strands (Fig. 7.31).

IF with emphysematous change was also noted (Fig. 7.32). Tuberuculous bacilli of bridging type were not found.

Case 6 (IF, asbestosis)

The patient was 60-year-old man who had worked as an arc welder for 21 years. He was a former smoker and died of virus infection.

PA chest radiographic findings were classified as s/s and category 3/3 in profusion, with honeycomb lung.

CR revealed numerous irregular opacities, reticular or reticulolinear, distributed densely and diffusely throughout the lungs, and honeycombing was seen in both lower lungs (Fig. 7.33).

CT demonstrated numerous honeycombing throughout the lungs, with distribution marked in the subpleural zones. These findings were of a pattern

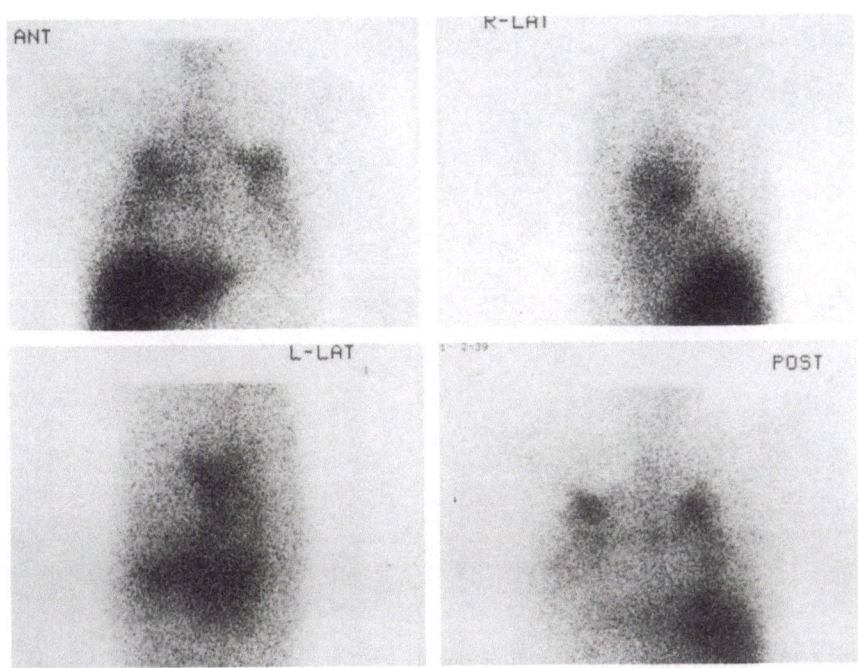

Fig. 7.28. Case 5. 67 Ga-citrate SG reveal marked uptake of radionuclide in the large opacities

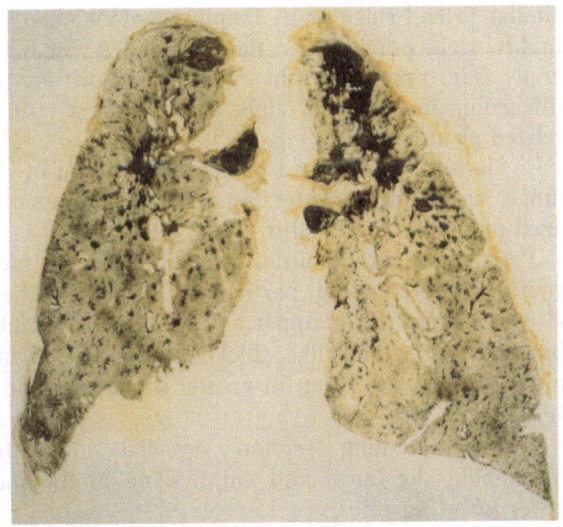

Fig. 7.29. Case 5. Whole lung section (G-W fixative) demonstrates massive fibrosis in the upper left lobe and in the right hilar portion, small numbers of individual pigmented fibrous nodules around the mass lesions and pigmented fibrous induration of both hilar lymph nodes. Fibrous pleural adhesions are presented. Tuberculous cavitary lesion was not noted

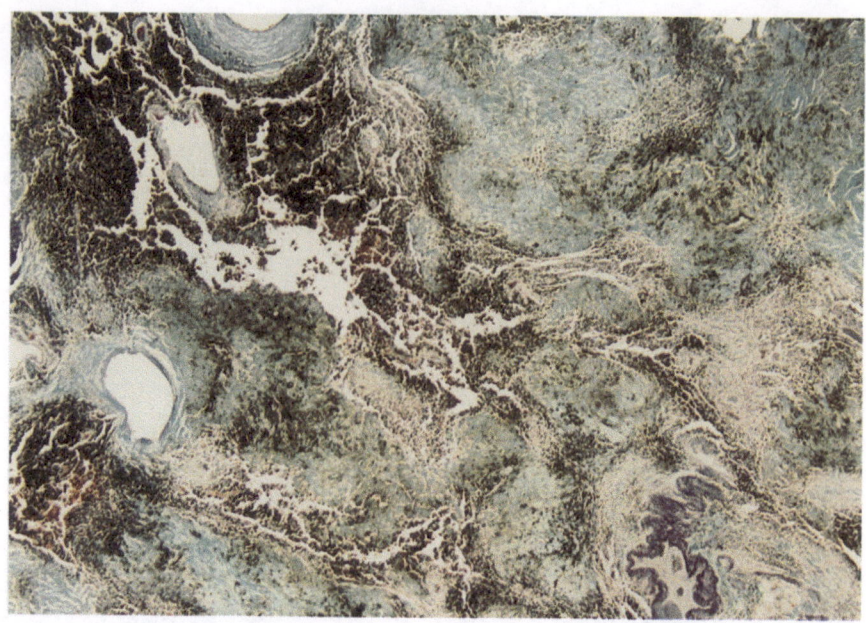

Fig. 7.30. Case 5. Histological section reveals PMF showing early cavitary degenerative change

similar to end-stage of IF. Emphysematous change was noted in the lower to middle right portion, and the pulmonary vasculature was not traced peripherally (Fig. 7.34). CT with soft-tissue algorithm revealed a localized pleural thickening in the upper right anterior chest wall, suggesting of an asbestos-related pleural plaque (Fig. 7.35).

^{99m}Tc-MAA SG showed patchy distribution of radionuclide throughout the lungs, suggesting considerably reduced pulmonary perfusion caused by damaged pulmonary vasculature (Fig. 7.36).

Pathological examination revealed extensive areas of diffuse IF with substantial honeycombing, particularly marked in the lower lobes and subpleural parenchyma of the upper and middle lobes and fibrous pleural adhesions, bilateral, with tumorlike thickening in the right anterior portion of the pleura, measuring 12 cm in greater dimension and up to 10 mm in thickness (Fig. 7.37).

G-W whole-lung section revealed substantial cystic honeycombing throughout the lungs and emphysema in the medial portion of the right lower lobe (Fig. 7.38).

Histological findings included end-stage changes of IF with asbestos body (Fig. 7.39a). This asbestos body was not refracted when exposed to polarized light (Fig. 7.39b). Iron dioxide dusts were found in the alveolar luminae stained by Berlin blue (Fig. 7.40). Marked air space dilatation was noted denoting honeycoming (Fig. 7.41).

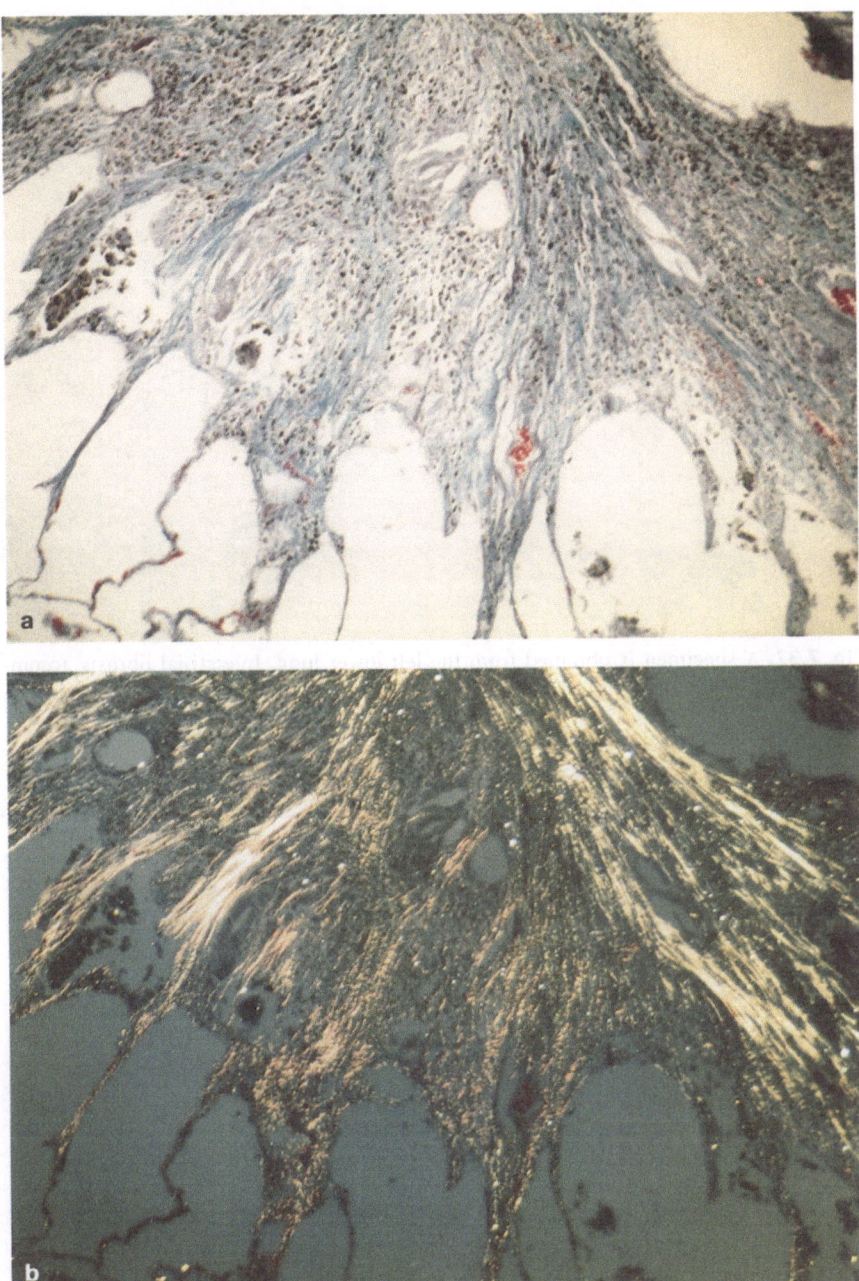

Fig. 7.31 a, b. Case 5. An MDF nodule is seen. Part of a MDF nodule, showing irregular-contoured fibrous tissue (stellate nodule) containing pigmented-laden macrophages is demonstrated. A small amount of birefringent dust particles in the nodule under the polarized light is observed

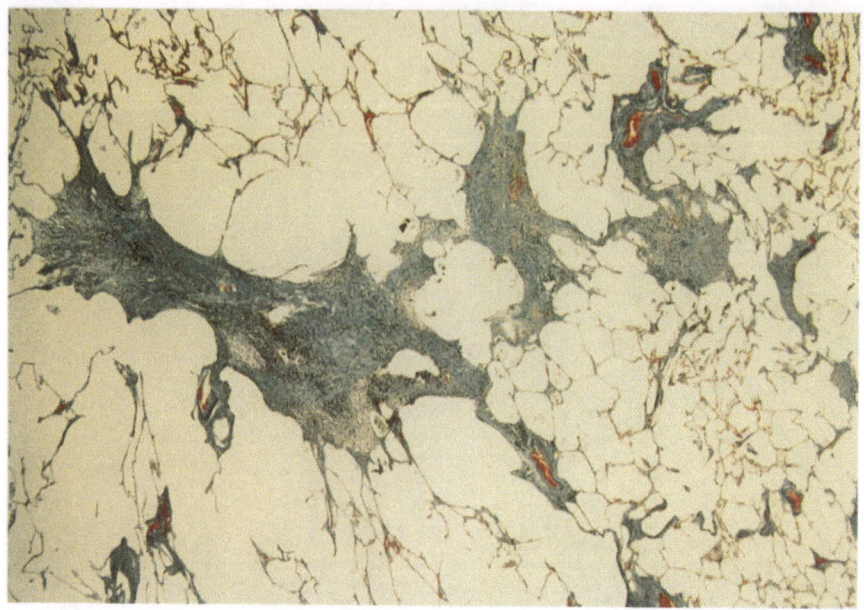

Fig. 7.32. A specimen is obtained from the left lower lung. Interstitial fibrosis accompanied by pulmonary emphysema is noted

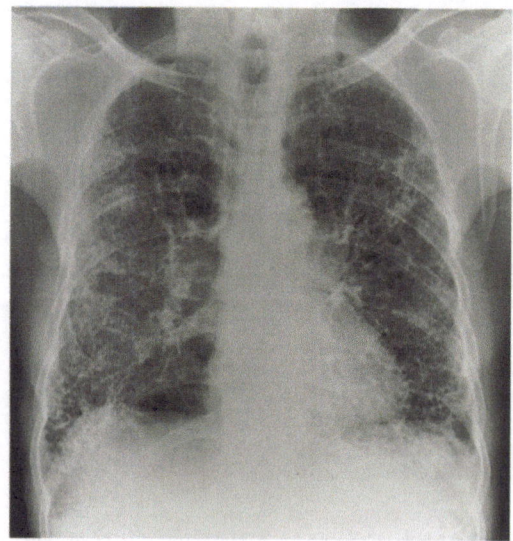

Fig. 7.33. Case 6. Posteroanterior CR chest image reveals numerous irregular opacities, reticular or reticulolinear, throughout the lungs and honeycombing are seen in both lower lungs

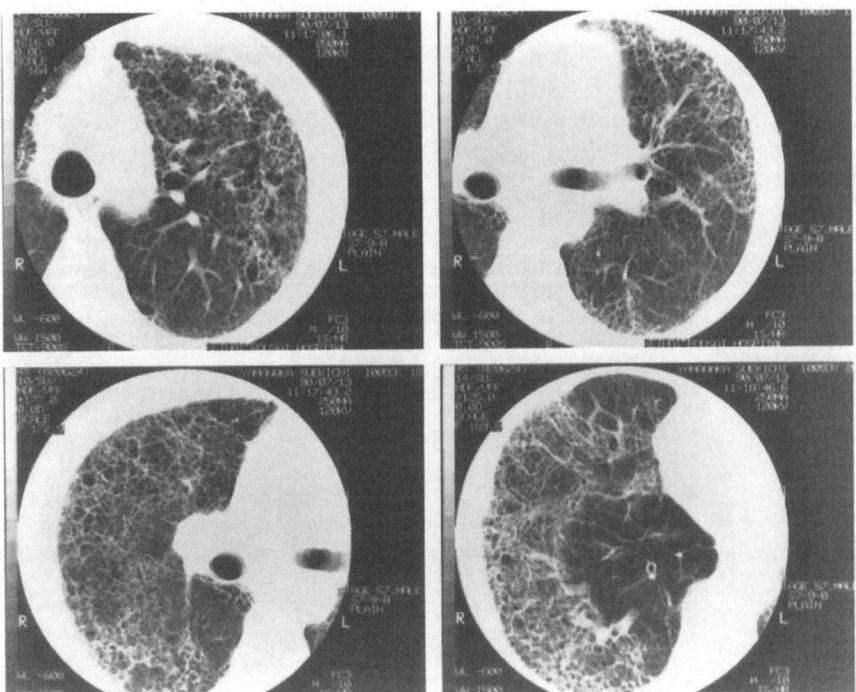

Fig. 7.34. Case 6. CT images (1-s scan time, 10-mm collimation, window width 1500, window level 600, FC3 filter) demonstrate numerous honeycombing throughout the lungs, with distribution marked in the subpleural zones. These findings are a resemble pattern of the end stage of IF change. Emphysematous change is noted in the lower right middle portion, and pulmonary vasculature is not traced peripherally

The patient's occupation was arc welder, but we confirmed typical asbestosis due to a presence of the pleural plaque on CT and asbestos bodies on histological findings.

Case 7 (MDF)

The patient was a 67-year-old man who worked in an activated carbon factory for 14 years and in a rubber factory for 5 years. He was a smoker and died of gastric carcinoma.

PA chest radiographic findings were small irregular opacities t/t in shape/size, and 3/3 in profusion.

CR revealed numerous, small irregular opacities 1.5–2.0 mm in width and associated with honeycombing throughout the lungs, and both hilar enlargements was noted. Pulmonary vasculature was blurred (Fig. 7.42).

CT demonstrated numerous fibrous strands, cystic bullae, and honeycombing. Findings were marked architectural disorder and damaged pulmonary vasculature (Fig. 7.43).

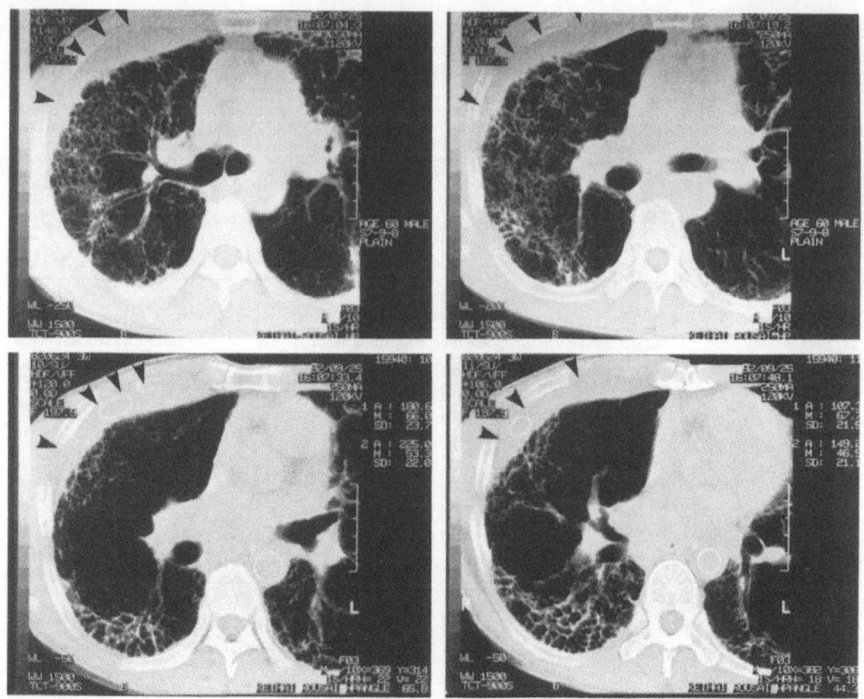

Fig. 7.35. Case 6. CT images (soft-tissue argorithm, window width 1500, window level 50, FC3 filter) reveal a localized pleural thickening in the upper right anterior chest wall, suggesting of an asbestos related pleural plaque

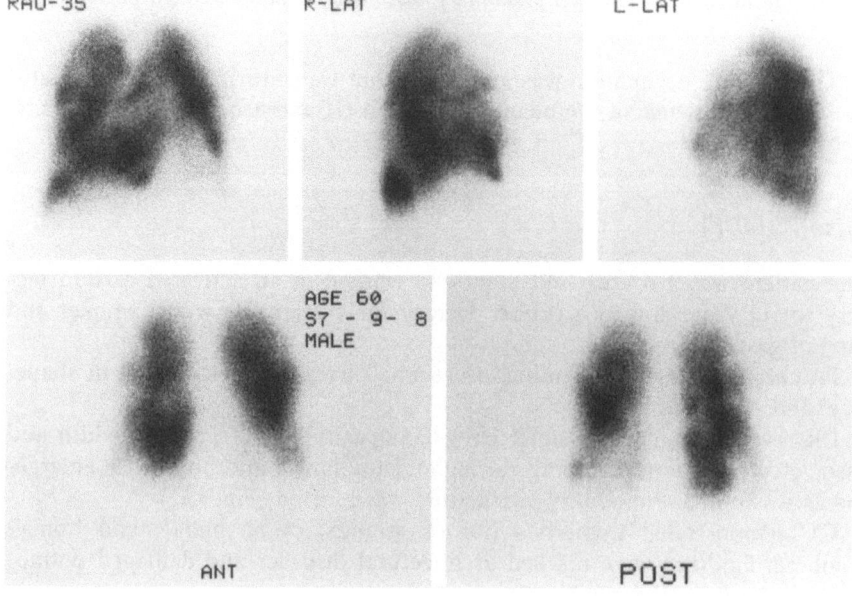

Fig. 7.37. Case 6. Cut surfaces specimen demonstrate extensive areas of diffuse IF with numerous honeycombing, particularly marked in subpleural parenchyma. Fibrous pleural adhesions, bilateral, with difference tumorlike thickening of the right anterior portion of the pleura

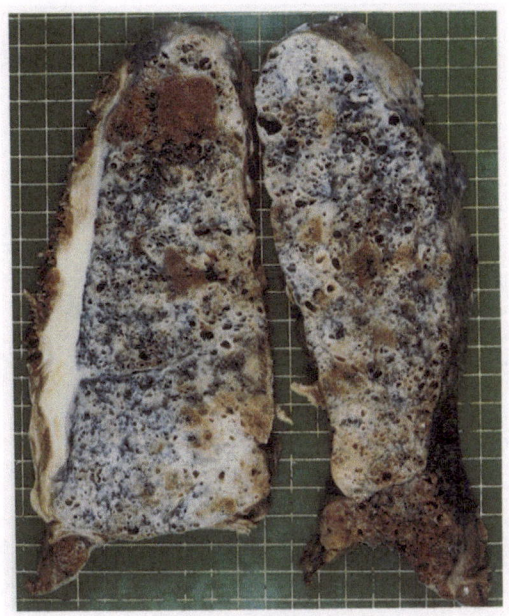

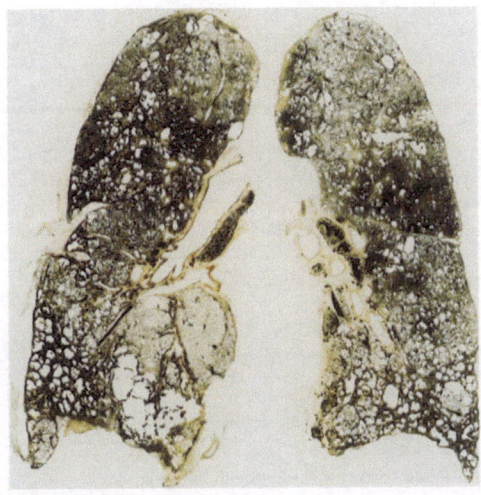

Fig. 7.38. Case 6. Whole lung section (G-W fixative) reveals numerous cystic honeycombing throughout the lungs and emphysema in the medial portion of the right lower lobe

Fig. 7.36. Case 6. ^{99m}Tc-MAA SG images show marked patchy distribution of radionuclide throughout the lungs

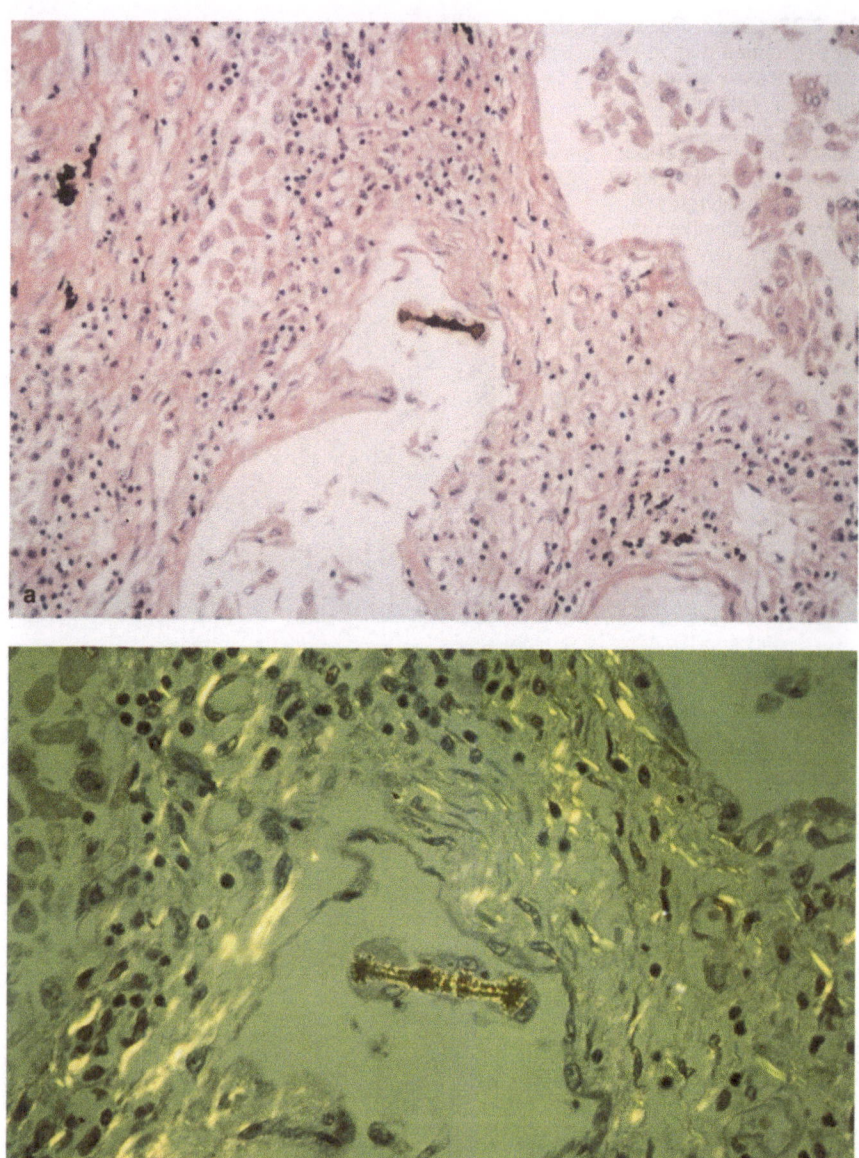

Fig. 7.39 a, b. Histological specimen obtained from an area of honeycomb lung, demonstrating an asbestos body (**a**) which is weakly birefringent under polarized light (**b**)

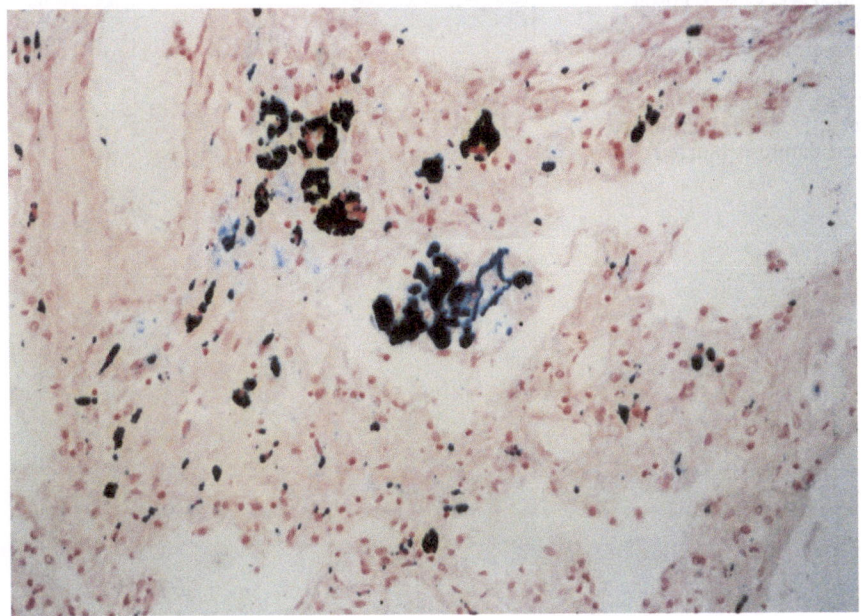

Fig. 7.40. Iron strain demonstrates evidence of siderosis

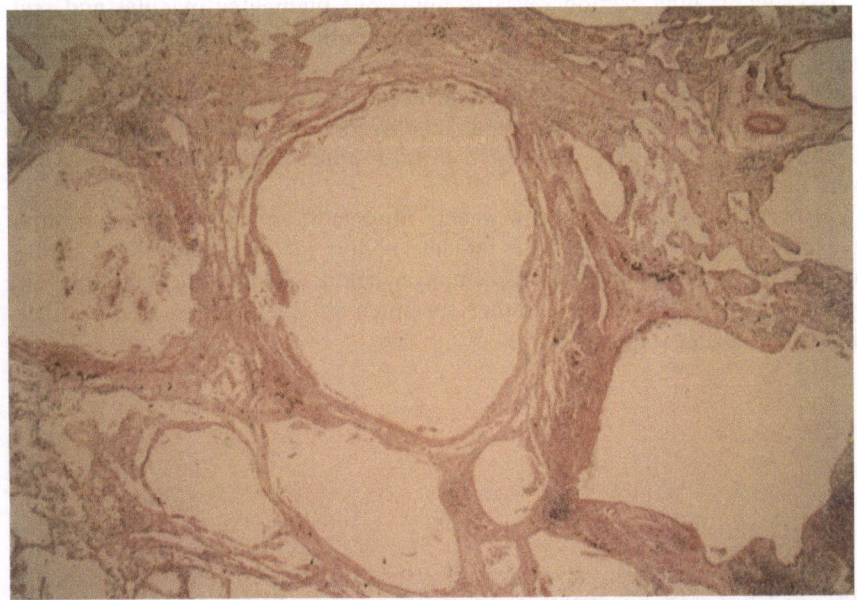

Fig. 7.41. Case 6. Low power micrograph demonstrates air space dilatation associated with interstitial fibrosis (honeycombing)

Fig. 7.42. Case 7. Posteroanterior CR image reveals
numerous small irregular
opacities throughout the
lungs, and hilar enlarge-
ment is noted. Pulmonary
vasculature is blurred

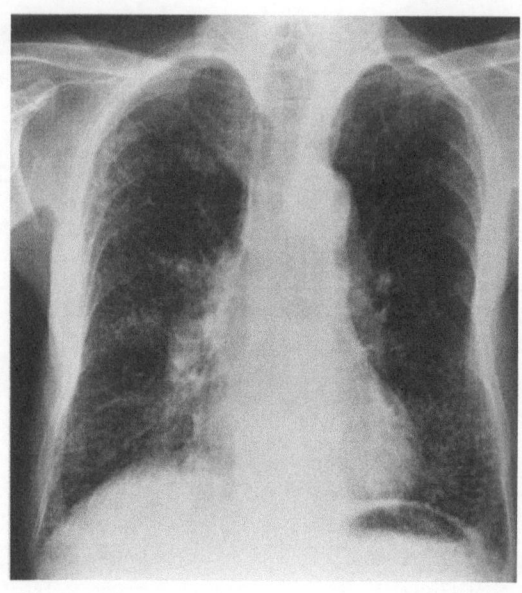

^{99m}Tc SG revealed marked patchy distribution of radionuclide throughout
the lungs and markedly reduced deposition of MAA in both middle anterior
and lower posterior zones, suggestive of considerably reduced lung perfusion
(Fig. 7.44).

G-W whole-lung section revealed numerous pigmented macules and scattered nodules of up to 5 mm in diameter in both lungs, associated with focal
emphysema (centrilobular emphysema), there was IF with marked honeycomb change, particularly intense and extensive in lower lobes and subpleural parenchyma, heavily pigmented. Emphysematous bullae, bilaterally, up to
5.0×2.5 mm in size were also noted in both upper subpleural regions. There
were no SN (Fig. 7.45).

At histological examination a weakly fibrogenic nodule was noted with an
irregular or star-shaped contour (stellate nodule [4] or medusa-head configuration [5]), and accompanied by emphysematous change. These findings are
typical of MDF (Fig. 7.46). Another specimen showed marked IF and dilatation of air spaces (Fig. 7.47).

Fig. 7.43 a, b. Case 7. CT images demonstrate numerous fibrous strands, bullae and
honeycombing, findings are marked architectural disorder and damaged pulmonary
vasculature

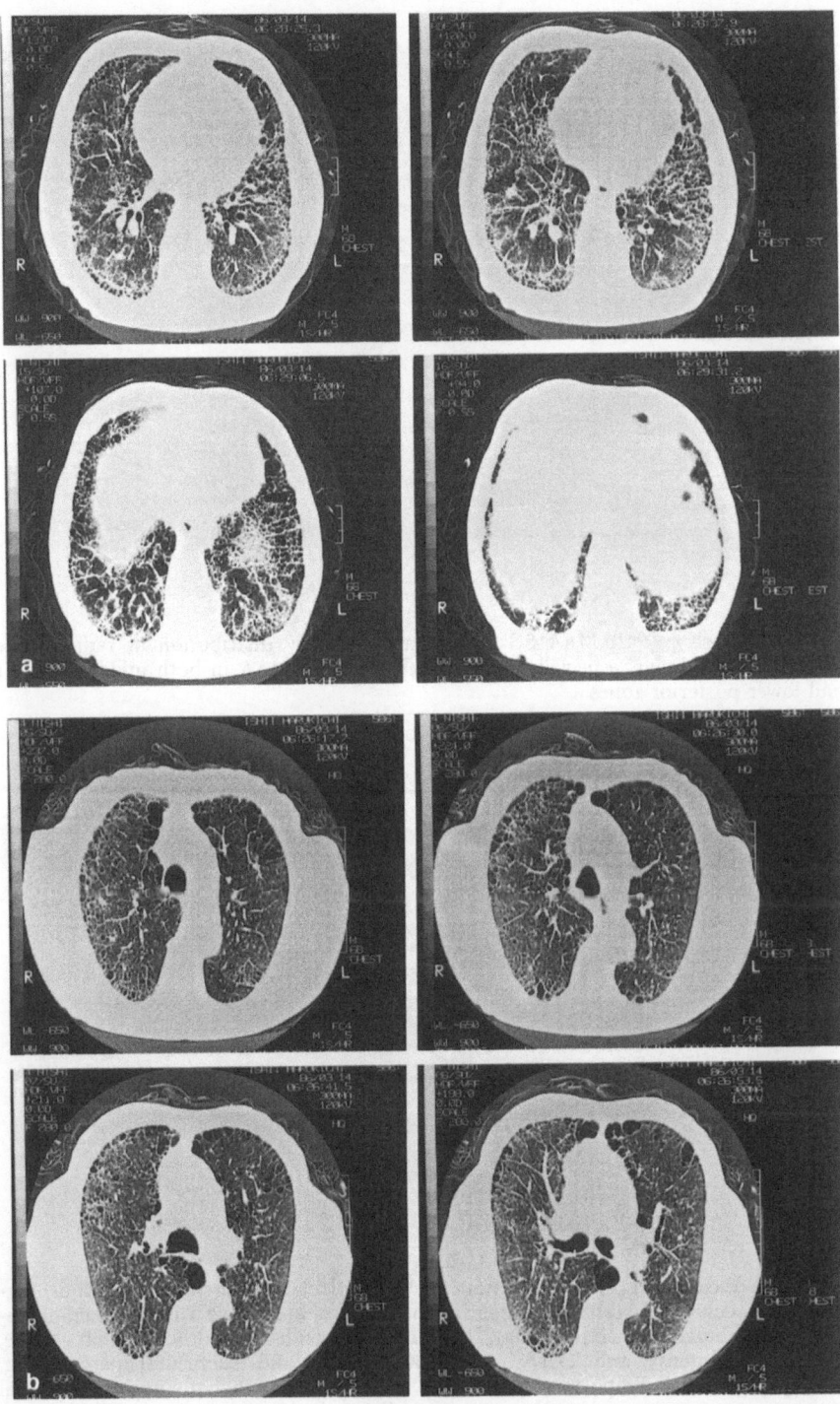

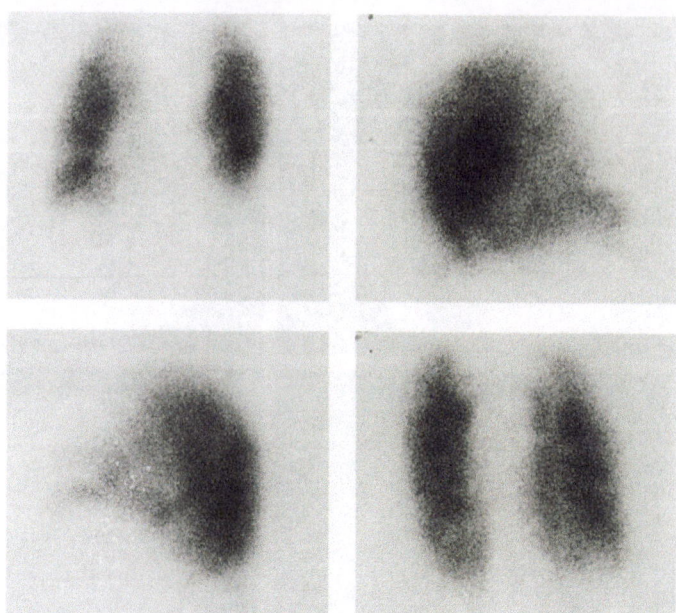

Fig. 7.44. Case 7. ^{99m}Tc-MAA SG show marked patchy distribution of radionuclide throughout the lungs, especially reduced deposition of MAA in both middle anterior and lower posterior zones

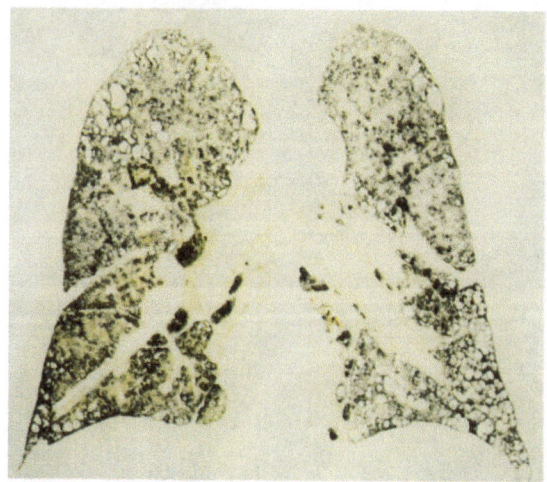

Fig. 7.45. Case 7. Whole lung section (G-W fixative) demonstrates numerous pigmented macules and scattered nodules in both lungs, associated with focal emphysema (centrilobular type emphysema), IF with marked with marked honeycomb change, particularly intense and extensive in lower lobes and subpleural parenchyma, heavily pigmented. Emphysematous bullae are also noted in both upper subpleural regions

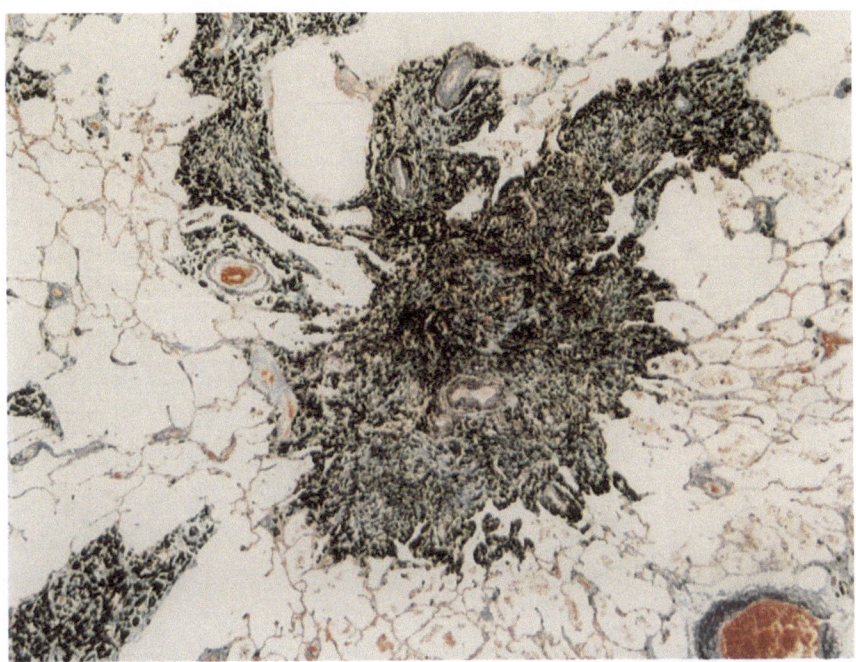

Fig. 7.46. Case 7. A photomicrograph shows a weakly fibrogenic nodule with irregular or star shaped contour (stellate nodule) or medusa-head configuration accompanied by emphysematous change, typical pattern of MDF

Discussion

Typical radiological findings of silicosis have been documented as small rounded opacity, but in many patients regarded as having silicosis the coexistence of small irregular opacities has also been reported.

Pathological characteristics of silicosis include combined patterns of typical SN, IF, and MDF [4, 5] associated with emphysematous change and honeycombing. The interpretation of conventional chest radiographs in pneumoconiosis may be limited in terms of radiological manifestations of pulmonary parenchyma or, especially, emphysematous changes and pleural abnormalities.

The new techniques with modalities such as CR, CT, and SG can provide more accurate diagnostic information than that obtained from conventional radiography and also may increase the efficacy in the diagnosis of pneumoconioses. Compared with the conventional screen-film system CR has the advantages of high-quality images, low radiation dose, easy interpretation, and wide dynamic range. This minimizes the radiation hazard [6].

The value of CT in the diagnosis of silicosis has been widely investigated [7-12] and has proved to be especially useful in visualizing fibrotic or em-

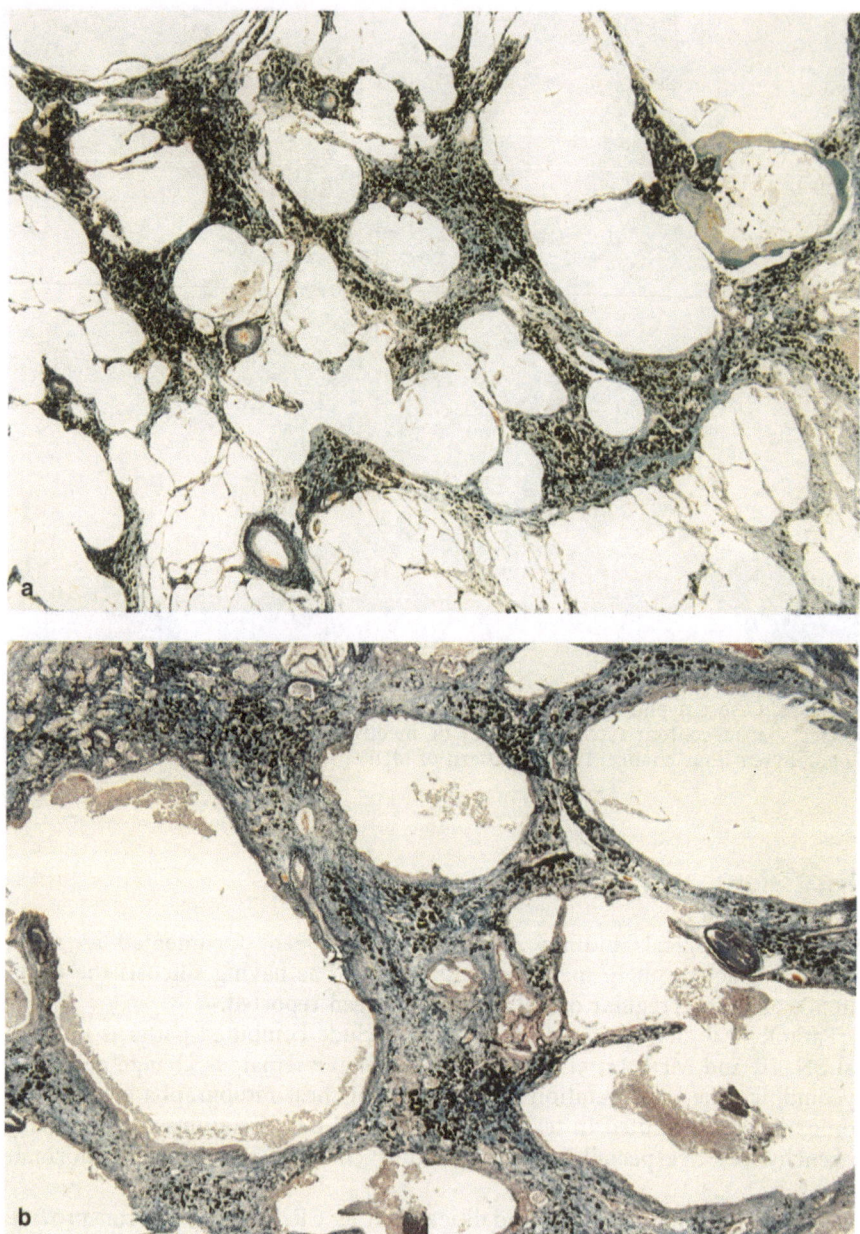

Fig. 7.47 a, b. Case 7. Specimens taken from the lower lobes show with advanced air space dilatation

physematous change, "rounded" atelectasis [13–16], and pleural abnormalities due to pneumoconioses. The detectable threshold of CT is 0.5 mm in diameter in nodules and 2 mm in diameter in emphysematous change. In addition, CT findings can be closely correlated with pathological characteristics.

In the present series ^{99m}Tc-MAA SG allowed some differentiation between different types of pneumoconioses. Predominantly small, rounded opacities show less tendency to decreased pulmonary perfusion, provided that there is no accompanying pulmonary emphysema. On the other hand, predominantly irregular opacities such as MDF that are usually accompanied by emphysematous and bullous changes have a tendency to marked decrease in pulmonary perfusion [19, 20].

^{67}Ga-citrate SG is not specific to any disease, for example, to lung cancer, silicotic PMF, or "rounded" atelectasis. The abnormal uptake of radionuclide is related not only to a malignant neoplasm lesion but also to fibrotic lesions with cellular activity or the area of inflammation [17–19].

In the diagnosis of pneumoconiosis the combined use of latest modalities should be stressed to integrate comprehensive information of the disease.

References

1. ILO (1980) International classification of chest radiograph of pneumoconioses. International Labour Office, Geneva
2. Fraser RG, Paré JAP (1976) PMF (progressive massive fibrosis). In: Fraser RG, Paré JAP (eds) Diagnosis of the chest disease silicosis with conglomeration, vol 3, 2nd edn. Saunders, Philadelphia, pp 1475–1528
3. Gough J, James WRL, Wentworth JE (1949) A comparison of the radiological and pathological changes in coal workers' pneumoconiosis. J Fac Radiol (Lond) 1:28–39
4. McLaughin AIG (1957) Pneumoconiosis in foundry workers. Br J Tubercul Dis Chest 51:297–309
5. Gibbs AR, Wagner JC (1988) Diseases due to silica. Mixed dust fibrosis. In: Churg A, Green FHY (eds) Pathology of occupational lung disease. Igaku-Shoin, New York, pp 155–175
6. Shida H (1987) Pneumoconiosis. In: Tateno Y, Iinuma T (eds) Computed radiography. Springer, Berlin Heidelberg New York, pp 164–173
7. Bégin R, Müller NL, Vedel S, Chan-Yaung M (1986) CT in silicosis: correlation within plain films and pulmonary function test. AJR 146:477–483
8. Akira M, Higashihara T, Yokoyama K, Yamamoto S, Kita N, Morimoto, Ikezoe J, Kozuka T (1989) Radiologic type p pneumoconiosis: high-resolution CT. Radiology 171:117–123
9. Remy-Jardin M, Kennedy T, Degreef JM, Beuscart R, Voisin Cyr, Remy J (1990) Coal worker's pneumoconiosis: CT assessment in exposed workers an correlation with radiographic findings. Radiology 177:361–371
10. Gamsu G. (1991) Computed tomography and high-resolution computed tomography of pneumoconiosis. J Occcup Med 34:794–796
11. Hosoda Y, Shida H, Hiraga Y (1991) Pneumoconiosis in developing countries: diagnosis and management. In: Lenfant C (ed) Lung biology in health and disease, vol 51: lung disease in tropics. Dekker, New York, pp 423–448
12. Remy-Jardin M, Remy J, Farre I, Marquette CH (1992) Computed tomographic evaluation of silicosis and coal worker's pneumoconiosis. Radiol Clin North Am 30:1155–1176

13. Hillerdal G (1989) Rounded atelectasis: clinical experience of 74 patients. Chest 95 (4):836–841
14. Chung-Park M, Tomashefski JF, Cohen AM, EL-Grazer M, Cotes EE (1989) Shrinkage pleuritis with lober atelectasis: a morphologic variant of 18 "round atelectasis." Hum Pathol 20:382–387
15. Honma K, Shida H, Chiyotani K (1995) Rounded atelectasis associated with silicosis. Wien Klin Wochenschr 107:585–589
16. Shida H, Chiyotani K, Honma K, Hosoda Y, Nobechi T, Morikubo H, Wiot JE (1995) Radiologic and pathologic characteristics of mixed dust pneumoconiosis. Radiographics 16:483–498
17. Shida H, Chiyotani K, Mishina M, Saito K (1973) Gallium 67-citrate scintigraphy in silicosis. In: Yasukouchi H (ed) Radiologic diagnosis in malignant neoplasms (in Japanese). Igaku-Shoin, Tokyo, pp 62–70
18. Siemen JK, Sergent N, Grebs SF, Siegfried FG, Winsor DW, Wenz D (1974) Pulmonary concentration of 67Ga in pneumoconiosis. AJR 120:815–820
19. Kammer RE, Berkman HW Jr, Rom WN, Tailor AT Jr (1985) 67Gallium citrate imaging in underground coal miners. Am J Ind Med 8:49–55
20. Bégin R, Bisson G, Boileau R, Massé S (1986) Assessment of disease activity by gallium-67 scan and lung lavage in the pneumoconioses. Semin Respir Med 3:271–280

8 Lung Cancer

E. E. KIM

Thoracic cancers are among the most common encountered by oncologists. Lung cancer continues to be a major health problem worldwide. In 1994, 172000 lung cancers were diagnosed in the United States, with 153000 deaths, and the incidence has been increasing in women [1]. It is now the second most lethal cancer in the world [9]. Non-small-cell lung carcinoma (NSCLC) accounts for about 75% of all lung cancers. Small-cell lung carcinoma (SCLC) generally has distant metastasis at the time of presentation and entails a 5 year-survival rate after surgical resection of less than 1% [9]. NSCLC has the potential for surgical cure if detected prior to metastases. The 5-year survival rate in stage No (no nodal metastasis) is 46%, in stage N1 (hilar nodes only) 33%, and in stage N2 (mediastinal nodes involved) only 8% [10]. The strongest prognostic factor for survival is whether complete resection is possible.

A frequent cause of therapeutic failure is local and distant nonresectable or residual disease. Patients with lung cancer who have metastases to the contralateral lung, involvement of the supraclavicular, cervical and/or contralateral mediastinal lymph nodes or to other organs are not considered candidates for surgery. Improved staging techniques may decrease the number of surgically treated patients and result in improved survival figures. Estimates of the percentage of patients whose disease is not resectable at presentation vary with criteria for resectability and patterns of referral; they range from 65% to 80% [9]. It is reasonable to attempt to evaluate patients with potentially operable disease to ensure that no detectable metastases preclude surgical therapy.

History, physical examination, serum chemistry, and chest radiography have a limited accuracy of 49%–51% for detection of metastases. Preoperative staging using chest X-ray and computed tomography (CT) is generally performed to identify the patients with a chance of cure and also to spare the risks of surgery in those who cannot be cured by surgery [9]. Chest CT has become the standard technique in the workup of patients with lung cancer, with 46%–91% sensitivity and 69%–89% specificity for the detection of mediastinal lymph nodes [14]. The use of radiopharmaceuticals and scintigraphic imaging permits detection of cancers in early stages and also the differential diagnosis of active residual or recurrent tumors from posttreatment changes. Gallium or ^{201}Tl scanning has been used for staging of patients with lung cancer (Fig. 8.1). CT is more sensitive than the gallium scan in detecting

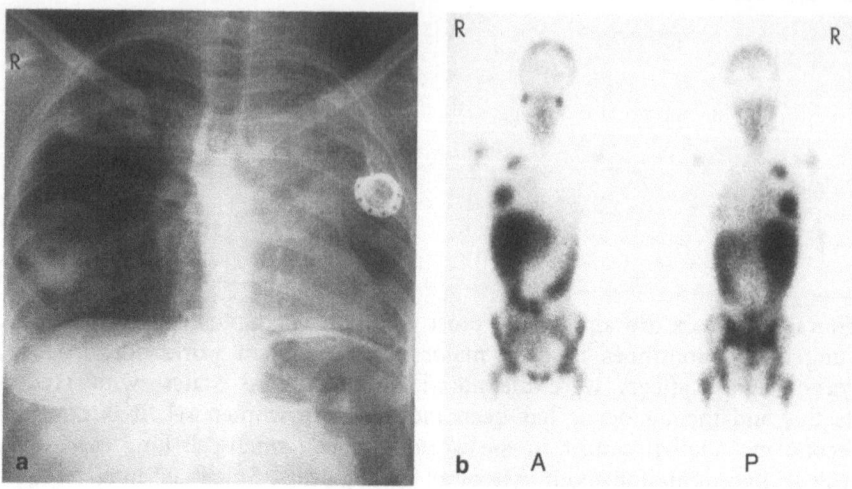

Fig. 8.1 a. Frontal view of chest X-ray shows nodular lesions of lung cancer in upper and lower right lung and atelectasis in upper left lung. **b** Anterior and posterior whole body images of ^{67}Ga scan show focal areas of markedly increased activity in upper and lower right lung. Note no significant uptake of ^{67}Ga in atelectatic upper left lung

tumor nodules within the pulmonary parenchyma. Abnormalities smaller than 1 cm are probably very difficult to detect with gallium scan, even when single photon emission computed tomography (SPECT) is used [13]. Furthermore, ^{67}Ga uptake is not necessarily tumor specific. ^{67}Ga scan, however, can be used to decide how to manage lung cancer or lymphoma after treatment in cases in which no other technique can provide the information about the nature of a residual mass [7]. Diffuse lung uptake of ^{67}Ga-citrate occurs after treatment in 16% of patients with lymphoma, and it is not indicative of lung involvement with lymphoma; this is probably the expression of a toxic effect of chemotherapy agents on the lungs [2] (Fig. 8.2).

Performing a test to evaluate the effect of a therapy is of value if it can be shown to contribute to improving the patient's quality of life or to lengthening his or her survival. Because gallium is a viability test agent, tumor response to treatment can be determined after treatment. A study of survival and disease-free survival treatment of lymphoma found a good correlation between ^{67}Ga uptake and prognosis [8]. Uptake of ^{201}Tl has been reported in lung cancer and lymphoma [4]. ^{201}Tl may be useful for evaluating tumor viability after treatment since its uptake is facilitated by the ATPase-dependent Na-K pump system in the tumor cell membrane. Positron-emission tomography (PET) using [^{18}F]fluoro-2-deoxy-D-glucose (FDG) may be clinically useful in detecting tumors and metastases.

Changes occurring after the treatment of primary lung cancer sometimes interfere with the radiological diagnosis of recurrent lung cancer (Fig. 8.3). Patz et al. [11] reported 97.1% sensitivity and 100% specificity of FDG PET in

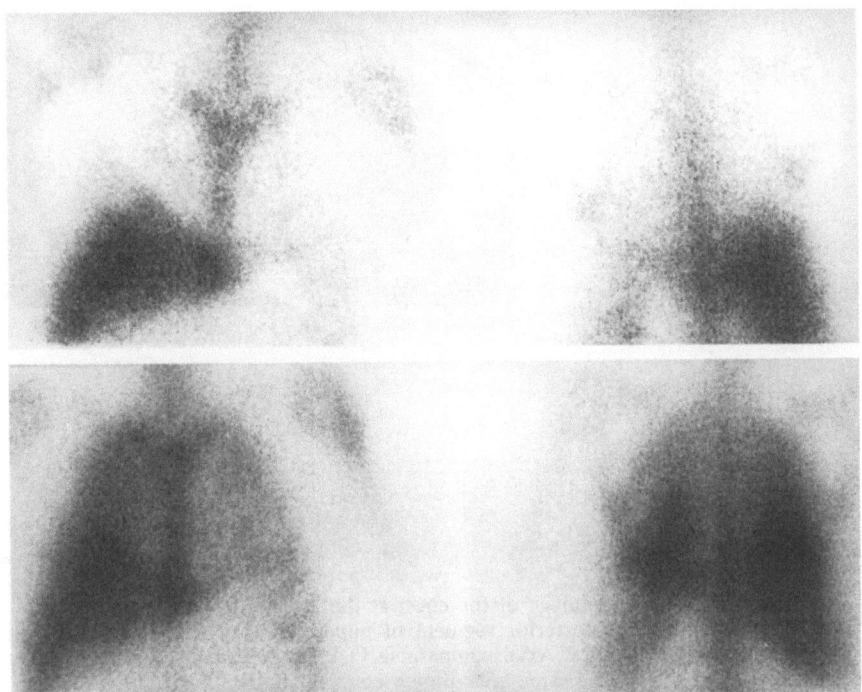

Fig. 8.2. Anterior and posterior static images of the chest before (*above*) and after (*below*) chemotherapy show diffusely increased uptake of ^{67}Ga-citrate in lungs due to toxic effects of bleomycin

detecting recurrent lung tumors with a threshold standard uptake value of 2.5. Inoue et al. [5] also found a high sensitivity but a lower specificity with a threshold SUV of 3.0. The CT + PET strategy in the conservative decision tree has been found to save U.S. $1154 per patient without a loss of life expectancy as compared to the alternate strategy of CT alone. The CT + PET strategy in the less conservative decision tree showed a savings of $2267 per patient [3]. The efficacy of radioimmunoimaging of lung cancer has been demonstrated. Tumor-associated antibodies labeled with ^{131}I or ^{111}In have shown primary and metastatic lung cancers (Fig. 8.4) [13]. ^{111}In-labeled octreotide or ^{99m}Tc-labeled P829 peptide has also revealed lung cancers on which somatostatin receptors are present [12].

Kaposi's sarcoma with pulmonary involvement must be considered in any patient with AIDS and respiratory symptoms [6]. Fever, cough, dysphea, and hypoxemia occur with both infection and Kaposi's sarcoma. The development of pulmonary Kaposi's sarcoma appears to be unrelated to the presence of mucocutaneous and nodal disease. However, the chest radiographic appearance of Kaposi's sarcoma is nonspecific, and differentiation from opportunistic infection may be difficult. Pulmonary parenchymal involvement in Kaposi's sarcoma tends to be diffuse, with linear infiltrates or nodular le-

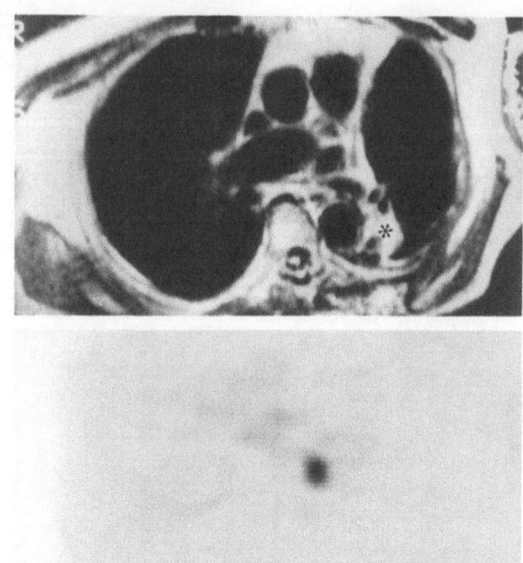

Fig. 8.3. Axial T1-weighted image of the chest at the level of aortopulmonic window shows a lesion (*) in the posterior segment of upper left lobe with atelectasis and postradiation fibrotic changes. Axial comparable PET image using [^{18}F]FDG shows a focal increased activity in the same area. Biopsy confirmed a recurrent lung cancer

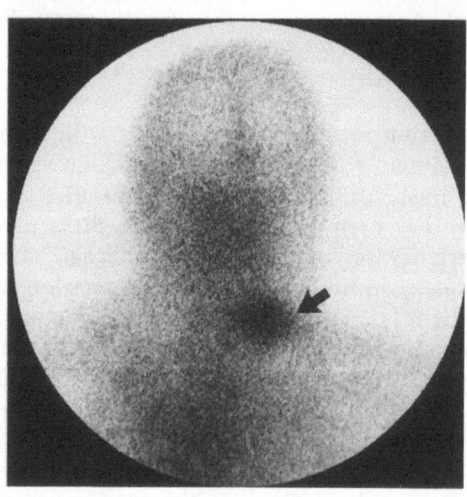

Fig. 8.4. Anterior image of head and neck using ^{111}In-labeled monoclonal antibody 96.5 shows a focal increased activity (*arrow*) in the left supraclaricular fossa. Biopsy confirmed a metastatic lung cancer

sions. Pleural effusions are common, and hemorrhagic mediastinal and hilar adenopathy occurs in up to 30% of patients with Kaposi's sarcoma. Gallium scintigraphy has been proposed as a potential method to help differentiate between active infection and pulmonary Kaposi's sarcoma since the lesions of Kaposi's sarcoma are not gallium avid [15]. In one study all premortem pathological diagnoses required open-lung biopsy, and pathological diagnosis may be difficult since the lesions are focal and scattered.

References

1. American Cancer Society (1994) Cancer facts and figures.
2. Bay-Shalom R, Israel O, Haim N, Levior M, Epelbaum R, Frenkel A, Ben-Haim S, Kolodny GN, Front D (1996) Diffuse lung uptake of Ga-67 after treatment of lymphoma. Radiology 199:473–476
3. Gambhir SS, Gupta P, Allen P, Hoh C, Maddahi J, Phelps ME (1996) A simulation tool for modeling cost effectiveness with applications for determing the cost effective role of nuclear medicine studies in lung and breast cancer. J Nucl Med 37:1428–1434
4. Hisada K, Tonami N, Miyamae T, Hiraki Y, Yamazaki T, Maeda T, Nakajo N (1978) Clinical evaluation of tumor imaging with Tl-201 chloride. Radiology 129:497–500
5. Inoue T, Kim EE, Komaki R, Wong FCL, Bassa P, Wong W-H, Yang DJ, Endo K, Podoloff DA (1995) Detecting recurrent or residual lung cancer with FDG-PET. J Nucl Med 36:788–793
6. Kaplan LD, Wofsy RB, Volberding PA (1987) Treatment of patients with acquired immunodeficiency syndrome and associated manifestations. JAMA 257:1367–1374
7. Kaplan WD, Jochelson MS, Herman TS (1990) Ga-67 imaging: a predictor of residual tumor viability and clinical outcome in patients with diffuse large-cell lymphoma. J Clin Oncol 8:1966–1970
8. King SC, Reiman RJ, Prosnitz LR (1994) Prognostic importance of restaging gallium scans following induction chemotherapy for advanced Hodgkin's disease. J Clin Oncol 12:306–311
9. Ginsberg RJ, Vokes EE, Raben A (1997) Non-small cell lung cancer. In: DeVita VT Jr, Heilman S, Rosenberg SA (eds) Cancer: principles and practice of oncology, 5th edn. Lippincott-Raven, Philadelphia, pp 858–910
10. Mountain CF (1989) Value of the new TNM staging system of lung cancer. Chest 96:47S
11. Patz EJ Jr, Lowe VJ, Hoffman JN, Paine SS, Harris LK, Goodman PC (1994) Persistent or recurrent bronchogenic carcinoma: detection with PET and F-18 2-deoxy-D-glucose. Radiology 191:379–382
12. Stokkel MP, Pauwels EK (1994) Octreotide scintigraphy for small cell lung carcinoma. Eur J Nucl Med 21:1276–1278
13. Waxman AD (1986) The role of nuclear medicine in pulmonary neoplastic processes. Semin Nucl Med 16:285–295
14. Webb WR, Gatsonis C, Zerhourni EA (1991) CT and MR in staging non-small bronchogenic carcinoma: report of the Radiological Diagnostic Oncology Group. Radiology 178:705–713
15. Woolfenden JM, Carrasquillo JA, Larson SM (1987) Acquired immunodeficiency syndrome: Ga-67 citrate imaging. Radiology 162:383–387

SPECT in Lung Tumors

H.S. Bom and J. Lee

Differentiation Between Malignant and Benign Lung Tumors

A study was performed by Tonami et al. [1] in 30 patients with suspected lung cancer, using SPECT imaging and a high dose of ^{201}Tl (296–370 MBq). Both early and delayed scans demonstrated abnormal accumulation in all of 23 malignant pulmonary lesions, including 21 lung cancer, one lung sarcoma and one metastatic lung cancer. Of seven patients with benign pulmonary lesions, including tuberculosis, bronchopneumonia, hemorrhagic infarction, and a pulmonary scar, the findings were abnormal in two (tuberculosis and bronchopneumonia).

There were significant differences in delayed ratio (uptake ratio of the lesion to the normal lung on delayed scan) and retention index (degree of retention in the lesion) between lung cancer and benign conditions, repectively ($p<0.01$, 0.05). The smallest lesion depicted was 1.5×1.0-cm adenocarcinoma of the lung. Two false negatives had small metastases less than 1.0 cm in diameter.

Despite these enthusiastically received early results subsequent reports have varied depending on the prevalence and the type of benign lung lesions in the studied population [2, 3]. Lee et al. [2] studied a larger group of patients (89 malignant, 44 benign) with a high prevalence of benign solitary pulmonary lesion. Benign lung conditions included 23 active and 5 inactive tuberculoses, 3 asperogillomas, 3 focal pneumonias, 2 thymomas, and 8 others. They were imaged using dual-headed SPECT at 15 min (early) and 3 h (delayed) after 222 MBq ^{201}Tl. Tumor-to-normal lung ratio (T/NL) was higher in malignant tumors; however, there was a large overlap between malignant and benign diseases. The retention index did not differ between the two groups. Although the sensitivity was high (92% with 15-min images and 93% with 3-h images), specificity was low (39% with 15-min images and 41% with 3-h images). They concluded that the value of ^{201}Tl SPECT is only marginal for lung cancer in a population with a high prevalence of the benign solitary pulmonary lesion.

Lee et al. [3] evaluated whether ^{201}Tl scintigraphy can differentiate central bronchogenic cancer from distal collapse consolidation in nine patients with squamous carcinoma with collapse confirmed by surgery and pathology. All nine patients studied underwent SPECT 1 h after an intravenous injection of 111 MBq ^{201}Tl; 24-h delayed SPECT was performed in five of the nine patients. The ^{201}Tl activity in tumor and collapse was assessed visually on the basis of the pathological findings. The specimens were prepared to have the same orientation and level with the SPECT image. The tumor activity appeared higher than that of the collapse in four patients, equal in three, and lower in two. Collapsed lung both with and without superimposed inflammation showed increased ^{201}Tl activity. Delayed SPECT aided in tumor detection within a collapsed lung in only two of five patients. They concluded that caution is needed to interpret ^{201}Tl scintigraphy in patients with central bronchogenic cancer and distal collapse.

In 1990 Tonami et al. reported that ^{201}Tl can be useful in the histological characterization of lung cancer [4]. However, in 1993 the same group reported on a larger group of patients [5] in whom there was no significant difference in uptake ratio in the lesion/normal lung on delayed scan between the various histological groups except between adenocarcinoma and large cell carcinoma. They also found that the retention index did not differ significantly between the different histological groups. Duman et al. [6] also did not find differences between histological types.

^{99m}Tc-MIBI has recently been evaluated in patients with lung tumors. Hassan et al. [7] reported that 10 of 11 (91%) patients with untreated carcinoma of the lung showed abnormal ^{99m}Tc-MIBI results. In the patients with tumors of the lung who had received chemotherapy two were negative and one was slightly positive. Of six patients with benign lesions two with fibrosing alveolitis were positive. Additional ^{99m}Tc-MIBI SPECT have been performed, and these consistently demonstrate high sensitivities of 91% (20/22) [8] and 96% (22/23) [9] for the detection of primary or metastatic lung cancer. However, specificity is of some concern. Onsel et al. [10] reported that 22 of 24 (92%) patients with active pulmonary tuberculosis and 4 of 5 (80%) relapsed patients showed increased focal uptake of ^{99m}Tc-MIBI. As with ^{201}Tl, the value of ^{99m}Tc-MIBI SPECT for lung cancer in a population with a high prevalence of tuberculosis was only marginal.

The accumulation of ^{67}Ga is very high in primary lung tumors. Both tumor histology and size affect the sensitivity of ^{67}Ga scan in detecting lung cancer. Undifferentiated carcinomas and squamous cell carcinomas demonstrate significantly greater ^{67}Ga accumulation than adenocarcinomas. Although abnormal ^{67}Ga accumulation is commonly seen in diffuse interstitial lung disease, ^{67}Ga accumulation in lung tumor is relatively specific. Rageb et al. [11] found that ^{67}Ga is more sensitive than ^{201}Tl in assessing the local extent of the disease in nonoperable NSCLC, with sensitivity of 100% for ^{67}Ga and 88% for ^{201}Tl in centrally located lesions. In peripherally located lesions the sensitivity of ^{67}Ga was 88% versus 64% for [201]Tl. In all, the ^{67}Ga ratios were higher than [201]Tl. In neither ^{67}Ga nor ^{201}Tl was there a significant difference between the three histological groups – squamous cell, adenocarcinoma, and anaplastic carcinoma. They found ^{67}Ga scintigraphy superior to the chest X-ray and CT in 49% and 6% of cases, respectively, whereas ^{201}Tl was superior to the chest X-ray and CT in 27% and 3% only in detecting the local extent of the disease. In these patients there was usually underlying collapse and/or pleural effusion that made the interpretation of the results on the CT or chest X-ray difficult. CT was superior to both ^{67}Ga and ^{201}Tl imaging for the initial evaluation of the extension of the disease. [67]Ga added useful information for radiotherapy planning in 54% of the chest X-ray-based planning versus 19% of CT-based planning.

Itoh et al. [12] prospectively compared ^{201}Tl, ^{67}Ga, and ^{99m}Tc-labeled hexamethylpropyleneamine-oxime (HMPAO) for differentiation of pulmary nodule in 50 patients. In their study ^{99m}Tc-HMPAO was concentrated in 62% of

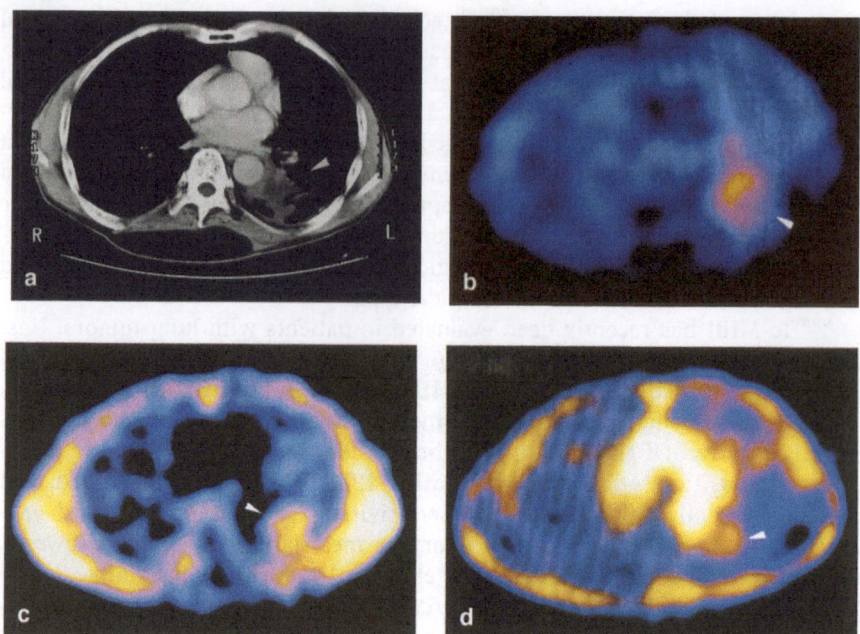

Fig. 8.5 a–d. Squamous cell carcinoma in the lower left lung in a 67-year-old man. CT (**a**) shows an irregular mass (*white arrowhead*) in the superior segment of lower left lobe. Transverse tomography of ^{201}Tl (**b**) and ^{99m}Tc-MIBI (**c**) shows hot uptakes (*white arrowheads*) in the tumor mass, while that of ^{99m}Tc-(V)DMSA (**d**) shows less hot uptake (*white arrowhead*) in the lesion

13 patients with malignant pulmonary nodules, which was slightly higher than ^{67}Ga in 54% of 28 patients. Sensitivity of early and delayed ^{201}Tl imagings was 88% and 91%, respectively. Specificity of both imagings was 85%. They therefore concluded that delayed ^{201}Tl SPECT images at 2 h postinjection are preferable for disclosing the malignant pulmonary nodule to early ^{201}Tl SPECT images at 15 min postinjection.

Hirano et al. [13] reported that ^{99m}Tc-(V)DMSA images demonstrated approximately 90% of the primary lung cancer in the study of 31 patients, and uptake ratios were higher in squamaous cell carcinomas than adenocarcinomas. Four cases incidentally revealed osseous metastatic lesions. Three benign lesions did not show increased uptake. In three cases there were false-negative results, and there were no false-positive cases for the primary lesions. However, evaluation of mediastinal tumor extension and nodal metastatic lesion was very difficult by high blood-pool activity in the major cardiovascular structures due to slow blood-pool clearance. Lee et al. [14] reported that diagnostic sensitivity and specificity of ^{99m}Tc-(V)DMSA in 41 subjects with lung cancer and 22 with benign solitary pulmonary lesion was 61% and 63.6%, respectively. The low sensitivity was due mainly to high blood pool activity obscuring the lesions near vascular structures in chest.

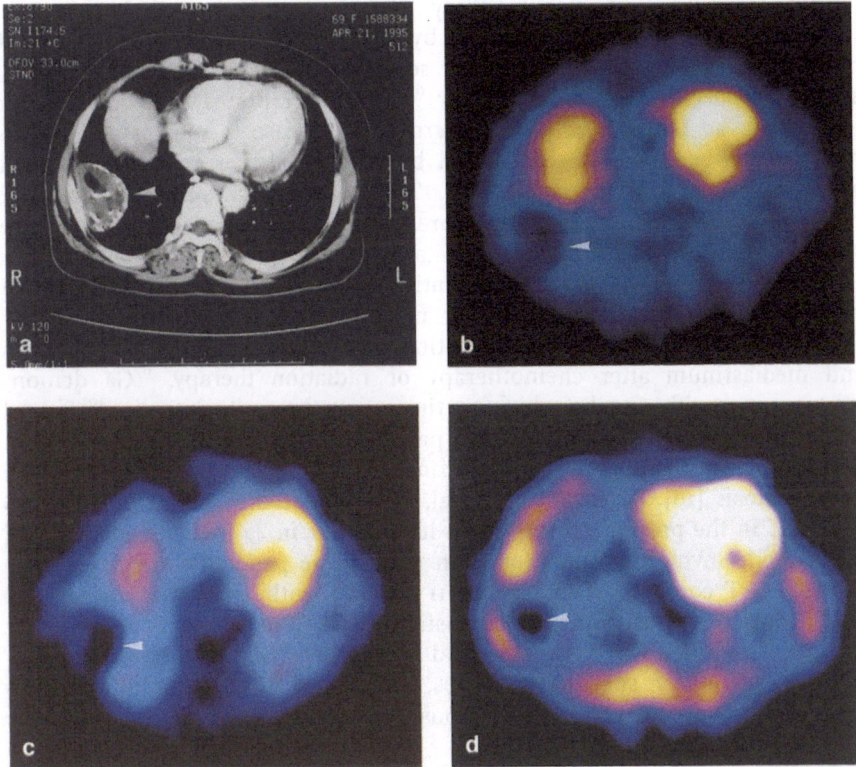

Fig. 8.6 a–d. Hamartoma in the lower right lung in a 69-year-old woman. CT (**a**) shows a round mass (*white arrowhead*) with popcorn calcification in the lower right lung. Transverse tomography of ^{201}Tl (**b**), ^{99m}Tc-MIBI (**c**), and ^{99m}Tc-(V)DMSA (**d**) show cold uptakes (*white arrowheads*) in the lesion

Evaluation of mediastinal tumor extension and nodal metastatic lesion is also difficult. However, it is useful in diagnosis of peripheral lung cancers and metastatic lesions to the osseous structures. Low specificity due to accumulation in some benign lesions, such as active healing bony reaction, young breast tissue, and active inflammatory lesion, warrant cautions in populations with a high prevalence of the benign solitary lesion. Comparative imagings of ^{201}Tl, ^{99m}Tc-MIBI, and ^{99m}Tc-(V)DMSA in patients with lung cancer and benign lung tumor are illustrated in Figs. 8.5 and 8.6, respectively.

Staging of Lung Cancer

^{67}Ga scans have been advocated for the evaluation of mediastinal metastatic disease because detection of hilar and mediastinal lymph node involvement is critical in determining prognosis and treatment for lung cancer patients

[15–17]. However, a prospective study [18] of 75 patients with lung cancer who underwent ^{67}Ga scans followed by thoracotomy with total mediastinal node dissection reported a very low sensitivity of 23%, specificity of 82%, and overall accuracy of only 63% for ^{67}Ga scintigraphy. The low sensitivity was due to an inability to detect microscopic disease in mediastinal lymph nodes. The specificity was decreased by ^{67}Ga uptake in enlarged inflamed nodes that contained no metastasis. Therefore conventional ^{67}Ga nuclear medicine techniques should not at present be relied upon for preoperative staging of mediastinal lymph node metastases in lung cancer patients.

Several publications suggest a potential use for ^{201}Tl and/or ^{99m}Tc-MIBI in patients being evaluated for hilar or mediastinal tumor [19–21]. Many patients develop a low-grade inflammation of the lymph nodes in the hilum and mediastinum after chemotherapy or radiation therapy. ^{67}Ga demonstrates nonspecific uptake which at times may be quite intense. ^{201}Tl and ^{99m}Tc-MIBI are generally negative in patients without residual tumor and in those in whom the adenopathy is secondary to other disease processes such as sarcoidosis [19]. Recently Chiti et al. [21] compared ^{99m}Tc-MIBI SPECT to X-ray CT in the presurgical staging of lung cancer in 47 patients. Mediastinal lymph node involvement was found in 11 of the 36 patients evaluated. ^{99m}Tc-MIBI SPECT correctly staged 10 of 11 patients with and 21 of 25 without mediastinal nodes, showing a diagnostic sensitivity of 91% and a specificity of 84%. CT yielded 8 true-positive and 15 true-negative results, with a sensitivity of 73% and a specificity of 60%. ^{99m}Tc-MIBI SPECT results were also better than those of CT regarding positive- and negative-predictive values and accuracy.

A study of [^{111}In-DTPA-D-Phe1]octreotide scintigraphy found the technique able to identify the primary tumor and its metastases in all of 34 patients with SCLC, whereas only the primary tumor could be visualized in all of 36 patients with NSCLC [22]. As somatostatin receptors are absent on most NSCLC investigated thus far, their in vivo visualization is probably due to uptake of radioactivity by activated lymphocytes or a hyperplasia of neuroendocrine cells. Bronchial carcinoid can be successfully localized by somatostatin receptor scintigraphy [23].

Follow-Up of the Response to Therapy

^{201}Tl can be of particular use in the follow-up of the response to radiation and/or chemotherapy. Rageb et al. [11] reported that planar ^{201}Tl imaging is not useful for evaluating response to therapy and is inferior to CT and ^{67}Ga; however, Miyagawa et al. [24] used SPECT images, uptake ratio, and retention index and found these parameters to decrease significantly after radiation therapy with good response, whereas in recurrent lung cancer there was an apparant increase in these parameters before the recurrence was detected by CT. Miyagawa et al. concluded that ^{201}Tl SPECT is useful for the follow-up of patients with lung cancer during and after radiation therapy. It should be noted that Rageb et al. used planar imaging with a dose of 74 MBq of ^{201}Tl with only early imaging within 30 min after injection, whereas Miyagawa et al. used SPECT, early 15-min and delayed 3-h imaging, and a higher dose of 148–222 MBq of [201]Tl. Bom et al. [25] reported that ^{99m}Tc-MIBI was useful in the assessment of radiotherapy in 11 patients of NSCLC. The concordance between radiological change (chest X-ray and CT) and change of ^{99m}Tc-MIBI uptake after radiotherapy was 9/11 (81.8%).

^{99m}Tc-MIBI Uptake in Small-Cell Lung Cancer: A Predictor of Response to Chemotherapy

Although patients with SCLC usually respond well to chemotherapy, failure of initial chemotherapy was observed in 15% of SCLC patients [26]. The failure of chemotherapy can be induced by the presence of P-glycoprotein (Pgp), a 170-kDa cytoplasmic membrane protein encoded by the *MDR1* gene, which pumps out cytotoxic drugs such as anthracyclines, vinca alkaloids, epipodophyllotoxins, cholchicine, and actinomycin D [27]. Recently it has been found that Pgp also recognizes ^{99m}Tc-MIBI as a suitable transport substrate [28]. A case report showed that the absence of ^{99m}Tc-sestabmibi uptake was associated with failure of chemotherapy [29]. Bom et al. [30] evaluated whether the degree of ^{99m}Tc-MIBI uptake in SCLC or its retention on delayed imaging is correlated with response to chemotherapy. Nineteen patients (13 men, 6 women, mean age 60.2±10.9) with biopsy-confirmed SCLC were underwent ^{99m}Tc-MIBI planar and tomographic imagings 3–7 days before starting chemotherapy. Images were acquired 1 and 4 h after injection of 740 MBq ^{99m}Tc-MIBI. Regions of interest were localized to the tumor mass and normal lung, and theT/NL was determined there. The percentage retention (%R) was measured as: %R=100×(T/NL at 4 h)/(T/NL at 1 h). Differences in T/NL and %R among the three groups were studied by analysis of variance.

Table 8.1. ^{99m}Tc-sestamibi uptake and response to chemotherapy

Parameters	Response to chemotherapy			
	CR ($n=6$)	PR ($n=8$)	NR ($n=5$)	p value
p(T/N)1	1.78±0.49	1.34±0.12	1.37±0.32	0.08
p(T/N)4	1.47±0.28	1.38±0.32	1.33±0.28	0.69
p(%R)	124.90±48.55	100.45±21.44	106.03±26.9	0.46
t(T/N)1	2.88±0.76	2.27±0.42	1.65±0.36	0.002
t(T/N)4	2.73±0.97	2.57±0.72	1.66±0.42	0.03
t(%R)	110.06±24.14	92.33±19.74	103.59±28.43	0.52

p(T/N)1, p(T/N)4, planar tumor-to-normal lung ratio at 1 and 4 h; p (%R), percentage retention calculated from planar images; t(T/N)1, t(T/N)4, tomographic tumor-to-normal lung ratio at 1 and 4 h; t (%R), percentage retention calculated from tomographic images.

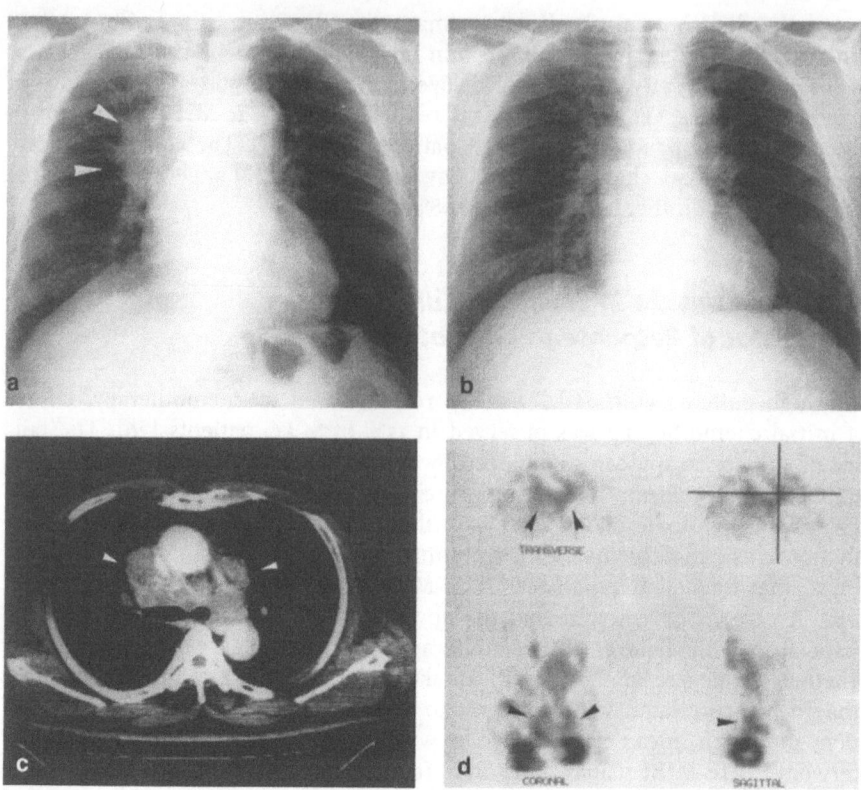

Fig. 8.7 a–d. Complete response. A tumor mass in the upper right lung (**a**, *white arrowhead*) was completely resolved after three courses of VAP chemotherapy (**b**), CT (**c**) and ^{99m}Tc-MIBI SPECT (**d**) were done before chemotherapy. CT shows a high density mass involving mediastinum (**c**, *small white arrowheads*). One-hour tomographic images of ^{99m}Tc-MIBI SPECT (**d**) shows hot uptakes (tumor-to-normal ratio=3.13) in the tumor mass (**d**, *black arrowheads*)

All patients received combination chemotherapy [etopside 100 mg/m², doxorubicin 40 mg/m², cisplatin 25 mg/m² VAP)] every 4 weeks for at least three times. Response to chemotherapy was classified according to the change in tumor size on chest X-ray and CT (WHO criteria) as complete response (CR; disappearance of all known disease), partial response (PR; 50% or more decrease in total tumor load), no change (NC; less than 50% decrease or less than 25% increase in total tumor load), and progressive disease (PD; more than 25% increase in total tumor load or appearance of new lesions) [31].

Among the 19 patients, 6 showed CR, 5 showed PR, 7 showed NC and 1 showed PD. NC and PD were classified as no response (NR) for statistical analysis. There was no statistical difference in age and sex between the three groups. Table 8.1 compares uptake and retention of ^{99m}Tc-MIBI according to the response to chemotherapy (CR, PR, and NR). T/NL of planar images

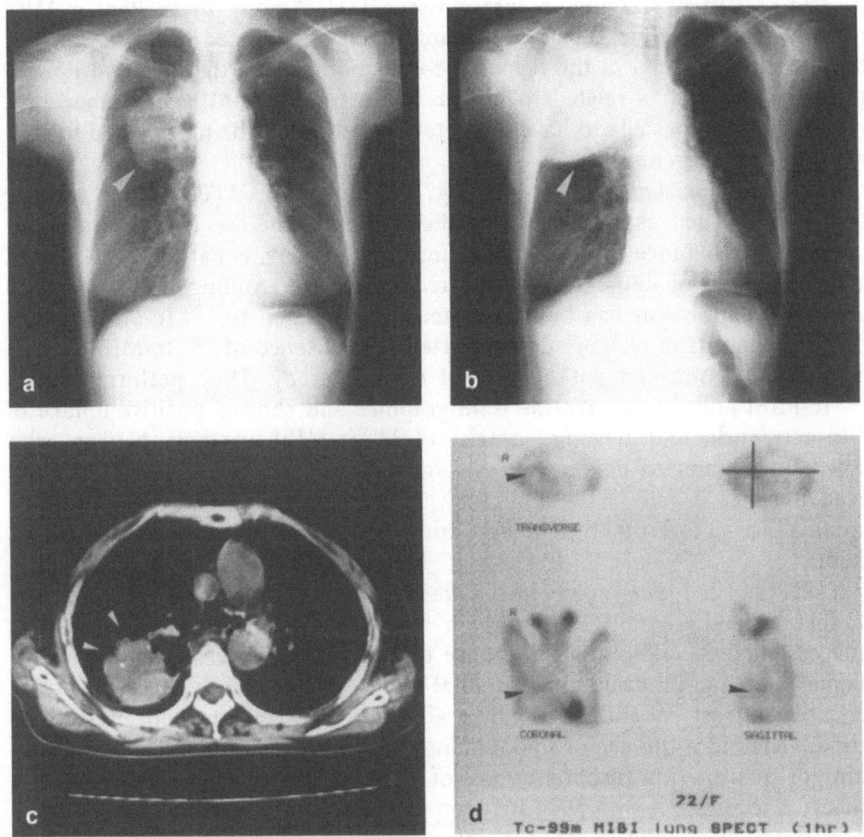

Fig. 8.8 a–d. Progressive disease. A tumor mass in the upper right lung (**a**, *white arrowhead*) was enlarged even after three courses of VAP chemotherapy (**b**, *white arrowhead*). CT (**c**) and ^{99m}Tc-MIBI SPECT (**d**) were done before chemotherapy. CT shows a high density mass in the upper right lung (**c**, *small white arrowheads*). One-hour tomographic images of ^{99m}Tc-MIBI SPECT (**d**) shows faint uptakes (tumor-to-normal ratio=1.55) in the tumor mass (**d**, *black arrowheads*)

showed no statistically significant difference between groups, while T/NL of tomographic images differed significantly between the groups ($p = 0.002$ on 1-h image, $p=0.03$ on 4-h image). The percentage retention between 1 and 4 h did not differ between the groups on either planar or tomographic images. Figures 8.7 and 8.8 illustrate patients with CR and PD, respectively. Indeed this was the first report that ^{99m}Tc-MIBI uptake is related to the response to chemotherapy in patients with SCLC. In other words, SCLC patients with higher uptake of ^{99m}Tc-MIBI are more likely to respond to chemotherapy than those with lower uptakes.

Factors related to ^{99m}Tc-MIBI uptake in tumors are blood flow, tissue viability, vascular permeability, tumor necrosis, metabolic demand, and mitochondrial activity of the tumor, and Pgp or multidrug resistance associated protein (MRP) expression in tumor tissue [32]. Among these Pgp or MRP expression is clearly associated with multidrug resistance. Blood flow to the tumor can be related to the response to chemotherapy. Higher blood flow to the tumor, which is related to higher uptake of ^{99m}Tc-MIBI in tumor [33], renders the tumor cells to have a greater probability of being exposed to chemotherapeutic agents.

Factors associated with multidrug resistance are ATP-binding cassette transporters such as Pgp or MRP, altered topoisomerase II, enhanced glutathione transferances and detoxification mechanisms, enhanced DNA repair, and low levels of cytochrome p450 reductase [34]. Among these only Pgp and MRP expression has been reported to be related to ^{99m}Tc-MIBI uptake [28, 35]. Moretti et al. [29] first reported that absence of ^{99m}Tc-MIBI uptake in SCLC is associated with failure of chemotherapy. They performed both ^{99m}Tc-MIBI and ^{111}In-octreotide scintigraphies and showed positive uptake of ^{111}In-octreotide and negative uptake of ^{99m}Tc-MIBI in their patient, who failed to respond to chemotherapy. Similar results were obtained when we used both ^{201}Tl and ^{99m}Tc-MIBI [36]. The association between ^{99m}Tc-MIBI uptake and factors other than Pgp and MRP expression has not been well studied.

T/NL on 1 h tomographic image was best in predicting response to chemotherapy followed by T/NL on 4 h tomographic image. T/NL on planar images failed to differentiate response groups. SPECT offers advantages over planar imaging in evaluating tumoral uptake in the body because of increased contrast enhancement which allows precise anatomic localization of tumor. Therefore the use of tomographic imaging is recommended for evaluating or quantitating tumoral uptake of ^{99m}Tc-MIBI in lung cancer. Although there was overlapping of T/NL between groups, there were statistically significant differences between groups, especially between responders and nonresponders. Patients who showed hot uptake (ratio >3.0) responded very well to chemotherapy (complete response) while those who showed faint uptake (ratio <1.7) did not responded to chemotherapy.

The time sequence of ^{99m}Tc-MIBI washout tumor cells expressing not expressing Pgp or is not well known, especially in vivo. Piwnica-Worms et al. [37] characterized multidrug-resistance Pgp transport function with ^{99m}Tc-MIBI, showing a rapid excretion of ^{99m}Tc-MIBI from Pgp-expressing Chinese hamster V79 lung fibroblast cell lines in vitro. The $t_{\frac{1}{2}}$ was less than 5 min. Although planar imagings could be acquired earlier (less than 15 min) after injection of ^{99m}Tc-MIBI [7], tomographic imaging of lung tumors using ^{99m}Tc-MIBI was usually performed 1 h after injection, and delayed imaging 2–3 h after injection [9]. In the present study we measured the retention of ^{99m}Tc-MIBI between 1 and 4 h, which might be too late. Late measurement may be one of the reasons why no relationship was found between %R and response to chemotherapy. Recently Yamamoto et al. [38] performed early and delayed imaging at 15 and 180 min after injection of ^{99m}Tc-MIBI in patients with SCLC. They found that responders to chemotherapy show higher tumor-to-normal lung ratio on the early images and higher retention index.

References

1. Tonami N, Shuke N, Kunihilo Y, Seki H, Takayama T, Kinuya S, Nakajima K, Aburano T, Hisada K (1989) Use of thallium-201 single photon emission computed tomography in the evaluation of suspected lung cancer. J Nucl Med 30:997–1004

2. Lee J, Ahn BC, Kim CH et al (1986) Can Tl-201 SPECT indeed differentiate a benign and malignant solitary pulmonary lesion? J Nucl Med 37:268P (abstract)

3. Lee JD, Lee BH, Kim SK, Chung KY, Shin DH, Park CY (1994) Increased thallium-201 uptake in collapsed lung: a pitfall in scintigraphic evaluation of central bronchogenic carcinoma. J Nucl Med 35:1125–1128

4. Tonami N, Yokoyama K, Taki J et al (1990) Tissue characterization of suspected malignant pulmonary lesion with Tl-201 SPECT. J Nucl Med 31:766 (abstract)

5. Tonami N, Yokoyama K, Shuke N et al (1993) Evaluation of suspected malignant pulmonary lesions with thallium-201 SPECT. J Nucl Med 34(S):139P (abstract)

6. Duman Y, Burak Z, Erdem S et al (1990) The value and limitations of Tl-201 scintigraphy in the evaluation of lung lesions and post-therapy follow-up of primary lung carcinoma. Nucl Med Commun 14:446–453

7. Hassan I, Sahweel C, Constantinides A et al (1989) Uptake and kinetics of Tc-99m hexakis 2-methoxy isobutyl isonitrile in benign and malignant lesions in the lungs. Clin Nucl Med 14:333–340

8. Muller SP, Reiners C, Pass M et al (1989) Tc-99m MIBI and Tl-201 uptake in bronchial carcinoma. J Nucl Med 30:845 (abstract)

9. Lebouthillier G, Taillefer R, Lambert R et al (1993) Detection of primary lung cancer with Tc-99m MIBI. J Nucl Med 34:140P (abstract)

10. Onsel C, Sonmezoglu K, Camsari G et al (1996) Technetium-99m MIBI scintigraphy in pulmonary tuberculosis. J Nucl Med 37:233–238

11. Rageb A, Elgazzar AH, Ibrahim AK et al (1993) A comparative study between planar Ga-67, Tl-201, chest x-ray and x-ray CT scans in inoperable non-small cell carcinoma of the lung. Eur J Nucl Med 20:838 (abstract)

12. Itoh K, Takekawa H, Tsukamoto E et al (1992) Single photon emission computed tomography using Tl-201 chloride in pulmonary nodules: comparison with Ga-67 citrate and Tc-99m-labeled hexamethylpropyleneamine-oxime. Ann Nucl Med 6:253–260

13. Hirano T, Otake H, Yoshida I, Endo K (1995) Primary lung cancer SPECT imaging with pentavalent technetium-99m DMSA. J Nucl Med 36:202–207

14. Lee J, Ahn BC, Kim CH et al (1996) Prospective comparison of Tl-201, Tc-99m MIBI and Tc-99m-(V)-DMSA in the same subjects with a solitary pulmonary lesion. J Nucl Med 37(s):267P (abstract)

15. Alazraki NP, Ramsdel JW, Talylor A et al (1978) Reliability of gallium scan, chest radiography compared to mediastinoscopy for evaluating mediastinal spread in lung cancer. Am Rev Respir Dis 117:415–420

16. Fosburg RG, Hopkins GB, Kan MK (1979) Evaluation of the mediastinum by Ga-67 scintigraphy in lung cancer. J Thorac Cardiovasc Surg 77:76–82

17. Lesk DM, Wood TE, Carrol SE, Reese L (1978) The application of Ga-67 scanning in determining the operability of bronchogenic carcinoma. Radiology 128:707–709

18. McKenna RJ, Haynie TP, Libshitz HI et al (1985) Critical evaluation of the Ga-67 scan for surgical patients with lung cancer. Chest 87:428–431

19. Waxman AD, Goldsmith MS, Greif PM et al (1987) Differentiation of tumor versus sarcoidosis using thallium-201 in patients with hilar mediastinal adenopathy (abstract). J Nucl Med 28:561

20. Matsuno S, Tanabe M, Kawasaki Y et al (1992) Effectiveness of planar image and single photon emission tomography of thallium-201 compared with gallium-67 in patients with primary lung cancer. Eur J Nucl Med 19:86–95

21. Chiti A, Maffioli LS, Infante M et al (1996) Assessment of mediastinal involvement in lung cancer with technetium-99m-sestamibi SPECT. J Nucl Med 37:938–942

22. Krenning EP, Kwekkeboom DJ, Reubi JC, Lamberts SW (1994) Somatostatin receptor scintigraphy with [In-111-DTPA-D-Phe1] octreotide. In: Murray IPC, Ell PJ (eds) Nuclear medicine in clinical diagnosis and treatment. Churchill Livingston, New York, pp 757–764

23. Orsolon P, Bagni B, Basadonna P, Geatti O, Talmassons G, Guerra-UP (1995) A case of bronchial carcinoid: diagnosis and follow-up with In-111-DTPA-octreotide. Q J Nucl Med 39:311–314

24. Miyagawa M, Watanabe K, Shiode M et al (1993) Tl-201 SPECT in the follow-up of patients with lung cancer during radiotherapy. J Nucl Med 34:222P (abstract)

25. Bom HS, Song HC, Kim JY et al (1994) The usefulness of Tc-99m MIBI SPECT in the localization and the assessment of radiotherapy in non-small cell lung cancer. Kor J Nucl Med 28:186–191

26. Ihde DC (1992) Chemotherapy of drug cancer. N Engl J Med 12:1434–1441

27. Deuchars KL, Ling V (1989) P-glycoprotein and multidrug resistance in cancer chemotherapy. Semin Oncol 16:156–165

28. Piwnica-Worms D, Chiu ML, Budding J, Kornauge JF, Kramer RA, Croop JM (1993) Functional imaging of multidrug-resistant P-glycoprotein with an organo-technetium complex. Cancer Res 53:977–984

29. Moretti JL, Cagler M, Boaziz C, Caillat-Vigneron N, Morere JF (1995) Sequential functional with technetium-99m hexakis-2-methoxyisobutylisonitrile and indium-111 octreotide: can we predict the response to chemotherapy in small cell lung cancer? Eur J Nucl Med 22:177–180

30. Bom HS, Kim YC, Song HC, Kim JY, Park KO (1996) Tc-99m sestamibi uptake in small cell lung cancer: A predictor of response to chemotherapy. J Nucl Med 37:67P (abstract)

31. Miller AB, Hoogstraten B, Staquet M, Winkler A (1981) Reporting results of cancer treatment. Cancer 47:207–214

32. Waxman AD (1996) Thallium-201 and technetium-99m methoxyisobutyl isonitrile (MIBI) in nuclear oncology. In: Sandler MP, Coleman RE, Wackers FJT, Patton JA, Gottschalk A, Hoffer PB (eds) Diagnostic nuclear medicine, 3rd edn. Williams and Wilkins, Baltimore, pp 1261–1274

33. Scopinaro F, Schillaci O, Scarpini M et al (1994) Technetium-99m sestamibi: an indicator of breast cancer invasiveness. Eur J Nucl Med 21:984–987

34. Harris AL, Hochhauser D (1992) Mechanisms of multidrug resistance in cancer treatment. Acta Oncol 31:205–213

35. Crankshaw C, Piwnica-Worms D (1996) Tc-99m sestamibi may be a transport substrate of the human multidrug resistance-associated protein (MRP). J Nucl Med 37:247P (abstract)

36. Kapucu CO, Akyuz C, Vural G et al (1996) The value of MIBI scintigraphy in predicting the prognosis in pediatric patients with lymphoma. J Nucl Med 37:139P (abstract)

37. Piwnica-Worms D, Rao VV, Kronauge JF, Croop JM (1995) Characterization of multidrug resistance P-glycoprotein transport function with an organotechnetium cation. Biochemistry 34:12210–12220

38. Yamamoto Y, Nishiyama Y, Fukynaga K, Satoh K, Takashima H, Tanabe M (1996) Evaluation of Tc-99m MIBI to predict chemotherapeutic response of patients with small cell lung cancer. Ann Nucl Med 10 [Suppl]:S137 (abstract)

9 Adult Respiratory Distress Syndrome

E. E. KIM and M. C. LEE

Adult respiratory distress syndrome (ARDS) is a severe, progressive pulmonary disorder that is associated with a variety of underlying etiologies [2]. The term was first used in the late 1960s to describe a recurring group of clinical, physiological, and radiological manifestations of acute respiratory failure in adults. Findings include tachypnea and dyspnea, hypoxia refractory to increasing concentrations of inspired oxygen, noncompliant lungs, normal pulmonary capillary wedge pressure, and widespread infiltrates on chest radiographs. It represents the pulmonary consequences of cellular and humoral mechanisms that are activated in the lungs of susceptible individuals. Disorders frequently associated with ARDS include pulmonary trauma, aspiration, intravascular coagulopathy, and sepsis.

Damage to the alveolar-capillary membrane is the fundamental parenchymal injury of ARDS [3]. In the earlier, exudative phase type I epithelial cells are severely damaged. Although initial findings may be limited to the interstitium, increased permeability eventually results in alveolar filling with protein-rich fluid and cells. Decreased production of surfactant probably contributes to microatelectasis. Fibrin precipitation and accumulation of cellular debris produce characteristic hyaline membranes. These are established within 4 days and apparently do not progress with assisted ventilation. Modern ventilatory support is provided with volume-cycled respirators and positive end-expiratory pressure (PEEP) to maintain adequate oxygenation while avoiding the risks of high inspired-oxygen concentrations for prolonged periods. Within 1–2 weeks the second phase supervenes, characterized by organization, fibrosis, and proliferation of type II alveolar cells. With time the proliferative type II cells can differentiate into the type I cells, partially restoring the normal epithelial lining.

The overall reported mortality rate remains at least 50% in most instances. When a patient first becomes symptomatic, chest radiographs often are normal. The latent period before radiographic changes appear may last for 12–24 h and occasionally for more than 72 h after the initial injury. Pulmonary emboli and respiratory obstruction are the major differential diagnostic considerations. Vascular indistinctness consistent with interstitial edema is an early radiographic change. The more severe cases progress to diffuse consolidation, with a tendency to spare the costphrenic angles and apices. Air bronchograms are usually evident, and pleural effusions are not common. Variations in the evolutionary pattern may reflect the underlying etiology.

Bicompartmental Model of Pulmonary Capillary Protein Leak

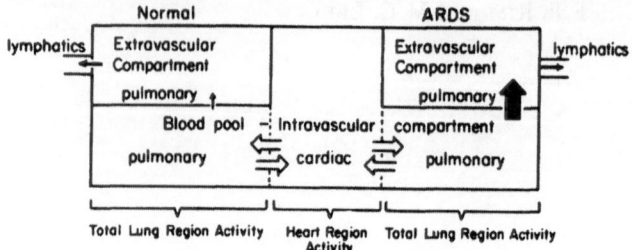

Fig. 9.1. Bicompartmental mel of pulmonary capillary protein leak. (Reprinted with permission from [5])

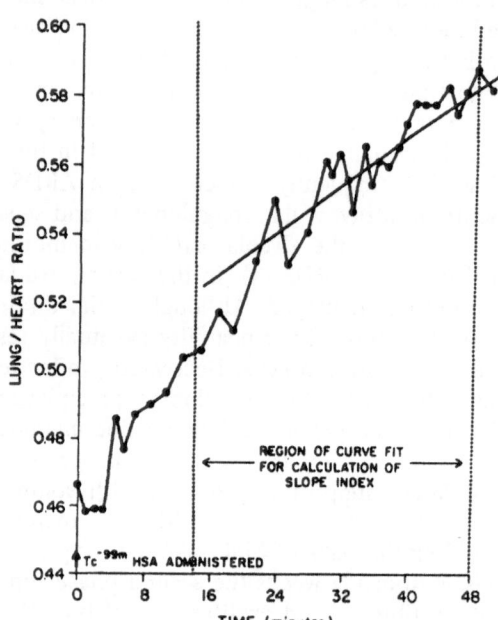

Fig. 9.2. Gradual leak of ^{99m}Tc-labeled human serum albumin from the lung capillaries in a patient with ARDS. (Reprinted with permission from [5])

Scintigraphic methods have been used to provide noninvasive evidence of alveolar-capillary membrane damage. Abnormally rapid clearance of pulmonary activity occurs after the inhalation of aerosolized ^{99m}Tc-DTPA, suggesting increased permeability of the alveolar-capillary membrane [1]. This is not specific to ARDS although it does occur quite early in patients with ARDS. One of the potential pitfalls of radioaerosol studies in patients with ARDS might be poor peripheral penetration of radioactivity. The pulmonary activity (relative to that in the cardiac blood pool) increases more rapidly in patients with ARDS than in those with many other pulmonary disorders such as congestive heart failure or pneumonia. This indicates that the endothelial portion of the alveolar-capillary membrane also is disrupted (Fig. 9.1).

Therefore it has allowed a large protein to leak from the vessels into the alveoli or interstitium [4] (Fig. 9.2). There has been little improvement in survival rates.

The effects of PEEP on the radiographic appearance and radioaerosol clearance rates must be considered whenever it is used as a supportive measure. High levels of PEEP can cause the lungs to expand and lead to recruitment of alveolar absorptive area and to artifactual increases in the rate of radioaerosol absorption. Corticosteroids have been widely used to treat ARDS, but there is no generally accepted documentation of their value. New therapeutic options include modulators of arachidonic acid metabolism, free-radical scavengers, and antibodies to endotoxins.

References

1. Butler SP, Alderson PO, Greenspan RL, Doctor DG, DeFilippi VJ (1990) The utility of Tc-99m DTPA aerosol inhalation scans in artificially ventilated patients. J Nucl Med 31:46–51
2. Greene RE (1987) Adult respiratory distress syndrome: acute alveolar damage. Radiology 163:57–66
3. Modig J (1986) Adult respiratory disease syndrome. Pathogenesis and treatment. Acta Chir Scand 152:241–249
4. Stokkel MP, Pauwels EK (1994) Octreotide scintigraphy for small cell lung carcinoma. Eur J Nucl Med 21:1276–1278
5. Tatum JL, Strash AM, Sugarman HJ, Hirsch JI, Beachley MC, Greenfield LJ (1981) Single isotope evaluation of pulmonary capillary protein leak (ARDS model) using computerized gamma scintigraphy. Invest Radiol 16:473–478

10 Mucociliary Clearance

T. Isawa

Experimental Studies in Dogs

When a single radioactive bolus is placed on the carina or the main bronchus of the normal dog through a vinyl tube under bronchoscopic guidance, the radioactive bolus is transported upward toward the vocal cord with the mucous blanket or the mucus layer along the main bronchus passing the carina or along the trachea at a nearly constant steady velocity. The transport can be well appreciated by sequential or follow-up imaging as shown in Fig. 10.1. The transport velocity is calculated by dividing the migrating distance of the radioactive bolus by time required for the transport. The transport velocity of the particular dog in Fig. 10.1 was 12 mm/min.

When dogs are forced to smoke cigarettes, the transport velocity tends to slow as the number of cigarettes smoked increases (Fig. 10.2). This indicates that the toxicity of the cigarette smoke acutely hinders mucociliary clearance in the normal dogs [1]. Cauterization of the airway mucosa in the normal dog can also damage mucociliary clearance [2]. Recovery of the normal mucociliary clearance from either cigarette smoke or cauterization takes about 2 weeks [1, 2]. Filtered cigarettes do not prevent the mucociliary clearance function from being damaged as the number of cigarettes smoked exceeds a certain level, say five cigarettes, on a normal dog's running [1].

Human Studies

Delayed Imaging

Because anesthesia of the oropharynx and the upper airways is absolutely necessary for bronchoscopic insertion, the placement of a radioactive droplet on the large airways under bronchoscopic guidance itself is not practical under clinical situations. Instead, inhalation of radioaerosol which is not absorbable from the mucosal surface becomes the method of choice in daily clinical practice.

When delayed imaging is repeated following radioaerosol inhalation in patients with bronchogenic carcinoma, some show a hot spot which either remains constant in size or grows larger than that on an image acquired im-

Fig. 10.1. Radioactive droplet (^{99m}Tc-MAA) placed on the large airway of a dog is transported upward with time. In this dog the transport velocity along the trachea was 11.3 mm/min

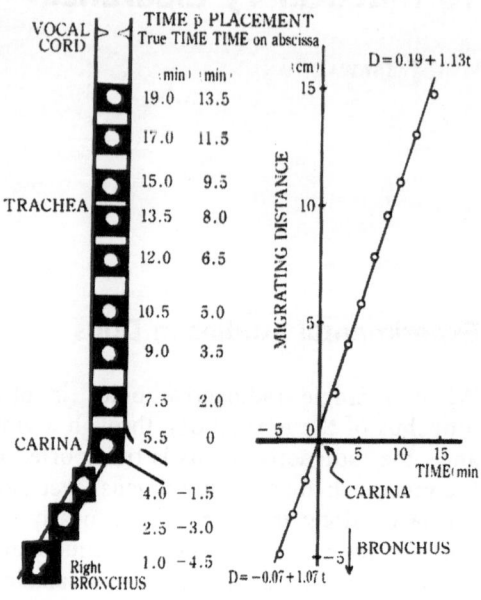

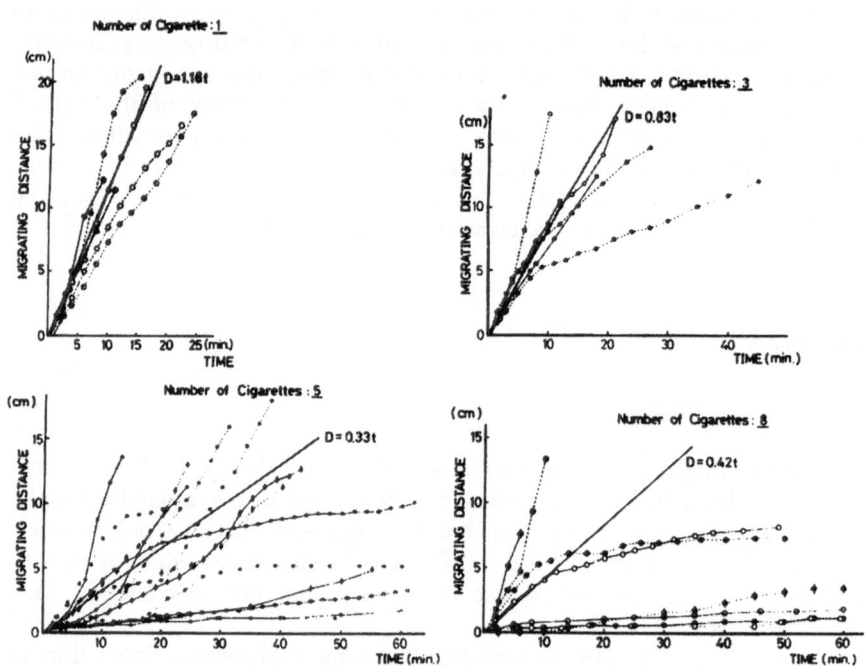

Fig. 10.2. Migrating or mucociliary transport distance versus time when the dog smokes 1, 3, 5, and 8 nonfiltered cigarettes. *Shaded band*, normal range. The transport velocity generally becomes slower as the number of cigarettes smoked increases

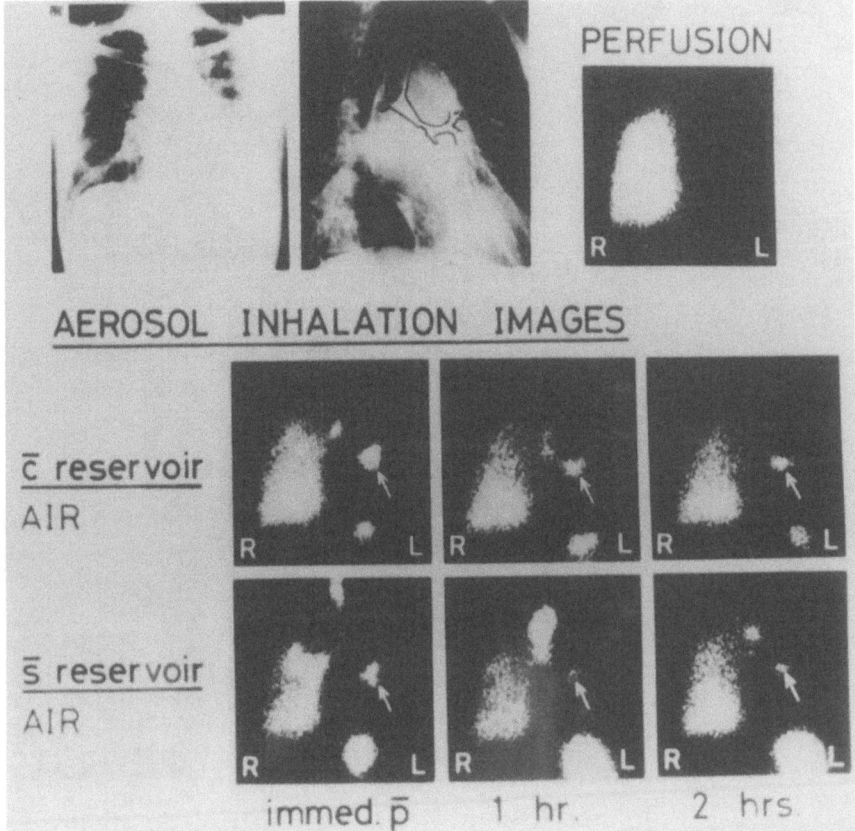

PERFUSION

R   L

AEROSOL INHALATION IMAGES

c̄ reservoir

AIR

R   L R   L R   L

s̄ reservoir

AIR

R   L R   L R   L

immed. p̄   1 hr.   2 hrs.

Fig. 10.3. A hot spot at the site of cancer invasion on the left main bronchus persists for 2 h or longer, indicating disturbed mucociliary clearance. A 55-year-old man with large cell carcinoma

mediately after inhalation (Fig. 10.3), while in others a hot spot observed on an immediate image disappears on delayed images (Fig. 10.4). The former indicates that the airway mucosa at the site of the hot spot is studded with cancerous invasion, while in the latter it is not invaded, indicating that the mucociliary clearance remains intact.

In studying mucociliary clearance function by repeated delayed imaging following radioaerosol inhalation, we were puzzled by the case shown in Fig. 10.5 regarding interpretation of the behavior of a mucous glob. Immediately after aerosol inhalation there was no radioactivity in the left main bronchus. Delayed imaging at 1 h showed a radioactive glob on the left main bronchus, which disappeared within 2 h following inhalation. If mucus is always transported cephalad toward the vocal cord, it is difficult to interpret the presence of radioactivity on the left main bronchus. This finding suggests that there must be some inherent defect in this method for studying

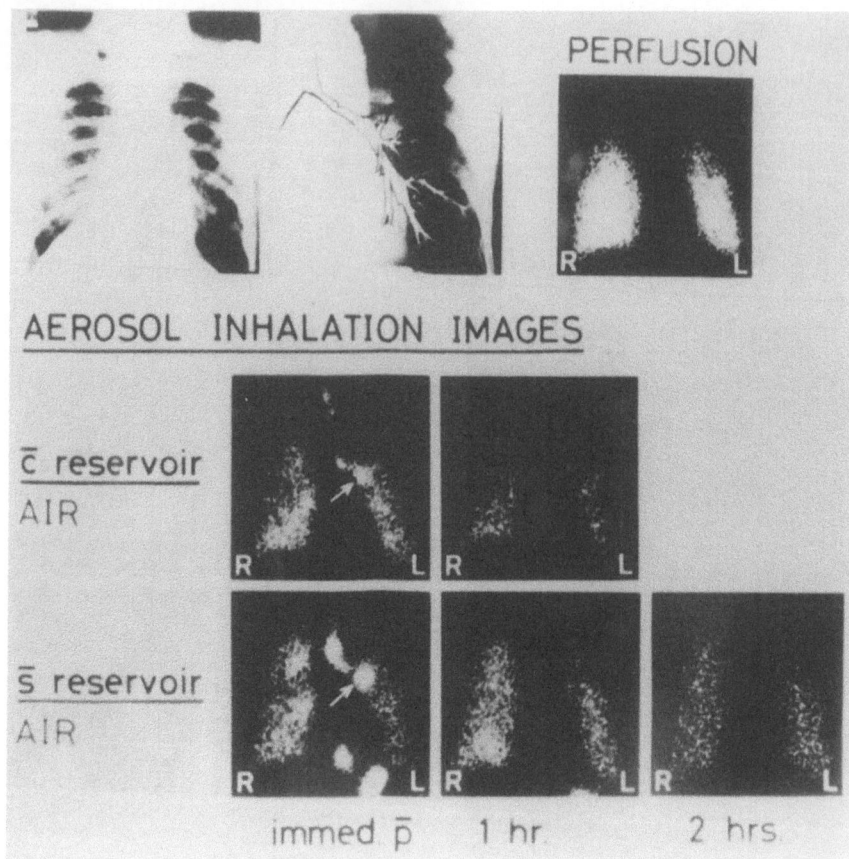

Fig. 10.4. A hot spot recognized immediately following radioaerosol inhalation at the site of cancer protrusion disappears by 1 h, indicating intact mucociliary clearance. A 46-year-old man with small-cell carcinoma

mucociliary clearance. Continuous measurement of radioactivity following radioaerosol inhalation instead of spotlike repeated delayed imaging is mandatory to determine precisely what happens to the inhaled aerosols in terms of mucociliary clearance.

Radioaerosol Inhalation Lung Cine-Scintigraphy

Following inhalation of ultrasonically generated ^{99m}Tc-labeled human serum albumin aerosol in tidal breathing through a mouthpiece with the nose clipped, a subject is placed either under or above a gamma-camera in the supine position, and radioactivity was measured over the entire thorax including the trachea for 120 min in sequential 10 s frame mode with 64×64 ma-

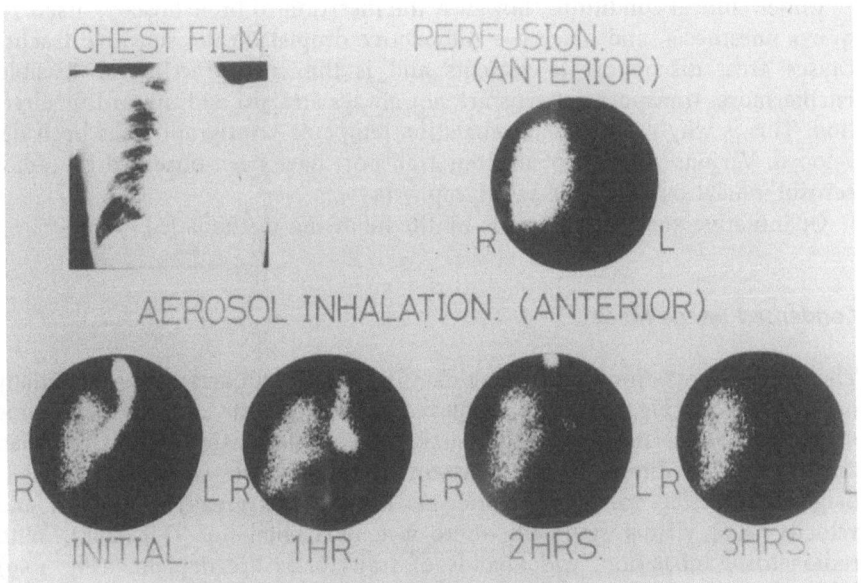

Fig. 10.5. Immediately after radioaerosol inhalation no radioactivity deposits in the left main bronchus, indicating no ventilation in the left lung. However, in 1 h a hot spot has appeared in the left main bronchus. By 3 h the hot spot has completely disappeared. A 50-year-old male with adenocarcinoma. The left lung shows a blackout on chest X-ray and absent perfusion on perfusion lung image

trices. The data were recorded and stored in a computer. The data were displayed in cine-mode on a cathode ray tube screen at the rate of 18 frames/s, and the cinematographic display was recorded in a movie camera. Dynamic mucous transport patterns on the large airways such as the trachea or the main bronchus were observed and evaluated by cinematographic display. This was in fact the first time for us to see the actual dynamic mucous transport in vivo in the human lungs [3–5].

Quantitative Evaluation

Extrapulmonary Airways

Under an experimental situation as described above (see "Experimental Studies in Dogs"), transport velocity of a radioactive droplet can be assessed by measuring peak radioactivity of the droplet at two different measuring points and the time required for transport between the two spots. The distance transported divided by the time required for the transport is equivalent to velocity of the mucociliary clearance. This is true only when transport is straight and upward in direction and constant in transport velocity.

Under clinical conditions, however, the insertion of bronchoscopy itself requires anesthesia, and placing a radioactive droplet on the sensitive trachea causes great discomfort to patients and is thus not practical or feasible. Furthermore, transport patterns are not always straight and upward in direction. This is why radioaerosol inhalation lung cine-scintigraphy has been developed. Various patterns of mucous transport have been observed by radioaerosol inhalation lung cine-scintigraphy [3–5].

Quantitative analysis was made by the following methods [6].

Condensed Image Mode

The tracheal portion of each frame data is selected and arranged sequentially on a computer (Fig. 10.6) and displayed on the cathode ray tube with time on the x-axis and distance on the y-axis. When mucous transport is cephalad and straight in direction and constant in velocity, the transport line is a diagonal line (Fig. 10.7). When mucous transport is greatly disturbed, and velocity is at virtual standstill, there is a horizontal line (Fig. 10.8). With radioaerosol inhalation, wide bands of trajectories are depicted (Fig. 10.9) [6].

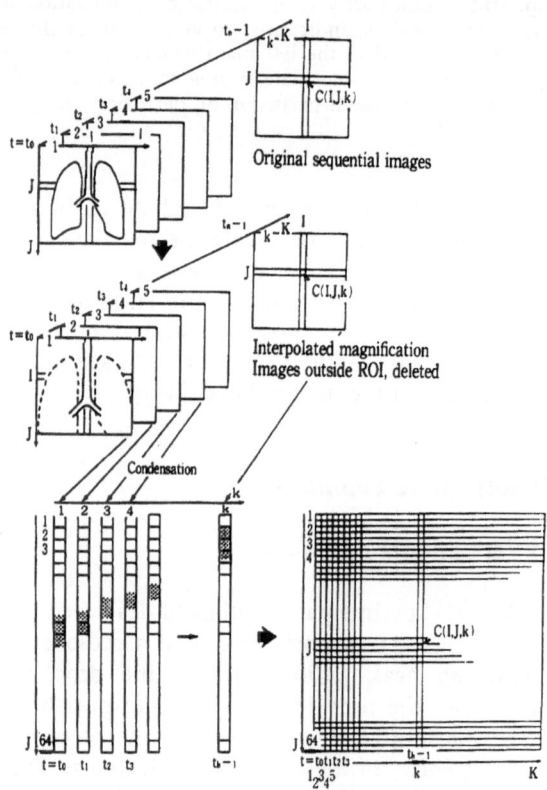

Fig. 10.6. Diagram of condensed image mode. Only the tracheal portion is arranged sequentially and the hot spot is imaged. (From [6])

Fig. 10.7. Transport of a radioactive droplet with mucus of a normal dog from the carina to the vocal cord. (From [6])

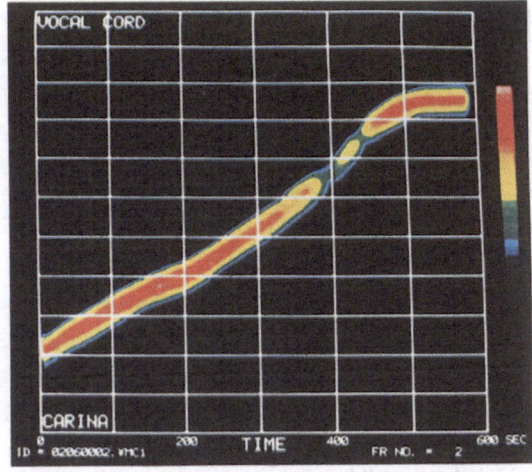

Fig. 10.8. Transport of a radioactive droplet with mucus of a normal dog forced to smoke five cigarettes. Mucus transport is greatly disturbed. (From [6])

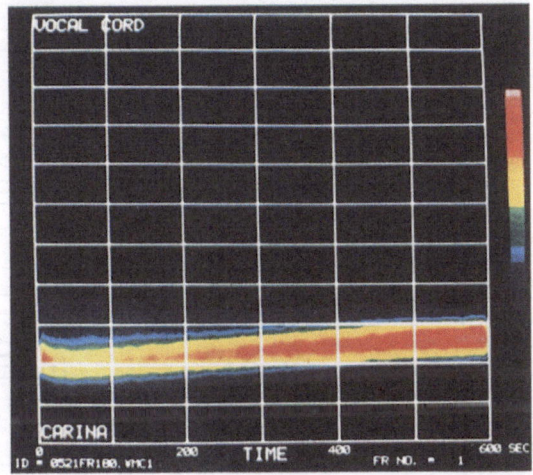

Trajectory Mode

In order to analyze the transport of a mucous glob more accurately and quantitatively, the following method was devised and termed "trajectory mode" [6]. First, a point of interest is set at a "hot spot" on a frame data magnified from the original 64×64 matrix data by interpolation, and its location is determined mathematically and recorded in a computer. On the next frame, also similarly magnified by interpolation, the change in hot spot location is measured mathematically and recorded. This procedure is repeated frame by frame, and each mathematical location is connected using B Spline function, which makes a trajectory of the transport of the hot spot

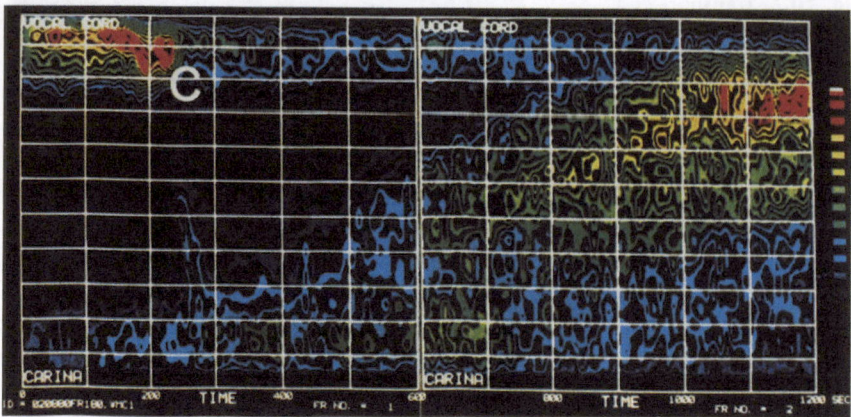

Fig. 10.9. Condensed image of a 29-year-old normal nonsmoker following radioaerosol inhalation. Wide bands in the upper right direction are seen. C, Mucus glob expectorated by cough at the vocal cord. (From [6])

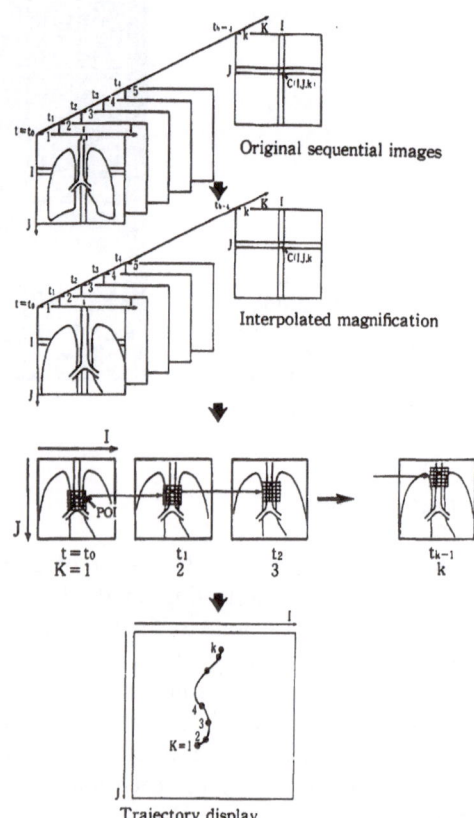

Fig. 10.10. Diagram showing the principle of the trajectory mode. The location of the point of interest is sequentially determined frame by frame, and each mathematical location is connected using B Spline function. (From [6])

Fig. 10.11. An example of the trajectory in a 29-year-old normal nonsmoker beginning at the lower cross (*red line*) to the upper cross (*blue line*). (From [6])

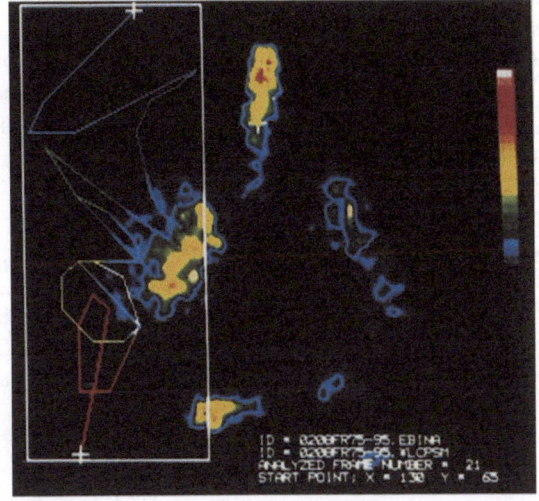

Fig. 10.12. Vector analysis of a trajectory. From START to END the actual pathway is comprised of s_1, s_2,.... S_N, although macroscopically it resembles a straight line between START and END. Each s_1, s_2,.... S_N is a vector and mathematical calculation is possible. (From 6])

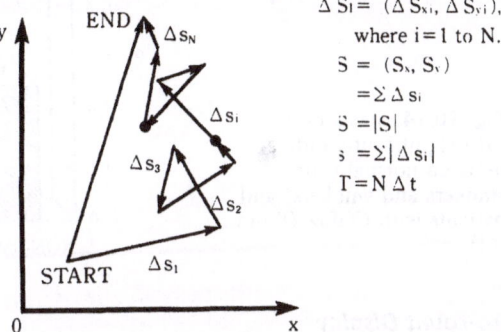

$$\Delta S_i = (\Delta S_{xi}, \Delta S_{yi}),$$
$$\text{where } i = 1 \text{ to } N.$$
$$S = (S_x, S_y)$$
$$= \Sigma \Delta s_i$$
$$S = |S|$$
$$s = \Sigma |\Delta s_i|$$
$$T = N \Delta t$$

(Figs. 10.10, 10.11). This trajectory enables a detailed analysis of mucociliary transport on the trachea [6].

Using this trajectory makes vector analysis possible, and various parameters can be calculated using various values indicated (Fig. 10.12). For example, Fig. 10.13 compares tracheal mucous transport in normal nonsmokers, smokers, and patients with chronic obstructive pulmonary diseases (COPD) regarding effective velocity and apparent velocity as defined below.

- Efective transport velocity (V_{eff}) = S/T
- Apparent transport velocity (V_{app}) = s/T
- Traveling pathway index (a) = s/S
- Stasis ratio (SR) = $\sum$ [no. of times ($\Delta s_i = 0$)/N)]

Fractions of forward transport, backward transport and stasis in mucous transport can also be easily calculated. Stasis ratios between healthy smokers, nonsmokers, and patients with COPD are shown in Fig. 10.14.

Fig. 10.13. Although there is no statistically significant difference in effective velocity (*Veff*) between nonsmokers, smokers and patients with chronic obstructive pulmonary disease (*COPD*), apparent velocity (*Vapp*) significantly differs between normal subjects (smokers and nonsmokers) and patients with COPD. (From [6])

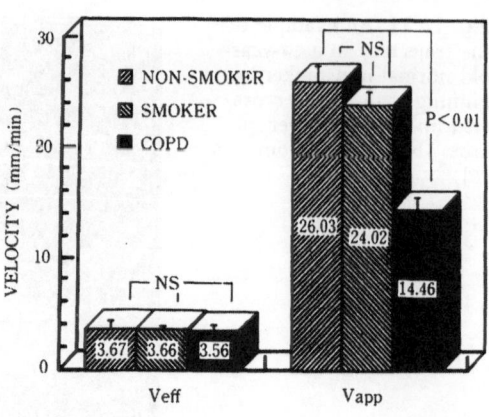

Fig. 10.14. Stasis ratio (*SR*) significantly differs between normal (nonsmokers and smokers) and patients with COPD. (From [6])

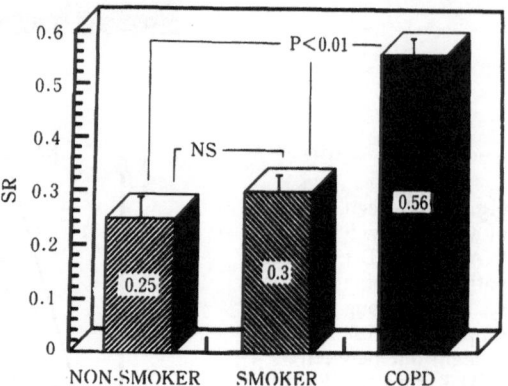

Iso-count Display

Iso-count display of a hot spot in sequential frames is also possible by delineating iso-count lines in each frame. The direction of transport can be assessed, but this method, too, is feasible only when a radioactive droplet is placed on the trachea. Thus this method is not practically applicable to aerosol inhalation studies [6].

Ciliated Airway in Lung Parenchyma

When radioaerosol is inhaled, radioactivity deposits in the extrapulmonary ciliated airways (A), intrapulmonary ciliated airways (B), in the nonciliated small airways including the alveolar space (C), and in the esophagus and the stomach or the gastrointestinal tract (D) as illustrated in Fig. 10.15 [4, 5].

Disregarding the radioactivity in the stomach and/or the gastrointestinal tract (D), the radioactivity at time zero or immediately after aerosol inhalation is finished can be written as follows:

Fig. 10.15. Diagram of deposition sites of inhaled aerosol such as the trachea and the proximal portions of the major bronchi (*A*), the intrapulmonary ciliated airways (*B*), the nonciliated small airways including the alveolarspace (*C*) and the digestive canal such as the mouth, the esophagus, the stomach, etc. (*D*)

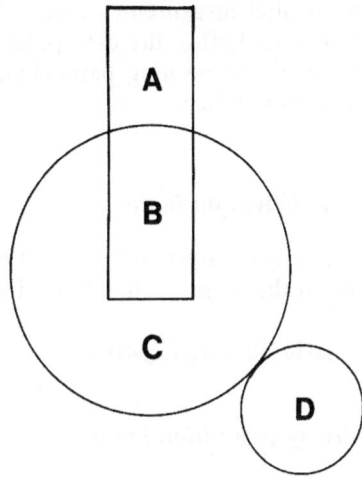

$$A_o + B_o + C_o = T_o \tag{1}$$

where A, B, C represent the compartments in Fig. 10.15 and T the total radioactivity in all three compartments. At time t, radioactivity at each compartment would be:

$$A_t + B_t + C_t = T_t \tag{2}$$

If radioactivity is corrected for physical decay, Eq. 2 becomes:

$$A_{tc} + B_{tc} + C_{tc} = T_{tc} \tag{3}$$

If we define the radioactivity remaining in the lung at 24 h later as the amount of radioactivity deposited in the nonciliated space of the lung, C_o, corrected for physical decay should be the same with C_{tc}: $C_o = C_{tc}$.

Practically speaking, it is extremely difficult to measure A_t without being contaminated by radioactivity in the esophagus behind the trachea that is being swallowed. In evaluating the clearance of radioactivity over time from the lung parenchyma, which is simply mucociliary clearance in the intrapulmonary ciliated airways, only radioactivity in the extrapulmonary airways should be taken into consideration. Radioactivity in the compartment A should be excluded from consideration. Thus the above formulae should be rewritten as follows:

$$B_o + C_o = T_o \tag{1'}$$

$$B_t + C_t = T_t \tag{2'}$$

$$B_{tc} + C_{tc} = T_{tc} \tag{3'}$$

Sequential measurements of radioactivity in the lung parenchyma or in the thorax excluding the extrapulmonary mediastinal region and the radioactivity in the same lung parenchyma at 24 h are required only to calculate the following indices.

Lung Retention Ratio

The lung retention ratio (LRR) expresses the amount of radioactivity remaining in the lungs at time t relative to the total radioactivity initially deposited:

$$LRR\ (\%) = T_{tc}/T_o \times 100$$

Airway Deposition Ratio

The airway deposition ratio (ADR) indicates the amount of radioactivity throughout the ciliated airways relative to the total radioactivity initially deposited in the lungs:

$$ADR\ (\%) = B_{tc}/T_o \times 100 = (T_{tc} - C_o)/T_o \times 100$$

Airway Retention Ratio

The airway retention ratio (ARR) measures the proportion of radioactivity initially deposited on the ciliated airways that still remains there at time t:

$$ARR\ (\%) = B_{tc}/B_o \times 100 = \{(T_o - T_{tc})/(T_o - C_o)\} \times 100$$

Airway Clearance Efficiency

Airway clearance efficiency (ACE) is the proportion of radioactivity initially deposited on the ciliated airways that has been cleared by time t:

$$ACE\ (\%) = (B_o - B_{tc})/B_o \times 100 = \{(T_o - T_{tc})/(T_o - C_o)\} \times 100$$

Alveolar Deposition Ratio

The alveolar deposition ratio (ALDR) indicates the proportion of total initial radioactivity remaining in the lung parenchyma at 24 h, or the proportion of radioactivity deposited in the nonciliated space of the lungs including the alveolar space at the completion of aerosol inhalation. The compartment C lacks mucociliary clearance:

$$ALDR\ (\%) = C_o/T_o \times 100$$

Table 10.1. Lung retention ratio (%) in the right and left lungs in normal nonsmokers, normal smokers, and normal subjects

Time (min)	Nonsmokers (n=13)		Smokers (n=15)		Normals (n=28)	
	Left	Right	Left	Right	Left	Right
10	100	100	100	100	100	100
20	93.9± 4.4	95.1±4.3	89.9±3.4	92.1±3.5	91.8±4.3	93.5± 4.1
30	90.0± 6.9	93.4±5.3	84.1±5.1	87.5±5.9	86.8±6.6	90.2± 6.3
40	87.3± 8.9	92.2±6.3	79.7±5.7	83.2±6.1	83.2±8.2	87.4± 7.6
50	85.2±10.4	90.8±6.7	77.4±6.9	80.5±7.0	80.9±9.3	85.3± 8.5
60	83.7±10.6	88.8±7.0	75.3±7.0	78.4±7.1	79.4±9.8	83.3± 8.7
70	82.6± 9.9	87.5±7.1	73.9±7.8	76.7±7.8	78.0±9.7	81.7± 9.2
80	82.0± 8.7	86.5±7.5	71.9±7.9	74.6±7.8	76.8±9.6	80.3± 9.6
90	80.8± 8.2	86.7±7.7	70.4±8.2	73.9±9.7	75.4±9.6	79.7±10.5

Table 10.2. Airway deposition ratio (%) in the right and left lungs in normal nonsmokers, normal smokers, and normal subjects

Time (min)	Nonsmokers (n=13)		Smokers (n=15)		Normals (n=28)	
	Left	Right	Left	Right	Left	Right
10	56.2±4.0	56.2±3.9	64.3±10.6	64.7±10.8	60.5± 9.1	60.7± 9.3
20	50.1±5.4	51.2±5.2	54.2±10.8	56.8± 9.9	52.3± 8.8	54.2± 8.4
30	46.2±6.7	49.5±5.3	49.1±13.2	52.1±10.4	47.7±10.6	50.9± 8.4
40	43.5±8.1	48.3±6.1	43.9±12.6	47.9±11.0	43.7±10.5	48.1± 8.9
50	41.3±9.3	46.9±6.5	41.5±12.9	45.2±11.1	41.4±11.1	46.0± 9.1
60	39.8±9.6	45.0±6.5	39.5±12.9	43.0±11.6	39.7±11.3	43.9± 9.5
70	38.8±8.9	43.7±6.6	38.1±12.7	41.3±11.5	38.4±10.9	42.4± 9.4
80	38.2±7.6	42.6±6.8	36.1±13.3	39.1±11.5	37.1±10.8	41.1± 8.9
90	36.9±7.0	42.8±7.0	34.5±13.9	37.6±12.0	35.7±11.0	40.1±10.0

Normal values using human serum albumin aerosol with an activity median aerodynamic diameter of 1.9 µm and geometric standard deviation of 1.7 are shown in Tables 10.1–10.4 [7]. The ALDR values may differ when differently sized aerosols are inhaled. The smaller the aerosol size, the higher is the ALDR [8]. It is ideal to establish the normal ranges of each parameter at each laboratory according to the aerosols used.

Mucociliary Clearance in Health and Disease

Large Airways: Trachea and Major Bronchi

Normal Subjects

In nonsmoking normal subjects the transport of inhaled radioaerosol deposited in the airways is always axial and cephalad in direction, and steady and constant in its transport velocity, showing no stagnation of radioactivity in

Table 10.3. Airway retention ratio (%) in the right and left lungs in normal nonsmokers, normal smokers, and normal subjects

Time (min)	Nonsmokers (n = 13)		Smokers (n = 15)		Normals (n = 28)	
	Left	Right	Left	Right	Left	Right
10	100	100	100	100	100	100
20	89.1± 7.9	91.2± 7.6	83.9± 5.5	88.0± 5.4	86.3± 7.1	89.5± 6.6
30	82.5±11.7	88.3± 9.0	74.8± 7.9	80.7± 9.1	78.3±10.6	84.2± 9.7
40	77.8±14.8	87.9± 8.9	67.3±10.1	73.6± 9.8	72.2±13.4	80.8±11.7
50	74.0±17.2	83.9±11.4	63.5±11.6	69.7±10.7	68.4±15.1	76.3±13.0
60	71.2±17.6	80.3±11.8	60.6±12.1	66.1±11.6	65.5±15.6	72.7±13.6
70	69.5±16.1	77.8±11.6	58.5±12.4	63.8±12.5	63.6±15.0	70.3±13.8
80	68.3±14.0	75.7±12.6	55.1±13.2	60.1±12.5	61.5±14.9	67.6±14.6
90	66.4±13.1	76.3±12.9	52.9±13.9	57.9±13.6	59.4±14.9	66.7±16.0

Table 10.4. Airway clearance efficiency (%) in the right and left lungs in normal nonsmokers, normal smokers, and normal subjects

Time (min)	Nonsmokers (n = 13)		Smokers (n = 15)		Normals (n = 28)	
	Left	Right	Left	Right	Left	Right
10	0	0	0	0	0	0
20	10.9± 7.9	7.3± 6.8	16.1± 5.5	12.0± 5.4	13.7± 7.1	9.8± 6.4
30	17.5±11.7	10.9± 8.7	25.4± 8.4	19.3± 9.1	21.7±10.6	15.4± 9.8
40	22.2±14.8	12.9±10.3	32.7±10.1	26.4± 9.8	27.8±13.4	20.1±12.0
50	26.0±17.2	15.2±11.0	36.5±11.6	30.3±10.7	31.6±15.1	23.3±13.1
60	28.8±17.6	18.8±11.3	39.4±12.1	33.9±11.6	34.5±15.6	26.9±13.6
70	30.5±16.1	21.3±11.2	41.5±12.4	36.2±12.5	36.4±15.0	29.3±13.9
80	31.7±14.0	23.6±12.4	44.9±13.2	40.1±12.6	38.5±14.9	32.1±14.8
90	32.8±14.3	23.0±12.6	47.1±13.9	42.1±13.6	40.3±15.6	32.9±16.1

the trachea or the bronchi. However, in smokers and some former smokers, although radioactive transport is still cephalad in direction and transport velocity nearly constant, temporary collection of radioactivity is seen over the bronchi near or over the carina [4]. Such stasis, however, never persists long. There is no visible retrograde transport or retreat, stasis, or stagnation of mucous globs, frequent up-and-down motions of radioactive globs in the trachea or bronchi, or migration into the other regions of the same lung or into the bronchus of the opposite lung, which are often observed in patients with obstructive airways disease [5].

By trajectory mode, however, the trajectory in a normal subject is tortuous and not a simple trajectory as shown in Fig. 10.11, indicating that there microscopically mixed forward and retrograde transports are mixed with stasis, but that the overall transport direction is oropharygeal [6].

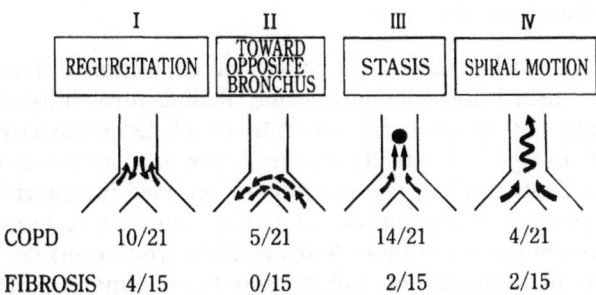

	I REGURGITATION	II TOWARD OPPOSITE BRONCHUS	III STASIS	IV SPIRAL MOTION
COPD	10/21	5/21	14/21	4/21
FIBROSIS	4/15	0/15	2/15	2/15

Fig. 10.16. Four abnormal mucus transport patterns on the trachea. Although steady transport cephalad in direction is seen in normal nonsmokers, the above four abnormal mucus transport patterns are observed in combination in pathological states. In straying only shuttling transport between the opposite bronchi is shown here, straying transport from one region to a different portion inside the same lung is also seen. The numbers below indicate frequency observed in 20 patients with COPD and 15 patients with idiopathic interstitial fibrosis

Obstructive Airways Disease

Transport of radioactivity over the trachea and the major bronchi is extremely protean in its direction and transport patterns. Of 21 patients with obstructive airways disease studied by radioaerosol inhalation lung cine-scintigraphy, 14 showed temporary but frequent stopping and starting of radioactivity in the airways in the course of lung clearance.

Even after radioactivity begins to migrate up the trachea, it tends to stop on the way. This stopping and renewed migration were repeated many times in the course of mucous transport. Migration is often accelerated by coughing and/or clearing the throat, with the radioactive mucus finally swallowed into the stomach or expectorated. Sometimes radioactivity remains at the same spot without migration until cleared by coughing. In this sense coughing appears to be the only means of upward propulsion of the mucus. In 10 patients there was reversal of mucus flow, in 5 migration or straying of radioactivity from one bronchus to that of the opposite lung, bypassing the trachea, followed by shuttling between the right and left main bronchus, finally coughed up upward. In 4 there was spiral or zigzag transport of radioactivity as shown in Fig. 10.16.

In other series of patients with obstructive airways disease radioaerosol inhalation lung cine-scintigraphy frequently showed not only the shuttling of mucus between the right and left main bronchus but also migration of mucus from one region of the lung into the different regions of the same lung [5].

By trajectory mode analysis the trajectory in patients with COPD is simpler in shape than that in a normal subject because stasis ratio becomes higher as shown in Fig. 10.14 [6].

Bronchiectasis

In bronchiectatic lung regions the deposition of inhaled radioaerosols is diminished and inhomogeneous. Radioaerosol inhalation lung cine-scintigraphy has revealed that transport of inhaled radioactivity from the bronchiectatic regions is greatly deranged. Regional stasis was observed in 12 of the 20 patients studied, regurgitation or reversed transport in 14, straying in 8, and spiral or zigzag motion in 1. The transport patterns were more or less the combinations of these four basic abnormal transport patterns. When coughs occur, regurgitation and straying become more marked in the bronchiectatic regions. Only coughs can squeeze out radioactive mucus from inside the bronchiectatic regions to outside. Mucociliary clearance from the bronchiectatic regions is very inefficient without the help of coughing. These regional abnormalities in mucociliary transport seem to be responsible for the development of infections and hemoptysis in the bronchiectatic regions [9].

Bronchogenic Carcinoma

Abnormal mucociliary transport patterns such as regurgitation, straying, stasis, and spiral or zigzag motions are seen in bronchogenic carcinoma especially when complicated by obstructive airways disease. Abnormal mucous transport patterns have nothing to do with the histological diagnosis of bronchogenic carcinoma but with the degrees of functional and anatomical airways obstruction.

Bronchial invasion or protrusion of cancer in the large airways is often recognized as "hot spots" which persist or disappear over time depending on the degree of mucosal damage. When a tumor is covered with intact ciliary mucosa, the hot spots disappear with time, but it persists there when the bronchial mucus is denuded of by the tumor [10].

Idiopathic Interstitial Fibrosis and Pulmonary Vascular Disease

Transport on the large airways does not differ from that in normal subjects unless complicated with obstructive airways disease. If complicated with COPD, similar transport patterns to those encountered in patients with COPD are observed [11, 12].

Ciliated Airways in Lung Parenchyma

Normal Subjects

The data in Tables 10.1–10.4 demonstrate the following:

■ LRR is 85%–90%, 80%–85%, and 75%–80% at 30, 60, and 90 min, respectively

- ALDR is equivalent to the LRR at 24 h and amounts to about 40%
- ADR immediately after inhalation is about 60% and decreases with time to 50%, 45%, and 40% at 30, 60, and 90 min, respectively
- ARR is 80%–85%, 65%–70%, 60%–65% at 30, 60, and 90 min, respectively
- ACE is 15%–20%, 30%– 35%, 35%–40% at 30, 60, and 90 min, respectively

Normal smokers show a slightly faster clearance than nonsmokers [7]. ALDR values are significantly larger in normal nonsmokers than in normal smokers (Table 10.5).

Table 10.5. Sex, smoking, age, pack-year (PY), alveolar deposition ratio (ALDR) and $FEV_{1.0}\%$

Case no.	Sex	Smoking	Age (years)	PY	ALDR	$FEV_{1.0}\%$
1	M	E	43	7	47	85.5
2	M	E	33	6	30	72.9
3	M	E	32	3	47	88.8
4	M	N	29	0	44	77.5
5	M	N	30	0	47	81.3
6	M	N	76	0	40	76.6
7	M	N	76	0	41	76.6
8	M	N	29	0	43	86.4
9	M	N	31	0	48	91.1
10	M	N	25	0	50	75.9
11	M	N	28	0	43	75.9
12	M	N	33	0	46	90.6
13	M	N	41	0	44	78
14	M	S	36	24	37	75.3
15	M	S	32	18	38	81.2
16	M	S	37	26	44	81.1
17	M	S	51	50	31	82.4
18	M	S	38	18	37	76.3
19	M	S	47	41	34	78
20	M	S	28	8	55	86.9
21	M	S	38	27	34	86
22	M	S	58	65	15	72.7
23	M	S	38	27	35	86
24	M	S	58	65	22	73.6
25	M	S	32	13	35	83.6
26	M	S	28	10	39	93
27	M	S	34	21	32	83.2
28	M	S	29	9	39	88.5
Nonsmokers ($n=13$)	–	–	38.9±17.2	0	43.8±5	81.3±6.3
Smokers ($n=15$)	–	–	38.9±10	28.1±18.8	35.1±9	81.9±5.8
Normals ($n=28$)	–	–	38.9±13.5	0	39.2±8.5	81.6±6

M, Male; E, exsmoker; N, nonsmoker; S, smoker

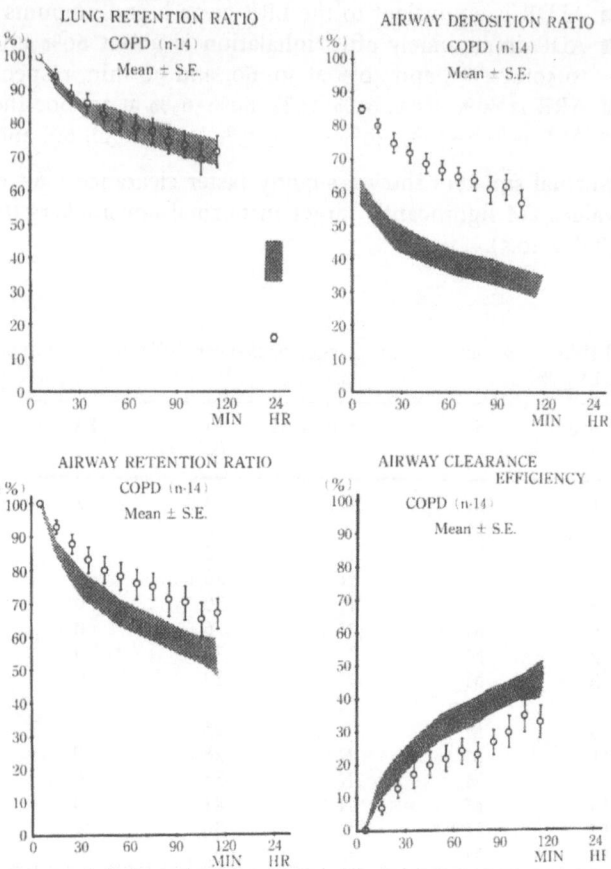

Fig. 10.17. Five parameters in patients with COPD. ALDR equivalent to LRR at 24 h and ACE are significantly decreased, and ADR and ARR, increased. LRR remains within normal limits. *Bands*, means and 95% confidence intervals

Obstructive Airways Disease

As shown in Fig. 10.17, LRR itself is not distinguishable from the normal range, but ALDR is significantly less than normal range. Both ADR and ARR are higher and ACC lower than the normal range, indicating a larger proportion of inhaled aerosol deposits in the ciliated airways and that mucociliary clearance is less efficient [5].

Idiopathic Interstitial Fibrosis and Pulmonary Vascular Disease

As shown in Fig. 10.18, all the parameters remain in the normal range [11, 12].

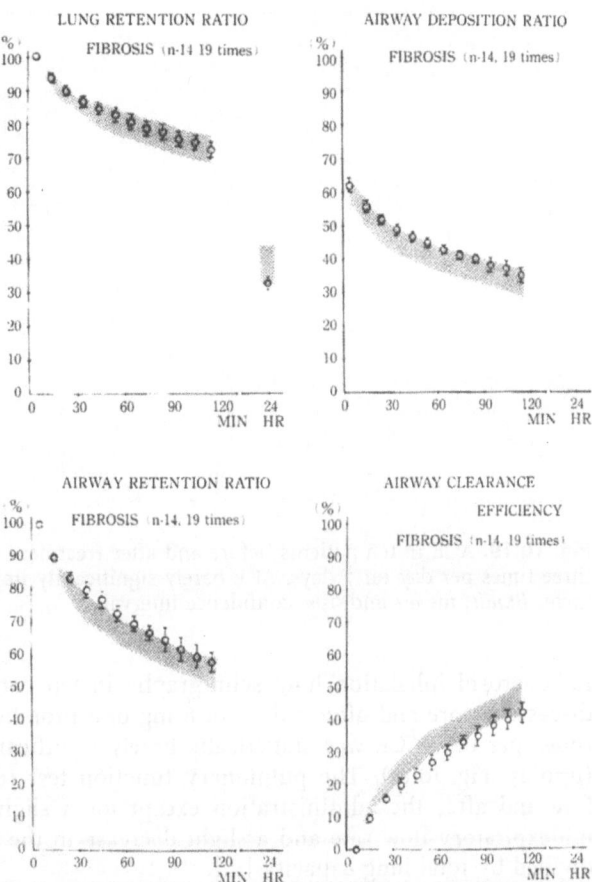

Fig. 10.18. Five parameters in patients with interstitial fibrosis. All five parameters remain within normal range in patients with interstitial fibrosis. *Bands*, means and 95% confidence intervals

Pharmacological Effects

Clinical effects of mucolytic agents and bronchodilators have been evaluated rather subjectively on the basis of patients' sense of clinical improvement. Quantitative evaluation is possible with the present methods of radioaerosol inhalation and subsequent sequential imaging and measurement of radioactivity of the lungs. Reports thus far regarding drug effects are rather conflicting [13–16].

Bromhexine

Bromhexine is claimed to liquefy mucus by breaking the mucopolysaccharide chains in the mucus, thus facilitating its removal. ACE was evaluated by

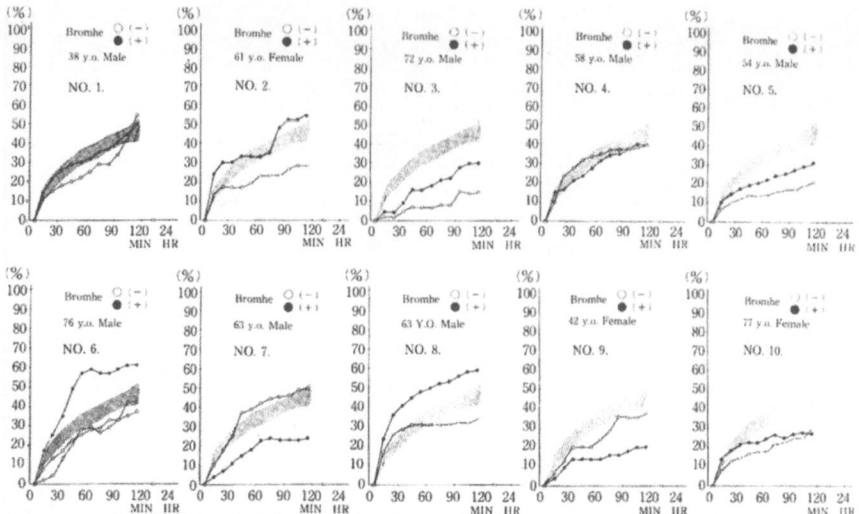

Fig. 10.19. ACE in ten patients before and after treatment with oral bromhexine 8 mg three times per day for 7 days. ACE barely significantly improved (*p*=0.05) after treatment. *Bands*, means and 95% confidence intervals

radioaerosol inhalation lung scintigraphy in ten patients with various chest diseases before and after 7 days of 8 mg oral bromhexine administered three times per day. ACE was statistically barely significantly improved by χ^2 test (*p*=0.05; Fig. 10.19). The pulmonary function test revealed little change before and after the administration except for a slight increase in maximum midexpiratory flow rate and a slight decrease in the ratio of residual volume divided by total lung capacity [17].

β_2-Stimulators

It is known that ciliary beat frequency in vitro is increased by the administration of salbutamol [18]. Oral administration of salbutamol 8 mg three times per day for 7 days did not change either radioaerosol inhalation lung images or quantitative parameters compared with baseline, although the pulmonary function test showed significant bronchodilation after 7 days' administration [19].

In the midst of radioactive measurement following radioaerosol inhalation the β_2-stimulator procaterol was inhaled to determine whether there is a change in shape of the time-activity curve. If the curve over the lungs becomes steeper, we could judge that the mucociliary clearance is accelerated by the medication. However, there was a significant acceleration neither in mucous transport by radioaerosol inhalation lung cine-scintigraphy, in the slope of time-activity curves, nor in any quantitative parameters in patients with bronchial asthma in remission, although spirometry indicated significant bronchodilation [20].

Aminophylline and β_2-Stimulator

Radioaerosol inhalation lung cine-scintigraphy and pulmonary function test were performed on ten patients with bronchial asthma in remission before and after 250 mg aminophylline infusion followed by inhalation of salbutamol. The bronchodilating effect of the combined treatment was significant; inhaled aerosol deposited more homogeneously and less centrally in the lungs. The penetration index increased from 31%±3% to 49%±7% and the alveolar deposition ratio from 29%±2% to 39%±1%. The ADR decreased from 72%±2% to 61%±1% immediately after the treatment. Spirometry indicated significant bronchodilation. However, there was little qualitative or quantitative improvement in mucociliary clearance after the treatment [21].

References

1. Isawa T, Hirano T, Teshima T, Konno K (1980) Effect of non-filtered and filtered cigarette smoke on mucociliary clearance mechanism. Tohoku J Exp Med 130:189–197
2. Hirano T (1988) Mucociliary clearance mechanisms. II. Acute effect of cigarette smoke with and without filter and recovery from its damaging effect on tracheal mucous velocity. Kohkenshi 40:115–127
3. Isawa T, Teshima T, Hirano T, Ebina A, Konno K (1981) Radioaerosol inhalation lung cine-scintigraphy: a preliminary report. Tohoku J Exp Med 134:245–255
4. Isawa T, Teshima T, Hirano T, Ebina A, Konno K (1984) Mucociliary clearance mechanisms in smoking and nonsmoking normal subjects. J Nucl Med 25:352–359
5. Isawa T, Teshima T, Hirano T, Ebina A, Motomiya M, Konno K (1984) Lung clearance mechanisms in obstructive airways disease. J Nucl Med 25:447–454
6. Teshima T, Isawa T, Hirano T, Anazawa Y, Miki M, Motomiya M (1989) Image processing for mucociliary transport system. Respiration 8:828–835
7. Isawa T, Teshima T, Hirano T, Anazawa Y, Miki M, Konno K, Motomiya M (1989) Normal values for quantitative parameters for evaluation of mucociliary clearance in lungs. Tohoku J Exp Med 158:119–131
8. Miki M, Isawa T, Teshima T, Anazawa Y, Motomiya M (1992) Difference in inhaled aerosol deposition patterns in the lungs due to three different sized aerosols. Nucl Med Commun 13:553–562
9. Isawa T, Teshima T, Hirano T, Anazawa Y, Miki M, Konno, K, Motomiya M (1990) Mucociliary clearance and transport in bronchiectasis: global and regional assessment. J Nucl Med 31:543–548
10. Isawa T, Teshima T, Hirano T, Ebina A, Konno K (1986) Mucociliary clearance mechanisms in lung cancer. Kohkenshi 38:147–157
11. Isawa T, Teshima T, Hirano T, Ebina A, Konno K (1986) Mucociliary clearance mechanism in interstitial lung disease. Tohoku J Exp Med 148:169–178
12. Isawa T, Teshima T, Hirano T, Ebina A, Anazawa Y, Konno K (1988) Mucociliary clearance in pulmonary vascular disease. Ann Nucl Med 2:41–47
13. Sackner MA (1978) Effects of respiratory drugs on mucociliary clearance. Chest 73 [Suppl]:958–964
14. Matthys H, Koehler D (1980) Effect of theophylline on mucociliary clearance in man. Eur J Respir Dis [Suppl] 109:98–102
15. Wanner A (1981) Alteration of tracheal mucociliary transport in airway disease. Effect of pharmacologic agents. Chest 80 [Suppl]:967–870
16. Pavia D, Sutton PP, Lopez-Vidriero, MT, Agnew JE, Clarke SW (1983) Drug effects on mucociliary function. Eur J Respir Dis 64 [Suppl 128]:304–317

17. Isawa T, Teshima T, Hirano T, Ebina A, Konno K (1984) Evaluation of mucociliary clearance mechanisms by radioaerosol inhalation lung scintigraphy - effect of oral bromhexine. J Jpn Soc Chest Dis 22:899–909
18. Van As (1974) The role of selective beta 2-adrenoreceptor stimulants in the control of ciliary activity. Respiration 31:146–151
19. Isawa T, Teshima T, Hirano T, Ebina A, Konno K (1986) Effect of oral salbutamol on mucociliary clearance mechanisms in the lungs. Tohoku J Exp Med 150:51–61
20. Isawa T, Teshima T, Hirano T, Anazawa Y, Miki M, Konno K, Motomiya M (1990) Does a beta 2-stimulator really facilitate mucociliary transport in the human lungs in vivo? Am Rev Respir Dis 141:715–720
21. Isawa T, Teshima T, Hirano T, Ebina A, Anazawa Y, Konno K (1987) Effect of bronchodilation on the deposition and clearance of radioaerosol in bronchial asthma in remission. J Nucl Med 28:1901–1906

11 Heart Scan

D. S. LEE and M. C. LEE

Myocardial Perfusion Scan

Myocardial blood flow can be evaluated either by myocardial perfusion scan or by single photon emission computed tomography (SPECT). Myocardial perfusion is the nutrient supply for myocardium – a muscle that has a reserve of about three to five times the normal level after stress [128]. Coronary arteries supply blood to the myocardium, and fixed stenosis of coronary arteries can limit the flow reserve of myocardium and even limit rest perfusion. Assessment of perfusion by myocardial perfusion scan and SPECT provides information about the clinical significance of fixed stenosis of coronary arteries.

Myocardial perfusion scan is used for diagnosis in patients suspected of having coronary artery disease. It is also useful for establishing a prognosis in patients with no known coronary artery disease and for risk stratification in patients with postmyocardial infarction, unstable angina, or postcatheterization, in postrevascularization patients, and for risk stratification of noncardiac surgery [10, 113].

Physiology and Pathophysiology of Myocardial Blood Flow

Blood flow in the entire human body is about 5–6 l min^{-1}; cardiac output is the source of this blood flow. If we assume that blood flow is distributed evenly all over body tissues, 1 g tissue has a blood flow of 0.07 ml min^{-1} (5 l/min divided by 70 kg). Blood flow in cardiac muscles is about ten times the average for the whole body. The resting level of blood flow of the myocardium is 0.6–0.8 ml min^{-1} g^{-1}.

Exercise is a common form of physiological stimulus for recruiting the perfusion reserve of the myocardium. Exercise increases cardiac output by increasing heart rate 300% and stroke volume 20%–30% [30]. The level of cardiac output reached after exercise is three or more times the normal level. An increase in cardiac output means an increase in the velocity of blood volume propelled by heart. Cardiac output, as blood flow throughout the body, must meet the demand of increased myocardial perfusion. A minimal dilation of coronary vessels meets the remaining portion of increase. In this sense coronary artery vasodilator is another term for myocardial blood flow enhancer.

Myocardial ischemia is the existence of a deficit of perfusion in relation to the demands of whole body. Fixed stenotic coronary arteries may limit the perfusion reserve although the resting flow is normal. Exercise causes demand ischemia in the myocardium supplied by stenotic arteries. Neurohumoral mediation is the link between the demand and the supply of blood flow to the myocardium. Some of its mediators or analogues such as adenosine and dobutamine may be used as an alternative enhancer of coronary blood flow. Dipyridamole, adenosine, nitrates, and papaverine are simultaneously coronary vasodilators and perfusion enhancers.

Exertional or stress-induced ischemia may either cause angina or remain silent. Reversible perfusion decrease or defect is observed in stress-redistribution or rest-stress myocardial SPECT.

Stress Test

Exercise Stress

Two types of stress are commonly used in most laboratories: the treadmill with modified Bruce protocol and supine bicycle exercise with ergometer. Exercise stress induces demand ischemia in patients who have significant stenosis in their coronary arteries. Dobutamine mimics exercise in that it increases heart rate and induces demand ischemia.

Treadmill Exercise

The modified Bruce protocol increases exercise every 3 min until the heart rate reaches 85% of anticipated maximal heart rate [30]. If patients tolerate the exercise without symptoms, we inject radiopharmaceuticals and have them exercise 60 or 90 s more. If patients complain of exhaustion or dizziness, or if hypotension, arrhythmia, or ischemic electrocardiographic changes are noted, radiopharmaceuticals are injected, and the study is then completed. ^{201}Tl images are acquired 5–7 min later. Images with ^{99m}Tc-labeled compounds are acquired between 30 min and 2 h later.

During treadmill exercise both stroke volume and heart rates are increased (Table 11.1).

Supine Bicycle Exercise

We use 25–50 W initially and increase by 25 W per 2–3 min. Some patients become so tired in their legs that they cannot finish the exercise in supine position. Stroke volume with this type of exercise is the same as that in the resting state [30], heart rate is increased.

Table 11.1. Comparison of characteristics of myocardial stress

Vasodilation	Increase in cardiac output	
	Increase in heart rate and stroke volume	Increase in heart rate
Exercise Dobutamine Coronary vasodilators	Treadmill exercise	Supine bicycle exercise Dobutamine Rapid atrial pacing

Table 11.2. Coronary vasodilators and their characteristics

	Dipyridamole	Adenosine	Dobutamine
Administered dose	0.14 mg min^{-1} kg^{-1} for 4 min	0.14 mg min^{-1} kg^{-1} for 6 min	40 µg min^{-1} kg^{-1}, incremental from 5 µg
Half-life	30 min	37 s	120 s
Contraindication	Asthma	Asthma	Same as exercise
Antidote	Aminophylline	Stop injection	–

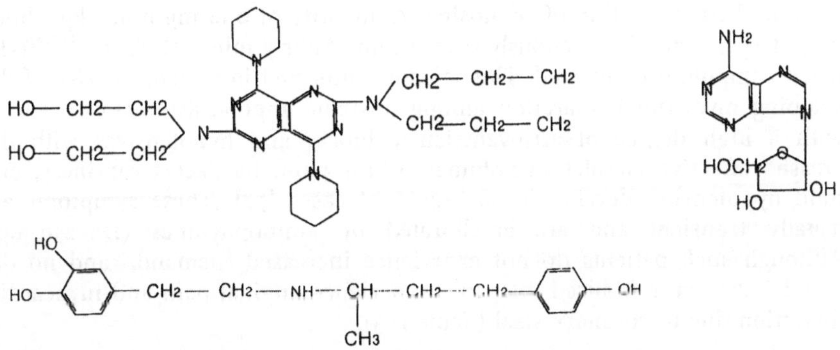

Fig. 11.1. Structure of coronary vasodilators: dipyridamole, adenosine, dobutamine

Pharmacological Stress

Coronary vasodilators are used to disclose the maximal capacity of a coronary vessel of interest (Table 11.2, Fig. 11.1). Myocardium supplied with stenotic artery shows less dilatation than myocardium supplied with normal artery. With pharmacological stress, cardiac output is not increased, in contrast to exercise stress, and coronary artery vasodilation is the major mechanism of increase in coronary blood flow (Table 11.1). Resistance vessels are the main sites of dilation.

Dipyridamole and adenosine may cause ischemic segments to experience coronary steal. Less perfusion at stress than at rest makes ischemic segments hypokinetic. Wall motion abnormalities disclosed by coronary steal are

Table 11.3. Side effects of dipyridamole

Mild		Severe	
Condition	Per 100 persons	Condition	Per 10 000 persons
Chest pain	9.7%	Death	0.95%
Headache	9.6%	Myocardial infarction	1.76%
Dizziness	9.6%	Sustained ventricular arrythmia	0.81%
Flushing	9.6%	Transient ischemic attack	1.22%
Nausea	9.6%	Severe bronchoconstriction	1.22%
Hypotension	0.1%		

exploited in pharmacological stress echocardiography. Nitroglycerine dilates coronary arteries but rarely causes coronary steal, probably because collateral vessels are also dilated [11].

Dipyridamole Stress

Dipyridamole blocks the clearance of endogenous adenosine and increases the blood concentration of adenosine. A quantity of 0.14 mg min^{-1} kg^{-1} body weight is injected intravenously over 4 min. After 3 min a ^{201}Tl- or ^{99m}Tc-labeled compound is injected. This is contraindicated in patients at risk of developing myocardial infarction among unstable angina, asthmatics, patients with a high degree of atrioventricular block, and hypotensives with decreased effective circulation volumes. Chest pain, headache, dizziness, and mild hypotension develop in 30%–40% of cases [77]. These symptoms are usually transient and are ameliorated by aminophyllines (125–250 mg). Although such patients do not experience increased "demand," and no demand ischemia is induced, they can experience anginal pain and myocardial infarction due to coronary steal (Table 11.3).

Adenosine Stress

Adenosine acts directly on coronary arteries [102]. A quantity of 0.14 mg min^{-1} kg^{-1} body weight is injected intravenously for 6 min. After 4 min a ^{201}Tl- or ^{99m}Tc-labeled compound is injected. Atrioventricular blocks, chest pain, headache, and hypotension may develop. As adenosine has a half-life of 37 s, it is sufficient to stop infusion when side effects develop.

Dobutamine Stress

Dobutamine is a β_1 stimulant and offers an alternative to exercise [40, 53, 87]. Heart rate, cardiac output, and myocardial perfusion are increased. This agent is not contraindicated in patients with asthma or hypotension. Dobutamine administration begins with the dose of 5 µg min^{-1} kg^{-1} body weight and increases to 40 µg. Rapid atrial pacing may increase heart rate, cardiac output, and myocardial blood flow. This may be used as another type of stress.

Methods of Myocardial Scintigraphy

Planar Scintigraphy

Anterior, left anterior oblique 30° or 45°, and left lateral or left anterior oblique 70° images are obtained after stress and at redistribution or rest. Right lateral decubitus or prone position is used to obtain left lateral images. Attenuation by breasts is easily discerned as the appearance of these artifacts is the same on stress and on rest images. We use this imaging method only when SPECT facilities are not available.

SPECT

Preparation

β-Blockers are not administered in the 48 h immediately before a study using stress to increase heart rates. Nitrates and calcium channel blockers are stopped for 24 h. Pharmacological stress can be used to test whether the patient's heart tolerates stress while the patient takes anti-ischemic drugs such as nitrates and potassium channel enhancers. Maintenance of antihypertensive drugs are recommended. No foods are allowed for 4 h before stress. Caffeine-containing beverages and drugs should be prohibited as these are antidotes against dipyridamole or adenosine.

Differences Between Radiopharmaceuticals

- The flow estimated by ^{82}Rb positron-emission tomography (PET) is best in relation to the flow measured directly with microsphere. ^{201}Tl uptake is somewhat less linear, and ^{99m}Tc-labeled methoxyisobutylisonitrile (MIBI) is more curvilinear.
- The area with decreased uptake of ^{201}Tl at stress is somewhat larger than that obtained with ^{99m}Tc-MIBI.
- The defect obtained by ^{201}Tl SPECT injected at rest is the same as the defect at rest shown by ^{99m}Tc-MIBI SPECT [92].

Net extraction fraction is not the only factor to consider in determining which radiopharmaceutical would yield us the most precise information about myocardial perfusion; the gamma-ray energy and penetrability, the resolution of the system, and the amount of radioactivity injected should also be taken into consideration. ^{99m}Tc-MIBI uptake may underestimate viability as ^{99m}Tc-MIBI uptake is less redistributed than ^{201}Tl uptake injected at rest [5, 18, 25]. Diagnostic accuracy does not differ between SPECT using ^{201}Tl and that using ^{99m}Tc-MIBI [17] (Table 11.4).

^{201}Tl Stress-Redistribution SPECT

At peak stress 74–111 MBq (2–3 mCi) ^{201}Tl is injected, and the stress image is acquired. After 4 h a redistribution image is obtained (Fig. 11.2 a, b). Upward creep of heart from its lower position just after exercise makes very early imaging undesirable. On the other hand, redistribution begins immediately after the completion of stress, and we therefore cannot wait long. We should use a window period to acquire the best stress images without artifacts due to either of the above factors.

Stress acquisition starts preferably 5–7 min after injection. The shorter the acquisition time, the more the images reflect the stress status. Stress perfusion observed with ^{201}Tl SPECT to represent coronary artery disease has a similar or slightly inferior capability than ^{82}Rb PET [37, 122]. Redistributed images are usually normal in mild stenosis with less ischemia. If the stenosis is more severe, and myocardium is hibernating, there is severely decreased perfusion or defect at redistribution. Reinjection or delayed acquisition of redistribution enables us to differentiate hibernating from nonviable myocardium among these segments [22, 105].

Rest-Stress or Stress-Rest ^{99m}Tc-MIBI SPECT

^{99m}Tc-MIBI is injected separately at rest and at stress (Fig. 11.2 c, d). The separate-day protocol can be used but the same-day protocol is that which is adopted in most laboratories. Either the rest or the stress image may be acquired first, that is, one can use either the rest-stress or the stress-rest protocol. The ability of the two protocols to detect ischemic areas is the same.

The first study is performed with 370 MBq (10 mCi) and the second with 1110 MBq (30 mCi). Fatty meals such as egg and milk facilitate the excretion of radioactivity from the liver. A rest defect is usually overestimated in the same-day/stress-rest protocol because half of the activity distributed at stress remains when another image is acquired at rest. Furthermore, stress perfusion is at least three times as great as rest perfusion. Therefore rest activity has an uneven background inherited from the stress study.

Some persistent defects found with stress-rest study are reversible with a rest-stress study [49], i.e., reversibility is underestimated by stress-rest study. On the other hand, because of the even background radioactivity ischemic segments cannot be detected in the same-day/rest-stress protocol [133].

Table 11.4. Diagnostic accuracy of ^{201}Tl, ^{99m}Tc-MIBI, and ^{99m}Tc-tetrofosmin myocardial perfusion SPECT

Method	Sensitivity	Specificity	Normalcy ratio	References
^{201}Tl SPECT	89% (1343/1500)	75% (275/344)	89% (265/297)	
Excercise redistribution ^{201}Tl SPECT	90% (938/1042)	70% (163/239)	89% (209/235)	[41, 57, 65, 67, 111]
Adenosine redistribution ^{201}Tl SPECT	87% (190/216)	89% (79/89)	–	[41, 102, 103]
Dobutamine/arbutamine redistribution ^{201}Tl SPECT	87% (150/172)	93% (15/16)	90% (56/62)	[53, 69]
Dipyridamole redistribution ^{201}Tl SPECT	93% (65/70)	–	–	[43]
^{99m}Tc-MIBI SPECT	87% (484/555)	73% (138/188)	–	
Rest exercise ^{99m}Tc-MIBI SPECT	87% (224/256)	72% (49/68)	87% (54/62)	[57, 65, 66, 110, 131]
Rest dipyridamole ^{99m}Tc-MIBI SPECT	87% (28/31)	–	–	[17]
Rest adenosine ^{99m}Tc-MIBI SPECT	90% (138/153)	74% (58/78)	92% (65/70)	[4, 87]
Rest dobutamine ^{99m}Tc-MIBI SPECT	84% (72/86)	74% (31/42)	95% (56/59)	[40, 87]
Attenuation corrected ^{99m}Tc-MIBI SPECT	84% (50/60)	–	–	[29]
Gated ^{99m}Tc-MIBI SPECT	87% (200/230)	69% (31/45)	92% (175/191)	[61]
Dual isotope separate acquisition	85% (202/237)	74% (28/38)	91% (181/199)	
^{201}Tl/exercise ^{99m}Tc-MIBI	85% (150/176)	74% (28/38)	91% (181/199)	[8, 50, 91]
^{201}Tl/dipyridamole ^{99m}Tc-MIBI	85% (52/61)	–	–	[138]

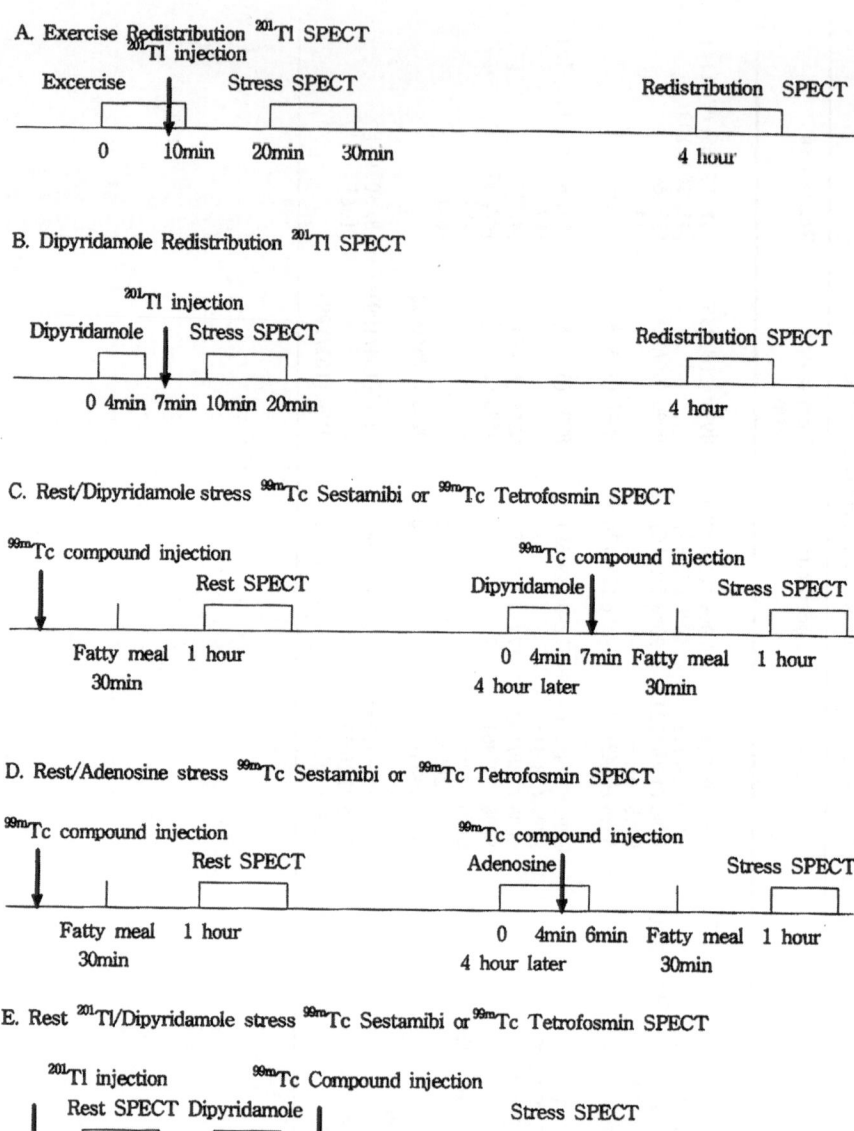

Fig. 11.2. Protocols for stress-rest or redistribution myocardial perfusion SPECT

Imaging and Reconstruction

A low-energy parallel-hole collimator is used for ^{201}Tl images. Projection images of 180° are used from 45° right anterior oblique to 45° left posterior oblique. Vertical, triple-head, or cardiofocal cameras are used.

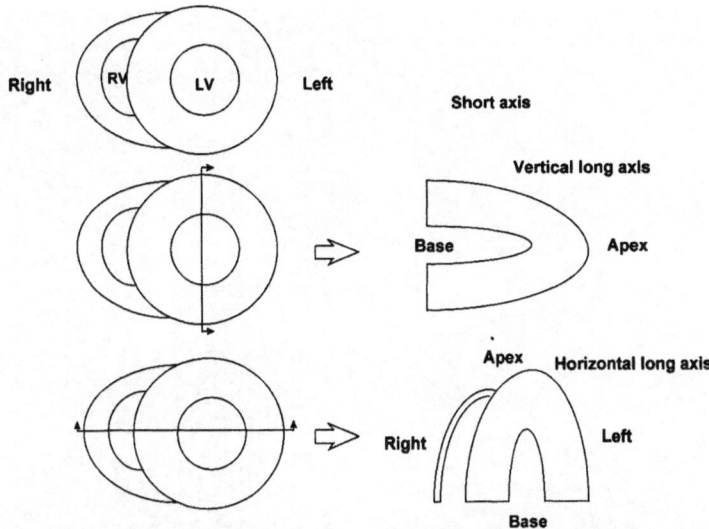

Fig. 11.3. Display for SPECT images. *RV*, right ventricle; *LV*, left ventricle. (Modified from ACC/AHA/SNM policy statement in J Nucl Cardiol 1994; 1:117–119)

A high-resolution parallel-hole collimator is used for ^{99m}Tc-labeled compounds. Projection images of 180° are acquired with the step-and-shoot method with 3° between them. Gated images with 8–16 frames can be acquired to calculate ejection fraction or determine wall motion.

Filtered backprojection or estimation maximization is used for reconstruction. Low-pass filters such as the Butterworth filter are used; alternatively the Metz or Wiener filter may be used. Reconstructed transaxial images are reoriented along the long axis of left ventricle. Short-axis and vertical and horizontal long-axis images are recorded on the monitor or color hardcopy according to Cardiovascular Council of Society of Nuclear Medicine, American College of Cardiologists, and American Heart Association (Fig. 11.3).

Normal Findings

Even homogeneous distribution is characteristic (Fig. 11.4). Inferior wall and septum have 15%–20% less activity. Myocardium of the right ventricle is faint or cannot be discerned. In men the diaphragmatic attenuation is so great that it cannot be differentiated from a real persistent decrease. In women with large breasts the anterior wall is attenuated to such an extent that it may be mistaken as persistent decrease. The apex is often so thin as to make a small persistent decrease. Focally increased activity is found in the direction of 2 and 7 o'clock on short-axis images because of papillary muscles.

Patients with left bundle branch block show decreased activity in the septum. It is believed that this is because septum lacks the time to be perfused

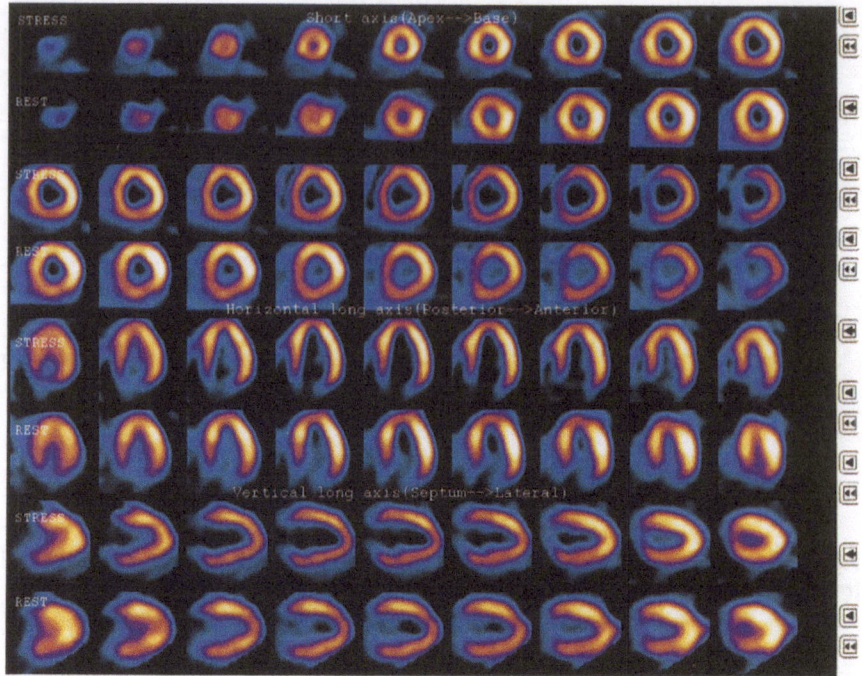

Fig. 11.4. Normal myocardial rest-stress perfusion SPECT

due to shorter diastole against wall stress generated by the right ventricle activated earlier.

Patients with long-standing hypertension usually show more uptake in the septum. The lateral wall may be misinterpreted to have decreased uptakes.

Dual Isotope Separate Acquisition
(Rest ^{201}Tl, Stress ^{99m}Tc-MIBI or ^{99m}Tc-Tetrofosmin SPECT)

One can perform a rest study first with ^{201}Tl and then study stress with ^{99m}Tc-labeled compounds [68, 83] (Fig. 11.2e). As rest images reveal rest perfusion and ^{201}Tl has lower energy, one can ignore crosstalk of the counts from ^{201}Tl to ^{99m}Tc energy ranges [68]. This method has been found to give the same accuracy in predicting significant stenosis of coronary arteries regardless of the stress method [8, 50, 91]. The study can be completed in less than 3 h [83, 138].

Quantitative Analysis

Semiquantitative Scoring

Apical, middle, and basal levels of short-axis images and vertical and horizontal long-axis images are divided into 12–27 segments. Normal, mild, and severe decreases and defects are scored. In comparing stress and rest images one notes persistent, reversible, or partially reversible perfusion decreases.

Polar Map Display and Quantitation

Circumferential profiles are calculated from apex to base and are arrayed side by side to make a circular shape. Anterior, septum, inferior, and lateral walls are displayed. Artery territories can be allocated for left anterior descending artery, right coronary artery, and left circumflex artery (Fig. 11.5). All the activities are normalized to the voxel having the maximal count.

Two methods are available for producing a circumferential profile: the maximal count and the average count for the relevant voxels. In making a circumferential profile we reduce the information by changing the counts of a layer of myocardium to that of a point. Although this means reduction in the quantity of information, polar display of the information helps us to identify what is wrong at a glance.

Stress, rest, delay, and reinjection images can be displayed on polar maps. With cumulative normal data in the system one can make a defect map by comparing each pixel data with a normal database to represent whether it is below the set limit derived from normal database.

Extent-weighted severity may offer a quantitative index to representing the significance of stenotic artery.

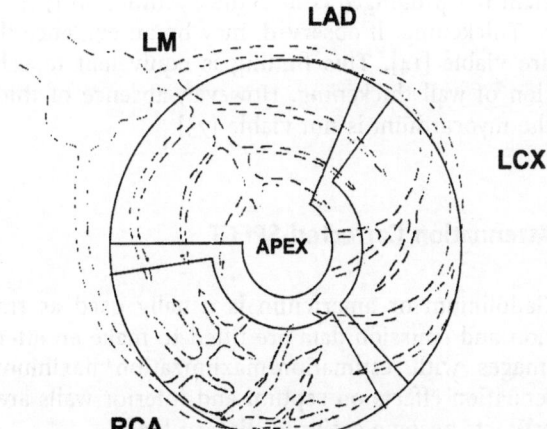

Fig. 11.5. Polar display of three artery territories and their supplying arteries. *LM*, left main artery; *LAD*, left anterior descending artery; *LCX*, left circumflex artery; *RCA*, right coronary artery

Gated Myocardial SPECT

Acquisition Method and Analysis

Either 8 or 16 frames are acquired as gated with electrocardiography. We use 370 or 1110 MBq (10–30 mCi) of ^{99m}Tc-labeled compounds. A period of 10–20 min is long enough to acquire a readable images [93]. Rest wall motion can be evaluated. With poststress gated SPECT images one is observing rest wall motion and stress wall perfusion [14]. Cine loops of images are run on the monitor. Automatically calculated ejection fraction was correct and reproducible [35].

The counts of myocardium are proportional to the wall thickness because the average thickness of myocardium is 10 mm at diastole and 16 mm at systole, and the usual resolution (full width half maximum) of SPECT cameras is 9–12 mm. Thickening is observed as a change in counts and as brightening during systole on the screen [15].

Advantages and Applications

Today's systems usually allow gated acquisition without increasing acquisition time as the system's sensitivity is sufficiently good. The existence of normal wall motions confirms that the wall is well perfused. Mild or severe persistent decrease in tissue perfusion despite normal wall motion should raise doubt as to whether it is artifact. Normal wall motion with persistent perfusion decrease helps to rule out artifacts [19].

Ischemia disclosed by adenosine or dipyridamole is accompanied by transient wall motion abnormality if ischemic segments experience coronary steal. These wall motion abnormalities are so transient that one find rest wall motion in most cases when acquiring stress perfusion gated SPECT images. There were reports of exceptions to these findings: some segments have transient but prolonged contractile dysfunction [74].

Thickening, if observed, may be an evidence that the myocardial segments are viable [14]. This finding is equivalent to echocardiographical confirmation of wall thickening. However, absence of thickening is not evidence that the myocardium is not viable [73].

Attenuation Corrected SPECT

Gadolinium or americium is usually used as transmission source. Attenuation and emission data are fitted to make an attenuation-corrected transverse images with estimation-maximization/maximum-likelihood algorithm. Attenuation effects on septum and inferior walls are compensated properly, and artifacts become easier to discern [29].

Diagnosis of Coronary Artery Disease

Ischemia

Increased blood flow of three to five times is a common flow reserve for normal myocardium. Fixed stenosis of coronary arteries first leads to shortage of reserves and then causes myocardium to lack rest perfusion. As noted above, there are two types of ischemia: stress-induced ischemia and rest ischemia. Rest ischemia is often confused with infarction and necrosis. Rest ischemia is accompanied by wall motion abnormalities. Decreased perfusion with contractile dysfunction is characteristic of rest ischemia.

Perfusion refers to tissue blood flow, and blood flow measured by Doppler means epicardial blood flow. Using intracoronary Doppler imaging, point velocity is measured and averaged, and multiplied by the cross-sectional area of the vessel to yield epicardial blood flow. Flow and perfusion, or flow reserve and perfusion reserve are interchangeable terms in this context.

Interpretation of Stress/Rest Perfusion

Myocardial SPECT can demonstrate which artery has significant stenosis. Reversible perfusion decrease is equivalent to stress-induced ischemia. With ^{201}Tl SPECT one observes redistribution; ^{99m}Tc-MIBI SPECT shows the difference between stress and rest images.

Infarcted myocardium is supplied with only 20%–30% of rest blood flow. A persistent perfusion defect is usually found. Myocardium supplied by a severely stenotic artery has severely decreased uptake at stress and also decreased uptake at rest. This area is said to have a partially reversible perfusion decrease. The cause may be ischemia surrounding infarct or ischemia intermixed with infarct. Very severely stenotic coronary arteries limiting tissue perfusion to this extent can cause a partially reversible perfusion decrease by itself without accompanying infarction. ^{201}Tl SPECT shows partial redistribution.

Reverse redistribution or reverse reversibility is sometimes observed. Washout is faster in these reverse-reversible segments in ^{201}Tl SPECT.

Disclosure of Stenotic Coronary Arteries

Segments of myocardial slices can be allocated to each large artery territory, and, using a polar map, software determines which territory belongs to which artery (Fig. 11.5). Among three vessels that are stenotic over 50% we can find the areas that are ischemic and thus which artery is significantly stenotic. The branch artery has its own location and supplying territory, and we can anticipate the causative artery.

Performance for Diagnosis of Coronary Artery Disease

The gold standard in diagnosing coronary artery disease is coronary angiography. A patient is considered to have coronary artery disease when there is more than 50% stenosis in one or more of the following arteries: left main, left anterior descending, left circumflex, right coronary, diagonal artery, first, second, or third septal branches, first, second, or third obtuse marginal arteries, or posterior descending artery [116] (Fig. 11.6).

Diagnostic performance is expressed as sensitivity and specificity of SPECT in determining single-, two-, or three-vessel disease patients with myocardial stress-rest SPECT. Sensitivity is 73%–83% for single-vessel disease, 87%–93% in two-vessel disease, and 95%–97% in three-vessel disease. Diagnostic sensitivity is 53%–87% for the left anterior descending artery, 30%–78% for the left circumflex artery, and 62%–92% for the right coronary artery [80].

Sensitivity levels substantially below 100% indicate that stenotic arteries sometimes do not always make a reversible or persistent perfusion decrease or defect on the corresponding artery territories. The characteristics of stenotic vessels (diffuse, tandem, concentric, distal, long-segment, etc.), the rapid or slow progress of the stenosis, compensation by collaterals, cooperation, and suffering of adjacent myocardium make this difference.

Low specificity is usually due to the postreferral bias in negative cases (Table 11.4). When SPECT results are negative, we do not perform angiography. This decreases the number of true-negative cases and thus specificity, as specificity is calculated by the formula: true negative/(true negative+false positive).

Acute Myocardial Infarction

Diagnosis

Typical chest pain, electrocardiographic changes, and elevated cardiac enzymes are the diagnostic triad for acute myocardial infarction. It is rare to use myocardial SPECT only to diagnose acute myocardial infarction. However, rest myocardial SPECT can be employed to assess infarcted myocardium at risk [119]. ^{99m}Tc-labeled compounds are injected upon arrival at the emergency room, and SPECT images are acquired after the patient's condition stabilizes [52].

Stress and rest images show similar perfusion defects. Over time the development of collateral circulation and revascularization allows the infarcted myocardium to take up ^{201}Tl- or ^{99m}Tc-labeled compounds. This reduces sensitivity if radiopharmaceuticals are injected later.

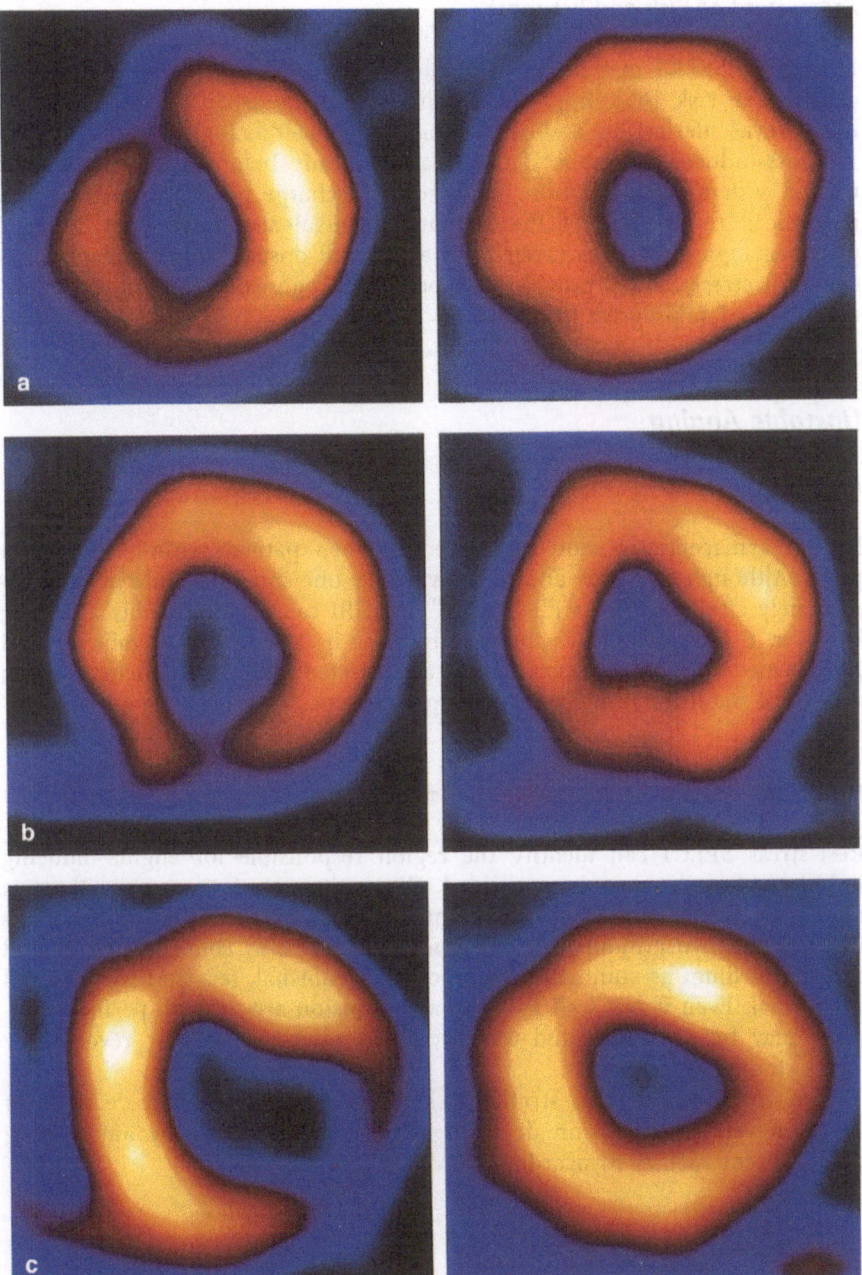

Fig. 11.6 a–c. Stress-rest myocardial SPECT findings. **a** Reversible perfusion decrease in the territory of left anterior descending artery. **b** Reversible perfusion decrease in the territory of right coronary artery. **c** Reversible perfusion defect in the territory of left circumflex artery. *Left*, stress; *right*, rest

Assessment of Risk and Prognosis

Myocardial SPECT in acute myocardial infarction can assess the size of myocardium at risk [99], improvement in myocardial perfusion after spontaneous revascularization, and development of collaterals [82].

Stress-induced ischemia, if found at the study before discharge, can be treated with revascularization. In these predischarge patients exercise stress is reduced to one-half of the metabolic equivalent (Met) value; however, pharmacological stress is carried out at the full dose. Predischarge pharmacological stress SPECT provides independent prognostic information for the recovery or late progress [81, 98].

Unstable Angina

Diagnosis

Radiopharmaceuticals should be injected when patients suffer from chest pains. Although ^{201}Tl may always be available, one should acquire images immediately after injection with ^{201}Tl. ^{99m}Tc-MIBI can also be readily available; however, this is not always the case because it takes about 30 min to label MIBI. Once ^{99m}Tc-labeled compounds are injected into these patients, we can wait until stabilization before acquiring an image.

Identification of Ischemia and Prognosis

Rest-stress SPECT can identify the region responsible for angina-inducing ischemia after the pain has subsided. When the pain is gone, and there is normal perfusion in the relevant region, we consider the event to be reversible and the myocardium viable. If contractility is also abnormal, we regard the myocardium as stunned. If contractility is normal, rest perfusion should be normal. Even if rest wall motion and perfusion are normal, perfusion reserve may be abnormal, and this decreased reserve is usually revealed by stress study.

Myocardial SPECT can stratify risk by assessing perfusion decrease at stress. Reversible perfusion decrease determines prognosis by anticipating cardiac event such as myocardial infarction and cardiac death.

Assessment of Revascularization

Revascularization of Coronary Arteries

Thrombolysis in patients with acute myocardial infarction, percutaneous transluminal coronary angioplasty, and coronary artery bypass graft in patients with chronic coronary artery disease can revive ischemic dysfunctional myocardium. Success of revascularization is usually documented by coronary angiography immediately after treatment. However, there is a period of discrepancy between improvement in tissue perfusion and patency of epicardial parts of large coronary arteries [85].

Contrast echocardiography recently confirmed the "no-reflow" phenomenon. Parallel to this finding, myocardial SPECT usually shows delayed improvement after reperfusion. Only 76% of the reperfused myocardial segments improve 1–2 days on exercise SPECT after angioplasty with or without residual stenosis [85]. Pharmacological stress SPECT better represents the improvement in myocardial perfusion after angioplasty [58]. Some defects improve after 3–4 weeks.

Restenosis is expected in 30%–40% of patients 6 months after angioplasty. Stent application decreases the restenosis rate to 10%–20%. One can find restenosis early after 4 weeks. Perfusion SPECT detects restenosis after successful angioplasty [97] (Fig. 11.7). The window period should be chosen between delayed improvement and development of restenosis in evaluating the effect of angioplasty.

Coronary artery bypass surgery is the definitive treatment for fixed stenosis. Initial technical failure in addition to perioperative myocardial infarction is reported to be between 4% and 40% (usually less than 20%). Underlying atherosclerosis cannot be cured with bypass surgery, and graft artery is affected by progressive process of atherosclerosis in these patients. Because myocardium suffers more during operation, including cardioplegic solution, improvement in tissue perfusion may be delayed somewhat. It is recommended to wait 3–6 weeks for delayed improvement in evaluating the effect of surgery by observing perfusion improvement (Fig. 11.8).

The patency of coronary bypass graft can be evaluated better with myocardial perfusion rest-stress SPECT than with exercise electrocardiography [72]. Late after surgery the myocardial SPECT findings add incremental prognostic value to the other variable [106].

Diagnosis of Viable Myocardium

Definition of Viability

Improved wall motion in the relevant area of myocardium after revascularization is evidence of viable myocardium. Ascertaining viable myocardium which could benefit from revascularization is one of the most important problems in cardiology clinics. This helps to guide clinicians in deciding whether a patient should be operated on. A good noninvasive method to find viable myocardium should have excellent positive and/or negative predictive values [56]. Without proper management patients having viable myocardium usually experience progressive worsening of cardiac function or eventual cardiac events [20, 127].

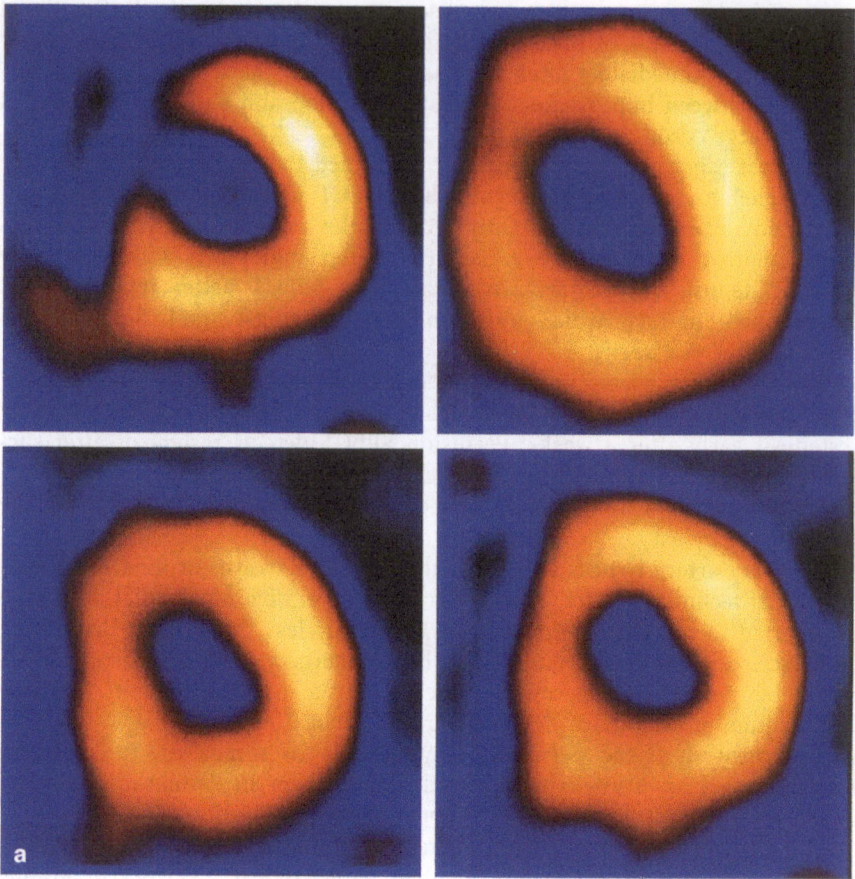

Fig. 11.7 a. Myocardial ischemia in the territory of left anterior descending artery improved after the first percutaneous transluminal coronary angioplasty (PTCA). Post-PTCA image was acquired 1 week after. *Upper row*, pre-angioplasty (1st); *lower row*, post-angioplasty; *left*, stress; *right* rest

Prediction of Viable Myocardium by SPECT

Myocardium showing normal perfusion at rest is definitely viable. Viable myocardium at risk often shows decreased perfusion at rest. Perfusion alone cannot predict viability as areas with decreased perfusion may be vital. However, there are reports that viability can be predicted to some degree by evaluating rest perfusion [38, 140]. This is because coronary blood flow is nutrient flow to myocardial muscle, and flow and oxygen metabolism are closely proportional in most cases [129]. Myocardial segments with mild rest decrease are generally viable.

Segments with severe perfusion decrease at rest should not be defined as nonviable. About 56% of myocardial segments with decreased rest perfusion

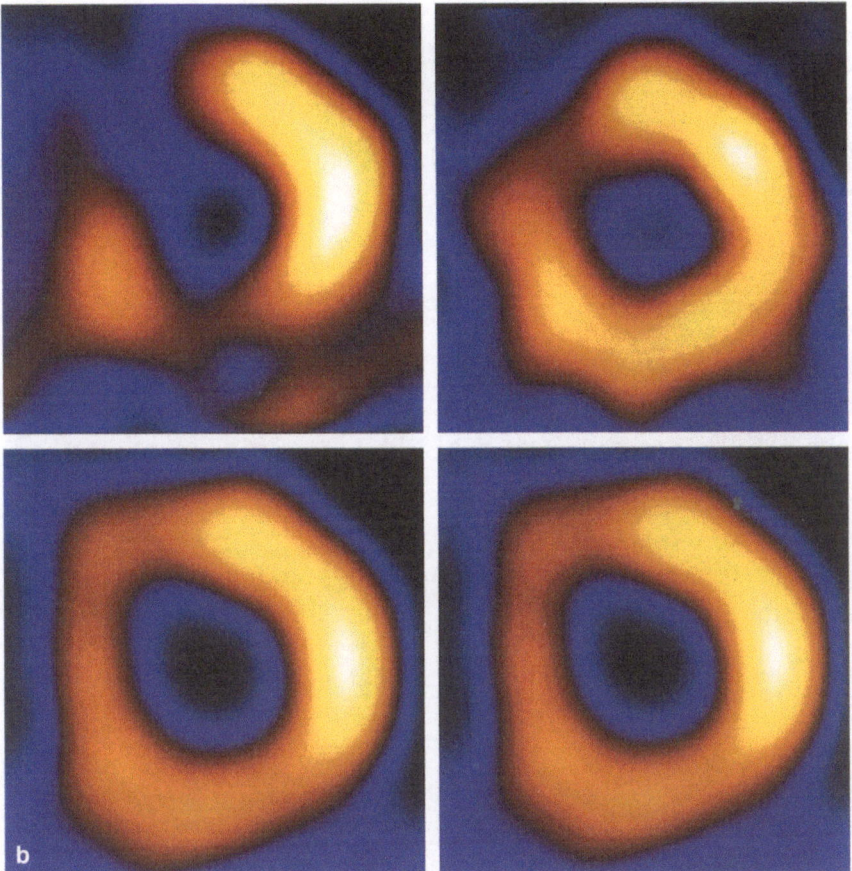

Fig. 11.7 b. Six months thereafter the patient suffered from recurrent chest pain. Follow-up SPECT showed the evidence of restenosis. After the second angioplasty, perfusion at stress normalized again. *Upper row*, pre-angioplasty (2nd); *lower row*, post-angioplasty; *left*, stress; *right*, rest

are metabolically active [120]. Less decrease in the uptake of both ^{99m}Tc-MIBI and ^{201}Tl at rest indicates viability [34].

Redistribution at rest of ^{201}Tl 4 or 24 h after injection can be expected in 15%–56% of segments [23, 24, 54, 124, 139] (Figs. 11.9 a, 11.10). Imaging 24 h after the resumption of cardiac drugs including nitrates [11, 46], and meal challenge reveals the highest prevalence of redistribution. Segments with perfusion defects can recover wall motion abnormalities if they are redistributed (Table 11.5).

Reinjection of ^{201}Tl can be an adjunctive tool to find viable myocardium when using stress-redistribution ^{201}Tl SPECT [62, 76, 115, 130] (Fig. 11.9 b). Reinjected ^{201}Tl increases the plasma concentration of ^{201}Tl and facilitates the filling of hypoperfused segments [22, 126]. After reinjection 15%–49% of segments with decreased uptake show more uptake than before. Wall motion is

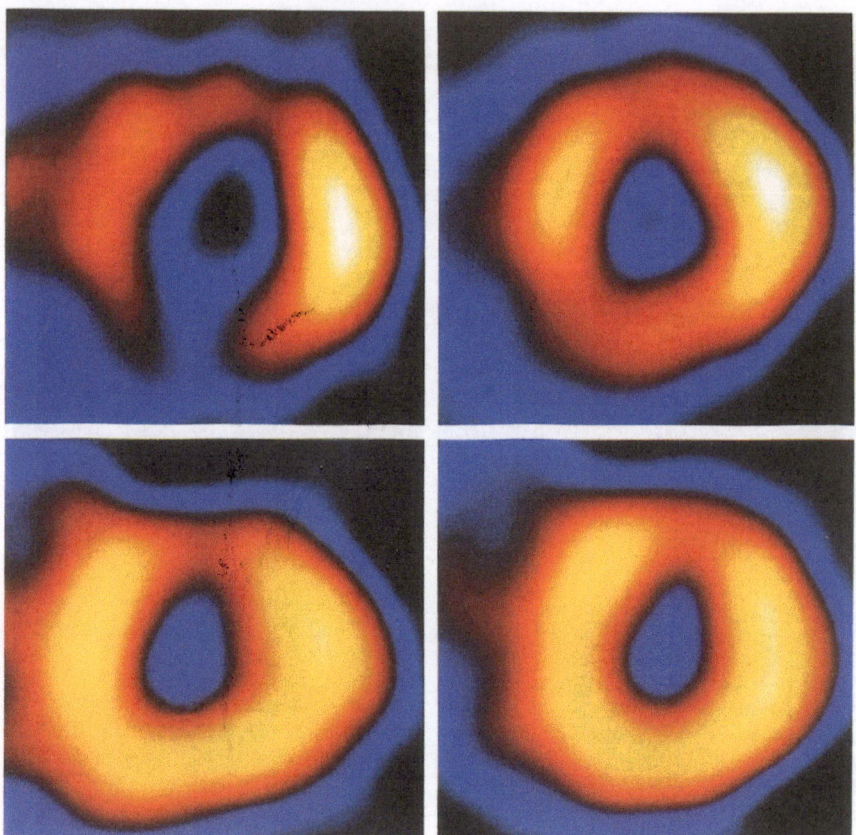

Fig. 11.8. Myocardial SPECT findings before (*above*) and after (*below*) coronary artery bypass graft (CABG) surgery. *Left*, stress; *right*, rest

Table 11.5. Predictive values of wall motion improvement (myocardial viability) after coronary artery bypass graft or angioplasty: rest redistribution ^{201}Tl SPECT

	Positive predictive value	Negative predictive value	Redistribu-tion	Revascular-ization	*n*
Mori [101]	11/14 (85%)	23/37 (62%)	4 h SPECT	CABG/ Angioplasty	17
Alfieri [2]	92/100 (92%)	14/20 (70%)	4 h SPECT	CABG	21
Ragosta [112]	81/141 (57%)	6/6 (100%)	4 h planar	CABG	14
Marzullo [88]	42/44 (95%)	24/31 (77%)	24 h planar	CABG/ Angioplasty	14
Yoon [140]	14/19 (74%)	17/37 (46%)	24 h SPECT	CABG	17
	240/318 (75%)	84/131 (64%)			

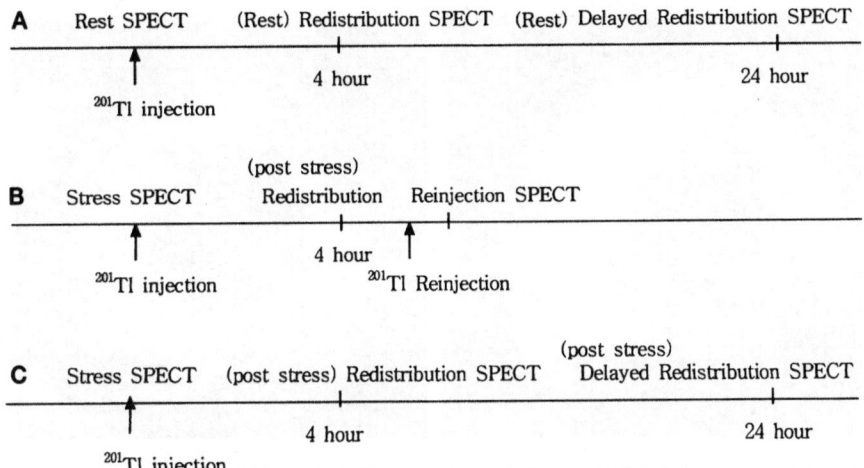

Fig. 11.9 A–C. Protocols for stress-redistribution-delay, rest-redistribution (4 and 24 h) and stress-rest-reinjection ^{201}Tl SPECT to delineate viable myocardium

Table 11.6. Predictive values of wall motion improvement (myocardial viability) after coronary artery bypass graft or angioplasty: reinjection after stress redistribution ^{201}Tl SPECT

	Positive predictive value	Negative predictive value	Revasculariza-tion	n
Dilsizian [22]	13/15 (87%)	8/8 (100%)	CABG/ Angioplasty	100
Ohtani [105]	23/31 (74%)	16/30 (53%)	CABG	24
Tamaki [126]	13/20 (65%)	8/32 (25%)	CABG	18
Arnese [6]	33/100 (33%)	62/67 (93%)	CABG	38
Haque [44]	33/39 (85%)	4/4 (100%)	Angioplasty	26
Schafers [115]	14/16 (88%)		CABG	32
	129/221 (58%)	98/141 (70%)		

improved in filled-in segments at reinjection after revascularization (Table 11.6). Imaging of reinjection has the drawback that it is literally equivalent to the mixture of perfusion of rest ^{201}Tl uptake (37 MBq) and of redistributed uptake of ^{201}Tl injected at stress (111 MBq). Delayed acquisition without reinjection until the day after stress imaging is possible and has been found to be equivalent to or somewhat inferior to a reinjection study in finding viable myocardium (Fig. 11.6c).

Persistent defects after delayed redistribution (4 or 24 h after rest injection) or reinjection (after stress redistribution) show a 15%–50% probability of having metabolic activity [24, 114, 126]. These segments should be evaluated with [^{18}F]fluoro-2-deoxyglucose (FDG) PET [3].

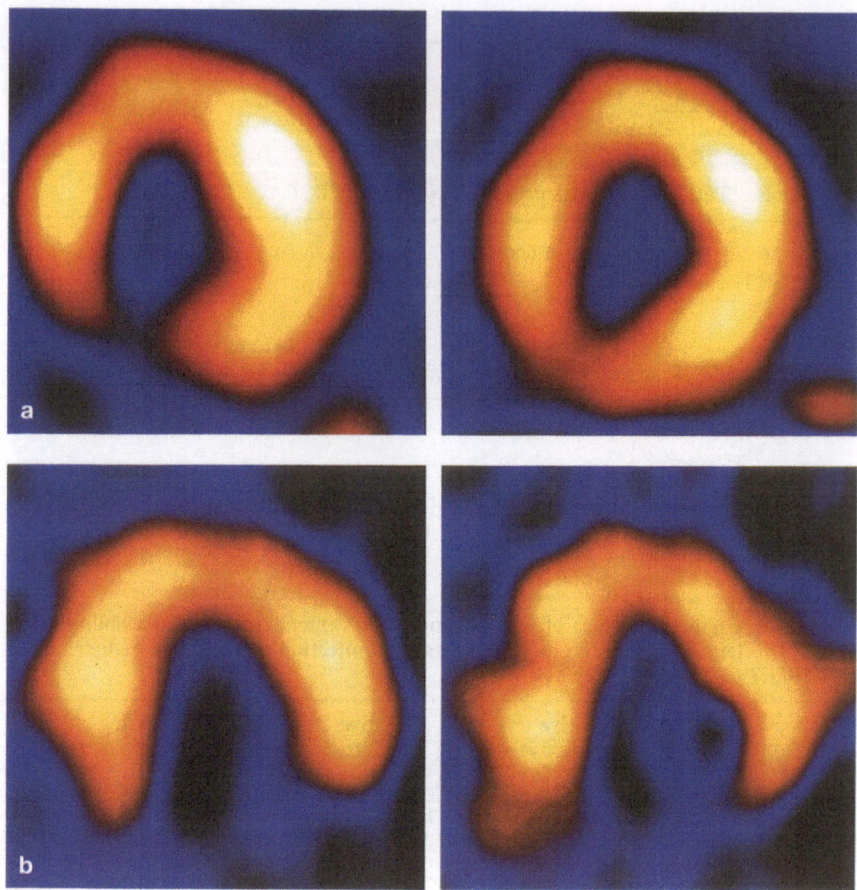

Fig. 11.10 a, b. Myocardial SPECT findings with rest 24-h redistribution ²⁰¹Tl SPECT. **a** Delayed uptake was found and inferior wall was considered viable. **b** Persistent defect at 24-h delay SPECT. *Left*, rest; *right*, 24-h redistribution

At redistribution in the rest-redistribution protocol some (10%–18%) of the segments reveal washout of activity taken up initially. Similar findings have been reported in stress-redistribution/delayed-redistribution studies. These segments were found to be still viable although the probability was somewhat lower than that of the segments improving at delay.

A relationship has been suggested between ²⁰¹Tl uptake and inotropic response to dobutamine [107, 118]. ²⁰¹Tl uptake appears to be prerequisite for sober inotropic reserve.

Stunned Versus Hibernating Myocardium

By definition, stunned myocardium has normal rest perfusion and decreased contractility. If one waits, contractility is improved. One can confirm stun-

Table 11.7. Stunned myocardium and hibernating myocardium

	Contractility	Rest perfusion	Glucose metabolism	Recovery of contractile dysfunction
Hibernating myocardium	Decrease	Decrease	Normal or increase	Possible after revascularization
Stunned myocardium	Decrease	Normal	Increase or decrease	Recover after follow up

ning by improved wall motion in the segment after follow-up. The limited resolution effect causes myocardium with less radioactivity to be confused with hibernating myocardium (Table 11.7).

By definition, hibernating myocardium has decreased rest perfusion and decreased contractility. This myocardium may recover function after revascularization. Hibernating myocardium is viable in that it can overcome long-standing hypoperfusion and contractile dysfunction after treatment (Table 11.7).

Stunned myocardium is known to have increased or decreased glucose metabolism [45, 51, 94, 95]. Stunned myocardium shows decreased oxygen or energy metabolism or at least preserved metabolism with poor contractile efficiency. Hibernating myocardium has increased glucose metabolism. Hibernating myocardium is thought to have preserved oxygen metabolism that is barely sufficient to maintain decreased muscular contractility. Increased extraction fraction of oxygen underlies the mechanism of preserved oxygen consumption of hibernating myocardium.

Energy production and consumption and the efficiency of work has not been well explained in these myocardial segments. Stunned myocardium requires observation, and hibernating myocardium calls for intervention.

Prognostication

Large defects with multiple-vessel areas, increased ^{201}Tl uptake in the lungs, and transient cavity dilatation indicate poorer prognosis according to the old criteria. Groups with high risk are those with high prevalence of cardiac events, such as cardiac death and nonfatal myocardial infarction. On the basis of SPECT data (Table 11.8) the prognosis of patients with coronary artery disease can be determined by the size and severity of perfusion decreases [59, 79, 86]. Normal study results are associated with benign prognosis [9, 42, 47]. Patients with ventricular dysfunction and redistribution on rest-redistribution ^{201}Tl SPECT have poorer prognosis [36]. Mismatch of [^{18}F]FDG and perfusion is another good predictor of cardiac events. Event-free survival was 50%–80% 1 year after follow-up [20, 127].

Table 11.8. Myocardial rest stress perfusion SPECT as prognosticator

Perfusion SPECT	n	Follow-up (months)	Rate of myocardial infarction or death				
			Normal	Abnormal			
Rest ^{201}Tl exercise ^{99m}Tc-MIBI	2200	17	0.3%	4.7% Mild		10% Severe	[42]
Exercise or dipyridamole [201]Tl	1926	33	1.08%		4%		[79]
Exercise ^{99m}Tc-MIBI	1702	20	0.25%		7.5%		[9]
Dipyridamole ^{99m}Tc-MIBI	512	18	1.7%		12.3%		[47]
Exercise [201]Tl	316	28	–[a]	5% Mild		25% Severe	[59]

[a] Included in "mild abnormality"

Patients undergoing elective noncardiac surgery can be evaluated with myocardial perfusion SPECT regarding their surgical risks [1]. For vascular surgery, perfusion SPECT predicts death or myocardial infarction [48]. For nonvascular surgery, rest-stress myocardial perfusion SPECT can be used as to predict late cardiac events [123]. The positive predictive value of dipyridamole SPECT is 4%–20% and its negative predictive value 99% [27].

Myocardial Infarction Scan

[99m]Tc-Pyrophosphate Scintigraphy

[99m]Tc-pyrophosphate seeks infarcted tissue from injured myocardium [16]. Its activity in infarcted tissue is about 20 times normal. Acute myocardial infarction is accompanied by membrane disruption, massive calcium influx, and precipitation on mitochondria. ^{99m}Tc-pyrophosphate is adsorbed to amorphous calcium phosphate or organic macromolecules.

[99m]Tc-pyrophosphate uptake is not linear to the decrease of blood flow [7]. When blood flow is decreased down 20%–40% of normal, ^{99m}Tc-pyrophosphate uptake is maximal. If blood flow is decreased further to near 5% of normal, uptake is reduced again.

Analysis

Uptake is graded by the amount of radioactivity localized in myocardium; grade 0, no radioactivity in myocardium; grade 1, faint uptake: grade 2, definite but less uptake than ribs; grade 3, uptake similar to rib activity; grade 4,

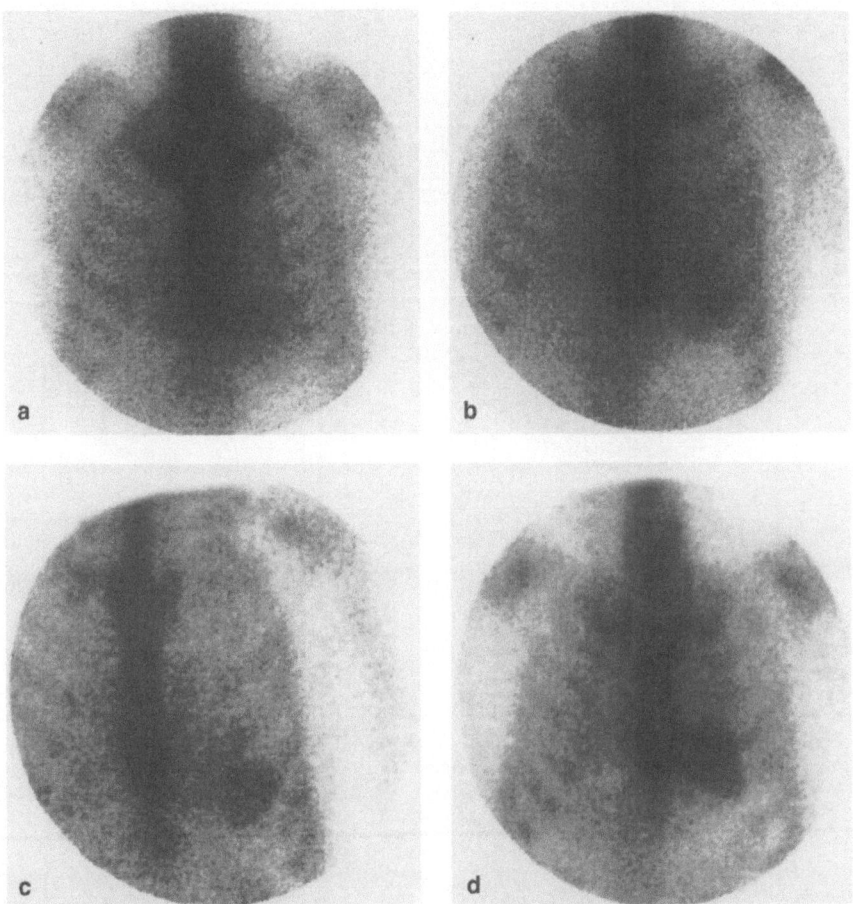

Fig. 11.11 a–d. Grades of ^{99m}Tc-pyrophosphate scan. **a** Grade 1. **b** Grade 2. **c** Grade 3. **d** Grade 4

prominent uptake more than ribs (Fig. 11.11). One often observes mild diffuse uptake over the entire heart area. Heart failure and poor labeling efficiency are the most common causes of this diffuse radioactivity. Localized uptake is significant.

Clinical Application

^{99m}Tc-pyrophosphate can help in diagnosing acute myocardial infarction when patients suffer from typical chest pains without typical electrocardiographic changes. ^{99m}Tc-pyrophosphate helps to localize the site of infarction (Fig. 11.12). Grade 3 or 4 or localized grade 2 uptake represents acute myocardial infarction.

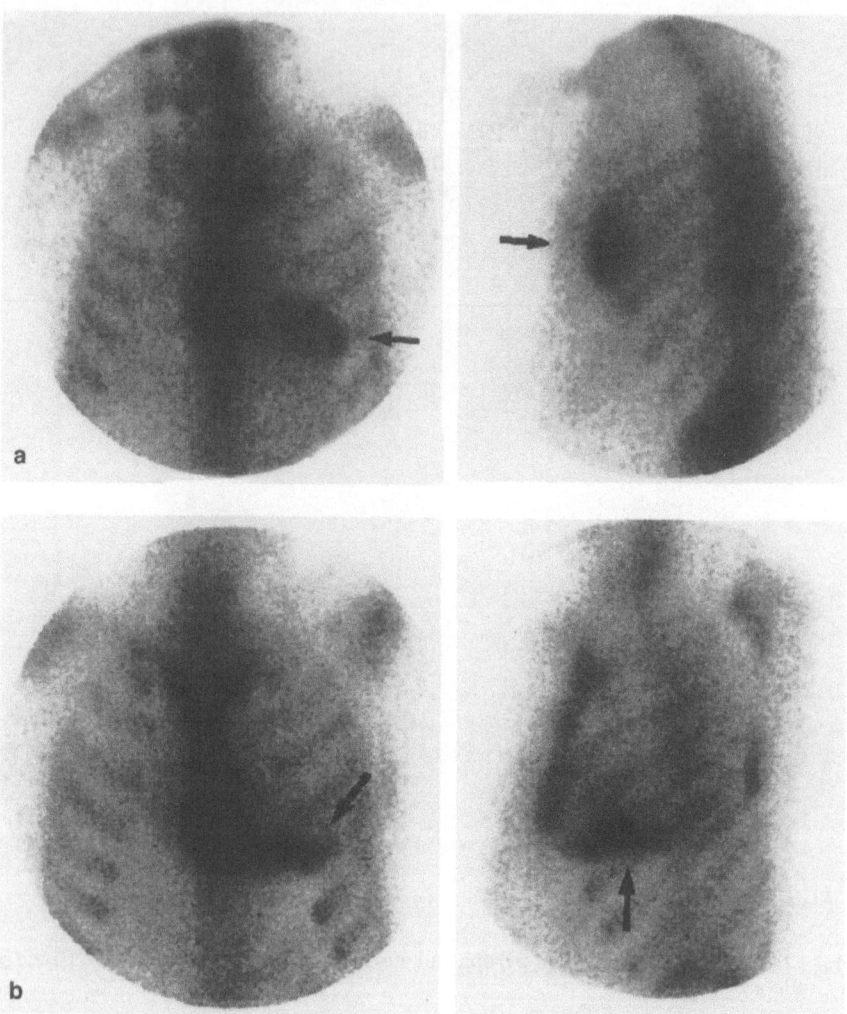

Fig. 11.12a, b. ^{99m}Tc-pyrophosphate scan findings in acute myocardial infarction. **a** Anterior and left lateral image in anterior wall infarction. **b** Anterior and left anterior oblique 70° images in inferior wall infarction

^{99m}Tc-pyrophosphate uptake can be positive at 12-h after infarction, strongly positive at 48–72 h after infarction, and fade away after 2 weeks. Sensitivity changes depending on the time course. Less sensitivity is reported in subendocardial myocardial infarction.

The doughnut sign (Fig. 11.13) indicates that a huge area of myocardium is involved, and that the center is nearly void of flow. This sign means an extensive, severe case and is associated with a grave prognosis. The size of the hot area in ^{99m}Tc-pyrophosphate scans is predictive of the course. Persistent

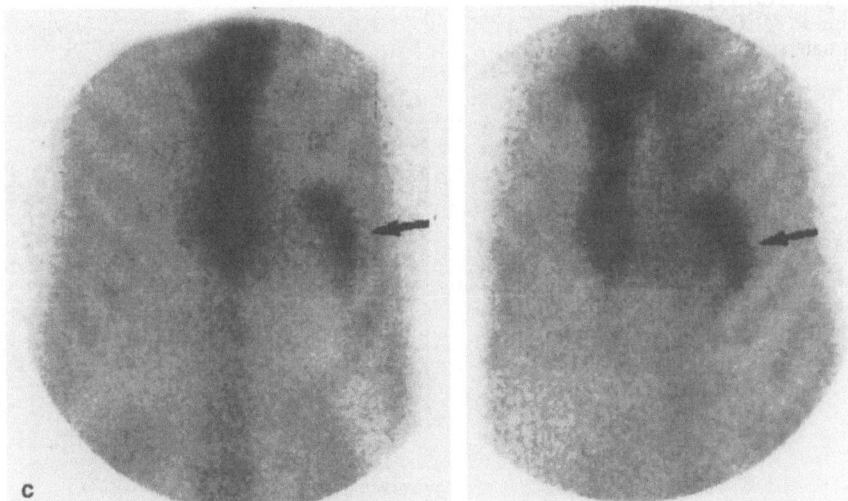

Fig. 11.12 c. Anterior and left anterior oblique 40° images in lateral wall infarction

^{99m}Tc-pyrophosphate uptake even 3 weeks after infarction suggests continuing injury to peri-infarct areas.

Right ventricular infarction can be diagnosed with ^{99m}Tc-pyrophosphate scan. Many cases can be diagnosed by ^{99m}Tc-pyrophosphate in which electrocardiographic changes or enzyme concentration provide no hint of right ventricular infarction.

^{111}In-Antimyosin Antibody Scintigraphy

Heavy chains of myosin proteins remain within damaged myocytes although light-chain proteins are released from infarct tissue. Antibodies cannot penetrate the cell membranes of normal myocytes. When cells are damaged by ischemic injury, antibodies penetrate into myocytes and bind to myosin heavy chains.

In contrast to ^{99m}Tc-pyrophosphate scans, the uptake of antimyosin antibodies is proportional to the nonstaining area of triphenyl tetrazolium chloride and inversely proportional to the decrease in blood flow [60].

Acquisition and Analysis

Antimyosin antibodies are labeled with ^{111}In or ^{99m}Tc [64, 117]. Fab fragment is usually used. ^{111}In-labeled antibodies can produce images at 6, 24, and 48 h after injection. ^{99m}Tc-labeled antibodies provide images at 4–6 h.

Fig. 11.13. Typical donut sign in ^{99m}Tc-pyrophosphate scan

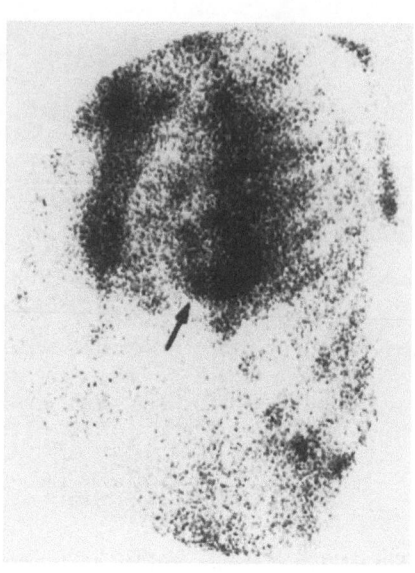

Clinical Application

Antimyosin antibody can assess the size of infarction and localize the site of infarction and its course [135]. However, it is taken up not only by infarct myocardium but also by injured and salvaged myocardium [100].

Antimyosin antibody can visualize injured myocardium in cardiomyopathy. Cardiomyopathy was once considered to be a diffuse process; however, recent evidence suggests that injury and damage are a regional process [104]. Image results with antimyosin antibody is one of the sources of this evidence.

[^{123}I]MIBG SPECT

[^{123}I]Metaiodobenzylguanidine (MIBG) can be used to visualize the presynaptic neuronal reuptake site of norepinephrine. [^{123}I]MIBG is unique in visualizing the autonomic nervous system in myocardium. First-pass extraction of [^{123}I]MIBG is high (0.89), and retension is believed to be related to a number of neuronal uptake sites and to the functional status of impairment.

Neuronal Uptake and Perfusion

After acute myocardial infarction the infarct center is void of [^{123}I]MIBG uptake. The area of [^{123}I]MIBG nonuptake is much larger than that in ^{201}Tl defect [121]. Remote myocardium has been found to have transiently decreased [^{123}I]MIBG uptake. Peri-infarct areas show uptake decreased at first, and then improve.

Clinical Application

Less uptake of [^{123}I]MIBG than of ^{201}Tl is reported to be related to arrhythmogenecity [134] and contractile dysfunction. Mismatched areas show variable outcome and are considered to be risk areas. Failure to accumulate [^{123}I]MIBG means loss of sympathetic innervation. Immediately after infarction the uptake of [^{123}I]MIBG is decreased earlier than that of ^{201}Tl. [^{123}I]MIBG uptake recovers later than ^{201}Tl uptake.

Diabetic neuropathy and idiopathic cardiomyopathy have been examined with [^{123}I]MIBG SPECT. Nonischemic myocardium in diabetics shows areas with decreased [^{123}I]MIBG uptake [84]. Idiopathic cardiomyopathy can be examined by [^{123}I]MIBG to assess regional damage and sequelae in apparent diffuse pathology of myocardium.

In heart failure either related to or not related to myocardial infarction [^{123}I]MIBG uptake is the same as in controls; however, washout is increased [137]. Increased sympathetic tone of heart failure seems to influence the status of presynaptic neurons. With advancing grades of heart failure, [^{123}I]MIBG uptake is decreased in addition to increased washout. This decrease is associated with poorer prognosis [96].

[^{123}I]BMIPP SPECT

[^{123}I]Betamethyliodophenylpentadecanoic acid (BMIPP) is an analogue of pentadecanoic acid and has a methyl residue in the beta position [70]. [^{123}I]BMIPP is taken up in myocardium along with myocardial blood flow. In contrast to [^{11}C]palmitate and [^{123}I]iodophenylpentadecanoic acid (IPPA), the oxidation of [^{123}I]BMIPP is hindered to some degree but not entirely. [^{123}I]BMIPP can be incorporated into the endogenous lipid pool or metabolized [33]. Alpha oxidation is the bypass to beta pathway.

[^{123}I]BMIPP may show initially low uptake and rapid washout, or initially high uptake and slow washout. Tissue is also found with initially high uptake and rapid washout. Myocardium rarely shows initially low uptake and retension. It is questionable despite earlier speculations that [^{123}I]BMIPP uptake can represent the metabolic rate of beta oxidation [63].

Substrate Metabolism Imaged by [^{123}I]BMIPP SPECT

Cardiac muscle devours any substrate available and has a mechanism of glucose–fatty acid switch. During fasting in humans myocardium takes up fatty acid and runs the oxidation cycle at mitochondria. Upon feeding, insulin and glucose aid cellular glucose uptake and catabolism.

[^{123}I]BMIPP can be washed out rapidly or trapped in the endogenous pool. [^{123}I]BMIPP uptake in myocardium represents both uptake and oxidation of fatty acid. Unlike [^{123}I]IPPA, which is used to show the metabolic rate of fatty acid, [123I]BMIPP, the beta-methylated analogue of [123I]IPPA, cannot be degraded this easily via the beta oxidation pathway. One may therefore obtain a static-image [123I]BMIPP SPECT. Rather slow but definite washout of [123I]BMIPP is considered to be due to initial back-diffusion and alpha oxidation [136].

Upon fasting, myocarium takes up and catabolizes more [11C]palmitate, but [123I]BMIPP uptake is higher upon feeding.

Clinical Application

Separate acquisition with dual isotope are possible in [123I]BMIPP imaging combined with 201Tl. In patients with acute myocardial infarction we find mismatched areas with more 201Tl uptake and less [123I]BMIPP [31]. These areas are thought to represent ischemic zones. Low uptake of both [123I]BMIPP and 201Tl means necrotic infarct.

In areas with less [123I]BMIPP uptake than 201Tl at rest, one may find redistribution of 201Tl at reinjection [90]. Areas with less [123I]BMIPP uptake than 201Tl after reinjection show impaired wall motion [125]. Mismatch (less uptake of [123I]BMIPP than of 201Tl) is associated with more [18F]FDG uptake [63]. These segments improve in patients with acute myocardial infarction.

[18F]FDG PET and SPECT

[18F]FDG is an analogue of deoxyglucose, and deoxyglucose is an analogue of glucose. Glucose, once taken up in myocytes, is catabolyzed through the glycolysis pathway and/or tricyclic acid cycle or is anabolyzed to glycogen. On the other hand, deoxyglucose is trapped in myocardium after its first phosphorylation at 6 carbon. Phophatase activity is virtually negligible with deoxyglucose-6-phosphate. 18F makes no difference when added to deoxyglucose molecule.

[18F]FDG can be used for images with both PET and SPECT cameras. With PET one acquires transmission images and make an attenuation map. Reconstruction is a deconvolution process using an emission and attenuation map in PET. For SPECT one can use a 511-keV collimator or molecular coincidence detection circuits.

[18F]FDG uptake can determine whether the relevant tissue is metabolically active, and thus viable. The wall motion of these segments can improve after revascularization [38, 71]. Classical mismatch is observed in segments with decreased perfusion at rest and preserved [18F]FDG uptake (Fig. 11.14).

[18F]FDG is really needed in ischemic cardiomyopathy patients [21]. About 90% of transplantation candidates can undergo revascularization after [18F]FDG study. The probability of patients with ejection fraction less than 30% benefiting from surgery is high only when 201Tl or [18F]FDG reveals viable myocardium [26].

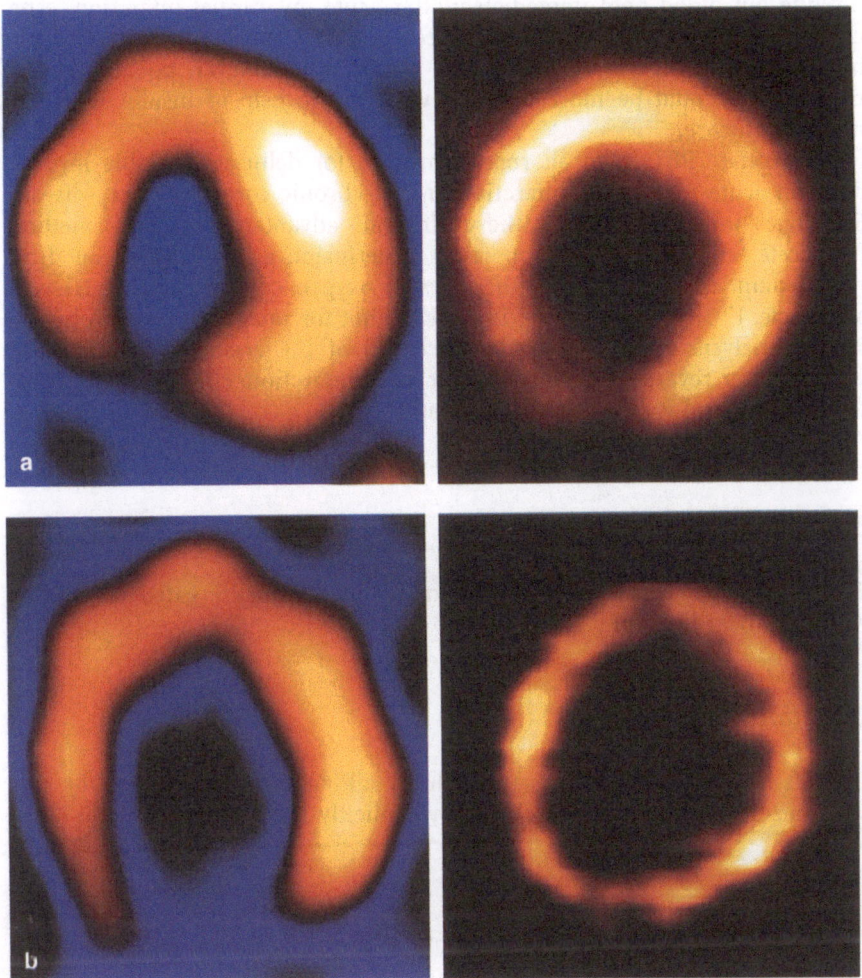

Fig. 11.14a, b. Match (**a**) and mismatch (**b**) of perfusion and metabolism in ^{201}Tl SPECT (*left*) and [18F]FDG PET (*right*)

After myocardial infarction there is decreased uptake of [18F]FDG in infarct myocardium (matched defect). Stunned myocardial segments may have decreased uptake, however, normal perfusion. Acutely hibernating segments show preserved glucose metabolism and decreased perfusion. Mismatched segments need treatment.

One-year mortality is 20%–50% in patients with ischemic cardiomyopathy and mismatched segments followed up under medical treatment [20, 127]. When operative mortality is around 10%, one needs to perform a bypass graft.

[18F]FDG uptake depends substantially on insulin sensitivity. Although we perform [18F]FDG PET in glucose-loaded conditions, we sometimes observe nothing but blood pool immediately after acute myocardial infarction, especially in diabetics. The contrast between ischemic myocardium and remote myocardium is highest when patients are fasting; however, poor images of myocardium could be more frequent without the help of insulin if we did not load glucose.

[^{11}C]Acetate PET is an alternative method for delineating viable myocardium in acute myocardial infarction and in chronic coronary artery disease. Substrate independence is the principal advantage of this method. [^{11}C]Acetate is taken up in proportion to perfusion and is washed out from myocardium in proportion to the rates of oxygen consumption or tricyclic acid cycle. [^{11}C]Acetate imaging is basically not for image observation but for kinetic analysis of clearance. Clearance (k_1) of [^{11}C]acetate is predictive of viability after revascularization in myocardial infarction, chronic coronary artery disease, and ischemic cardiomyopathy [39].

Blood Pool Scan

Blood pool is used to depict myocardial wall motion by gated acquisition with electrocardiography and cine loop display.

Quantification

The left ventricle is freed from the right by taking a vertical view to the septal plane. The left atrium is excluded by explicitly indicating the region of interest.

Left Ventricular Volume Curve and Ejection Fraction

A count-based method is usually adopted [78, 89]. Stroke volume is represented as counts by subtracting the number of endsystolic counts from the number of enddiastolic counts. Ejection fraction is calculated by dividing stroke count by (enddiastolic counts minus background counts). Normal ejection fraction is 50%–70%. Reproducibility is usually less than 5% of the coefficient of variation. The reproducibility of measurement contributes greatly to the routine use of this method. Individual variability over 6 weeks is reported to be 7% (ejection fraction) in rest and 10% (ejection fraction) in exercise in stable patients [80].

Regional Ejection Fraction

The geometric center is determined rather arbitrarily. This arbitrariness derives from the fact that the heart rotates and moves toward a base in three-

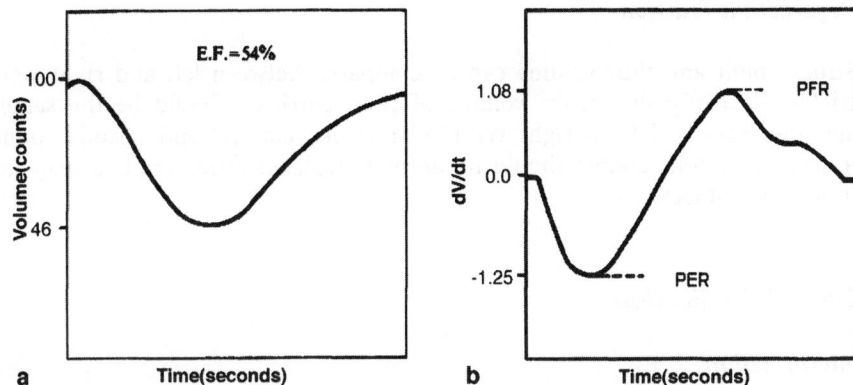

Fig. 11.15 a, b. Normal left ventricular time activity (volume) curve (**a**) and its first derivative (**b**; dV/dt vs. time). *PER*, Peak ejection rate; *PFR*, peak filling rate

dimensional space within the chest cavity, and that we view a planar projection of cardiac movement. Radial rays are drawn to make six or nine "pies." Disregarding valvular planes, regional motions of five or seven pies are represented. Septal motion is underestimated, and posterior wall motion is exaggerated.

Ejection and Filling Rate

The first derivative over time of the time-volume (activity) curve gives us a function dV/dt over time (Fig. 11.15). The ejection period discloses rapid and slow ejection, and filling discloses rapid and slow filling. The ejection rate can be averaged and represented by peak values (peak ejection rate). The filling rate can also be averaged and represented by peak rates. The ejection rate reflects systolic function, and the filling rate reflects diastolic function.

Phase Image

Time-volume curves can be represented by Fourier-transformed cosine function. Wall motion abnormalities can be found as delayed phase angles. Paradoxical motion or dyskinesia is expressed as a delay of about 180°. This parametric representation of cardiac motion is operator independent. Full-width/half-maximum of histograms of phase angles explain the concordance of movements of each left ventricular pixel. Intraventricular conduction abnormalities can show regional phase differences.

Right Ventricular Assessment

The volume curve and ejection fraction can be calculated. We can use the same position as the left ventricle; however, it is more desirable to adopt less oblique and caudally tilted projection image.

Regurgetant Fraction

Stroke count and thus volume can be compared between left and right ventricles. Normally the stroke volume of two ventricles should be the same, and the ratio of left to right ventricular stroke counts (enddiastolic count minus endsystolic count) should be unity. Calculated ratios are less than 1.2 in normal subjects.

Clinical Application

Interpretation

Chamber sizes and wall movements are evaluated on the monitor using left anterior oblique, anterior, and left lateral images. Wall motions are assessed as normal, hypokinesia (mild and severe), akinesia, and dyskinesia. Anterior, apex, septum, anterolateral, posterolateral, and inferior walls are representative walls on the projection images.

Quantitative indices are reproducible and can reflect regional and global performance of both ventricles. Among the indices ejection fraction is the most popular one and the best sole predictor of outcome of coronary artery disease [12, 108]. Ejection fraction, including regional ejection fractions, peak and average ejection rates and filling rates, normalized filling rate to ejection fraction, and phase angles are often used to assess left ventricular function.

Coronary Artery Disease and Cardiomyopathy

Regional wall motion abnormality and ejection fraction can help assess coronary artery disease with or without myocardial infarction. After acute myocardial infarction, regional walls can be dyskinetic or stunned. Adjacent or remote myocardium are often hyperkinetic in a compensatory fashion. Ejection fraction needs to be followed up for at least 6 weeks if it is to be stabilized. Improvement in abnormal wall motion can be analyzed after revascularization with this method.

Global hypokinesia with decreased ejection fraction of markedly enlarged chamber is characteristic of cardiomyopathy. When doxorubicin (Adriamycin) is administered to the limit dose for chemotherapy, global ejection fraction should be evaluated serially with this method.

Exercise Gated Blood Pool Scan

Bicycle exercise can be combined with gated blood pool scan. Exercise should increase ejection fraction about 5%. Cardiac drugs, advanced age, and female sex can lessen this increase. In addition, setting strict criteria with exercise gated blood pool scan requires caution as normal subjects with rest ejection fraction greater than 70% have little chance to show an increase in ejection fraction of more than 5%. Exercise ejection fraction measured with gated blood pool scan is a powerful means for predicting subsequent mortality in patients with heart failure [55, 132].

Regional wall motion abnormality can show up after exercise. Ischemic segments can be disclosed by new wall motion abnormality. However, supine bicycle exercise is a fairly difficult technique for patients to perform, and acquisition during exercise is also cumbersome in terms of patient logistics.

Single-Pass Scintigraphy

Study and Analysis

The external jugular vein is the preferred route of bolus injection. Success of bolus injection is checked by the time-activity curve at the superior vena cava. The injected activity should pass the superior vena cava within 3 s. Two cuts per second are acquired for 60 s. Images are stored on computer and made on film.

Activity appears in the superior vena cava, right atrium, ventricle, and then lungs. When the left ventricle appears, pulmonary activity should be cleared, and then aortic activity appears. Transit times are calculated. Transit times are 2.8±0.3 from the right ventricle to lungs and 3.9±0.4 from lungs to the left ventricle. Right to left ventricle transit times are 6.1±0.5.

Ejection Fraction

Images are stored in a computer per 40- to 50-ms sequence (20–25 frames per second). Ventricular and background regions of interest show time-activity curves that have peaks and troughs. Peaks are enddiastolic counts, and valleys are endsystolic counts. Ejection fraction can be calculated as the stroke count divided by the enddiastolic count [32]. When the bolus was good, one obtains three to five beat-equivalent peaks in the right ventricle and five to seven peaks in the left ventricle.

Reproducibility is excellent, with fewer than 5% errors [109]. Right ventricular ejection fraction is especially precise in comparison to echocardiography and gated blood pool scan.

Diagnosis and Quantification of Shunt

Left to right shunt is characterized by persistent pulmonary activity (Fig. 11.16). Pulmonary recirculation through intracardiac shunts leads to this

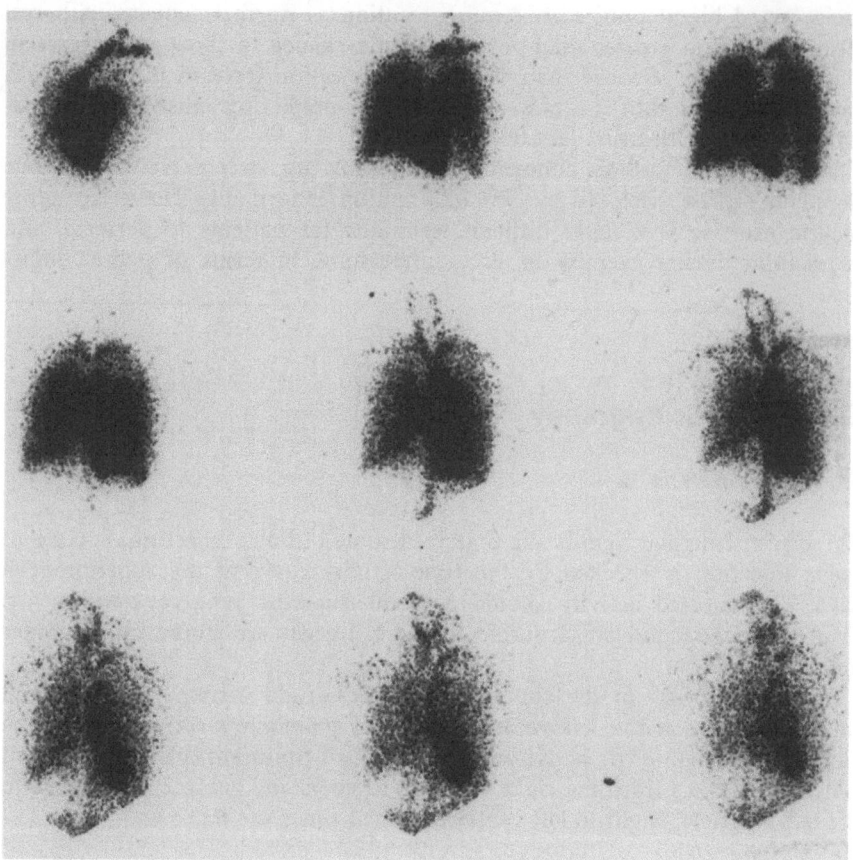

Fig. 11.16. Single pass scintigraphy of ventricular septal defect. Persistent visualization of pulmonary activity after aorta appeared. Right ventricle is empty

activity. However, this characteristic is seen only when the Q_p/Q_s value is greater than 1.6. A smudged appearance of atrial septal defect can be differentiated from ventricular septal defect (Fig. 11.17).

Pulmonary time-activity curves usually show small peaks due to recirculation at the descent phase. The gamma-variate model, which assumes no shunts, predicts a new descent curve and overlaps it upon the original curve. The area under model curve reflects pulmonary flow (Q_p). The area difference between the original curve and the model-based curve reflects the shunt flow (Q_{shunt}). Systemic flow is calculated by subtracting Q_{shunt} from Q_p. Thus Q_p/Q_s is calculated by $Q_p/(Q_p-Q_{shunt})$. Shunt fraction is well correlated ($r>0.9$) with oxymetric measurements. Q_p/Q_s measured by this method is accurate in the range of 1.2–3.0. Small amount of shunt cannot be detected at less than 1.2. If the shunt is too great, the calculated shunt underestimates reality. The quality of bolus is the most important factor.

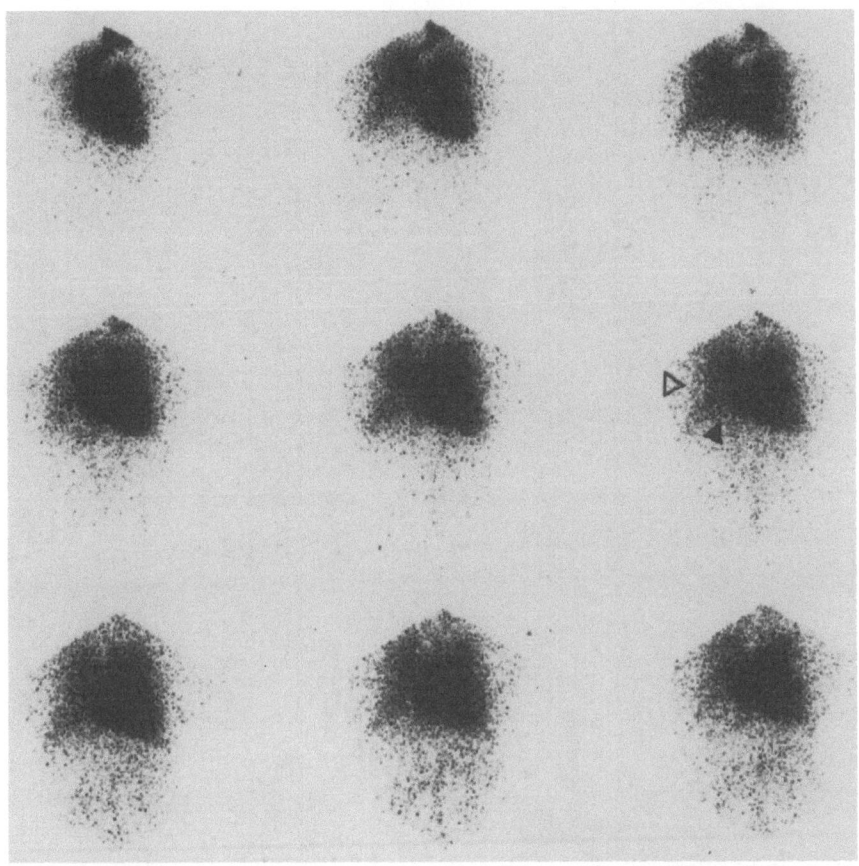

Fig. 11.17. Single pass scintigraphy of atrial septal defect. Right ventricle cannot be discerned from left ventricle (smudge appearance)

Right to left shunt is characterized by earlier appearance of activity at the left ventricle and aorta (Fig. 11.18). The shunt amount is calculated with ^{99m}Tc-labeled macroaggregated albumin (MAA). When injected, ^{99m}Tc-MAA should not appear in systemic circulation. Brain and kidneys are prominent organs which reveal trapped ^{99m}Tc-MAA in the systemic circulation. The amount of radioactivity at the kidneys and brain is measured in anterior and posterior positions. The count in these organs is divided by 0.32 to calculate systemic flow, assuming that brain has 12% of systemic flow and kidneys 20%. The geometric mean is compared with pulmonary counts measured on anterior and posterior views and averaged geometrically.

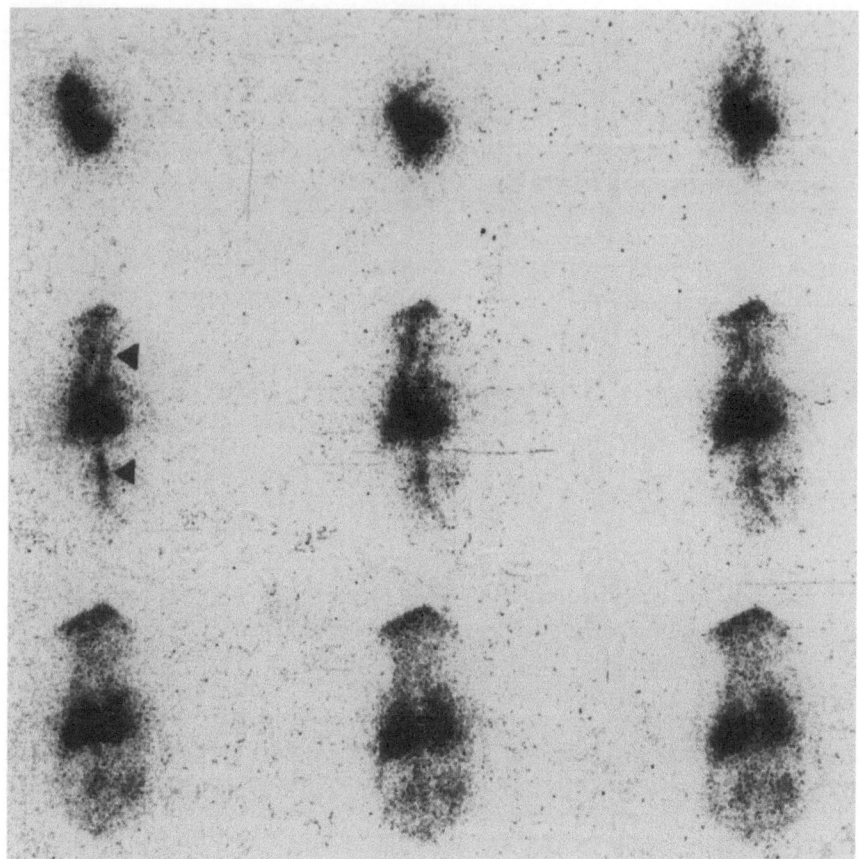

Fig. 11.18. Right to left shunt. Aorta and carotid arteries showed up very early in single pass study

Clinical Application

In congenital heart disease Q_p/Q_s can be used to quantify the shunt amount and to predict outcome. Atrial septal defects are diagnosed by the smudged appearance of right and left ventricles. Ventricular septal defect or persistent ductus arteriosus differentiates the right and left ventricles very easily, as the right ventricle lacks radioactivity. This is because the ventricular septal defect lies in the upper parts of the septum, principally in membranous portion, and the shunt flow is even stream.

In valvular heart disease after mitral commissurotomy Q_p/Q_s can be calculated with this method. Some of the iatrogenic shunt does not close once a catheter has been passed. Assessment of right to left shunt is helpful in cases of pulmonary arteriovenous fistula.

In coronary artery disease the ejection fraction can be evaluated with this method, and it has proven a good prognosticator [28]. Exercise study measuring ejection fraction can also stratify further risks of cardiac mortality [75].

References

1. Abraham SA, Eagle KA (1994) Preoperative cardiac risk assessment for noncardiac surgery. J Nucl Cardiol 1:389–398
2. Alfieri O, Canna GL, Giubbini R et al (1993) Recovery of myocardial function. The ultimate target of coronary revascularization. Eur J Cardio-thorac Surg 7:325–330
3. Altehoefer C, Hans-Jurgen K, Dorr R et al (1992) Fluorine-18 deoxyglucose PET for assessment of viable myocardium in perfusion defects in Tc-99m MIBI SPECT: a comparative study in patients with coronary artery disease. Eur J Nucl Med 19:334–342
4. Amanullah AM, Kiat H, Friedman JD, Berman DS (1996) Adenosine technetium-99m sestamibi myocardial perfusion SPECT in women: diagnostic efficacy in detection of coronary artery disease. J Am Coll Cardiol 27:803–809
5. Anagnostopoulos C, Laney R, Pennell D et al (1995) A comparison of resting images from two myocardial perfusion tracers. Eur J Nucl Med 22:1029–1034
6. Arnese M, Cornel JH, Salustri A et al (1995) Prediction of improvement of regional left ventricular function after surgical revascularization. A comparison of low-dose dobutamine echocardiography with ^{201}Tl single-photon emission computed tomography. Circulation 91:2748–2752
7. Beller GA, Chow BA, Haber E et al (1977) Localization of radiolabeled cardiac myosin-specific antibody in myocardial infarcts-comparison with technetium-99m stannous pyrophosphate. Circulation 55:74–77
8. Berman DS, Kiat H, Friedman JD et al (1993) Separate acquisition rest thallium-201/stress technetium-99m sestamibi dual-isotope myocardial perfusion single-photon emission computed tomography: a clinical validation study. J Am Coll Cardiol 22:1455–1464
9. Berman DS, Hachamovitch R, Kiat H et al (1995) Incremental value of prognostic testing in patients with known or suspected ischemic heart disease: a basis for optimal utilization of exercise technetium-99m sestamibi myocardial perfusion single-photon emission computed tomography. J Am Coll Cardiol 26:639–647
10. Berman DS, Kiat H, Friedman JD, Diamond G (1995) Clinical applications of exercise nuclear cardiology studies in the era of healthcare reform. Am J Cardiol 75:3D–13D
11. Bisi G, Sciagra R, Santoro GM et al (1995) Technetium-99m-sestamibi imaging with nitrate infusion to detect viable hibernating myocardium and predict postrevascularization recovery. J Nucl Med 36:1994–2000
12. Bonow R (1994) Prognostic assessment incoronary artery disease: role of radionuclide angiography. J Nucl Cardiol 1:280–285
13. Cecil MP, Kosinski AS, Jones MT et al (1996) The importance of work-up (verification) bias correction in assessing the accuracy of SPECT thallium-201 testing for the diagnosis of coronary artery disease. J Clin Epidemiol 49:735–742
14. Chua T, Kiat H, Germano G et al (1994) Gated technetium-99m sestamibi for simultaneous assessment of stress myocardial perfusion, postexercise regional ventricular function and myocardial viability. J Am Coll Cardiol 23:1107–1114
15. Cooke C, Garcia E, Cullon S et al (1994) Determining the accuracy of calculating systolic wall thickening using a fast Fourier transform approximation: a simulation study based on canine and patient data. J Nucl Med 35:1185–1192
16. Corbett JR, Lewis M, Willerson JT et al (1984) Technetium-99m pyrophosphate imaging in patients with acute myocardial infarction: comparison of planar images with single photon emission computed tomography with and without blood pool overlay. Circulation 69:1120–1128

17. Cramer M-J, Verzijlbergen JF, Van der Wall EE et al (1994) Head-to-head comparison between technetium-99m-sestamibi and thallium-201 tomographic imaging for the detection of coronary artery disease using combined dipyridamole-exercise stress. Coron Artery Dis 5:787–791

18. Cuocolo A, Maurea S, Pace L et al (1993) Resting technetium-99m methoxyisobutylisonitrile cardiac imaging in chronic coronary artery disease: comparison with rest-redistribution thallium-201 scintigraphy. Eur J Nucl Med 20:1186–1192

19. DePuey GE, Rozanski A (1995) Using gated technetium-99m-sestamibi SPECT to characterize fixed myocardial defects as infarct or artifact. J Nucl Med 36:952–955

20. Di Carli MF, Davidson M, Little R et al (1994) Value of metabolic imaging with positron emission tomography for evaluating prognosis in patients with coronary artery disease and left ventricular dysfunction. Am J Cardiol 73:527–533

21. Di Carli MF, Asgarzadie F, Schelbert HR et al (1995) Quantitative relation between myocardial viability and improvement in heart failure symptoms after revascularization in patients with ischemic cardiomyopathy. Circulation 92:3436–3444

22. Dilsizian V, Rocco TP, Freedman NM et al (1990) Enhanced detection of ischemic but viable myocardium by the reinjection of thallium after stress-redistribution imaging. N Engl J Med 323:141–146

23. Dilsizian V, Perrone-Filardi P, Arrighi JA et al (1993) Concordance and discordance between stress-rest-reinjection and rest-redistribution thallium imaging for assessing viable myocardium. Comparison with metabolic activity by positron emission tomography. Circulation 88:941–952

24. Dilsizian V, Arrighi JA, Diodati JG et al (1994) Myocardial viability in patients with chronic coronary artery disease: comparison of ^{99m}Tc-sestamibi with thallium reinjection and [18F]fluorodeoxyglucose. Circulation 89:578–587

25. Dondi M, Tartagni F, Fallani F et al (1993) A comparison of rest sestamibi and rest-redistribution thallium single photon emission tomography: possible implications for myocardial viability detection in infarcted patients. Eur J Nucl Med 20:26–31

26. Dreyfus GD, Duboc D, Blasco A et al (1994) Myocardial viability assessment in ischemic cardiomyopathy: benefits of coronary revascularization. Ann Thorac Surg 57:1402–1408

27. Eagle KA, Brundage BH, Chaitman BR et al (1996) Guidelines for perioperative cardiovascular evaluation for noncardiac surgery: report of the American College of Cardiology/American Heart Association task force on practice guideline (Committee on perioperative cardiovascular evaluation for noncardiac surgery). J Am Coll Cardiol 27:910–948

28. Emond M, Mock MB, Davis KB et al (1994) Long-term survival of medically treated patients in the Coronary Artery Surgery Study (CASS) registry. Circulation 90:2645–2657

29. Ficaro EP, Fessler JA, Shreve PD et al (1996) Simultaneous transmission/emission myocardial perfusion tomography. Diagnostic accuracy of attenuation-corrected ^{99m}Tc-sestamibi single-photon emission computed tomography. Circulation 93:463–473

30. Fletcher GF, Balady G, Froelicher VF et al (1995) Exercise standards: a statement for healthcare professionals from the American Heart Association. Circulation 91:580–615

31. Franken PR, De Geeter F, Dendale P et al (1994) Abnormal free fatty acid uptake in subacute myocardial infarction after coronary thrombolysis: correlation with wall motion and inotropic reserve. J Nucl Med 35:1758–1765

32. Friedman JD, Berman DS, Kiat H et al (1994) Rest and treadmill exercise first-pass radionuclide ventriculography: validation of left ventricular ejection fraction measurement. J Nucl Cardiol 4:382–388

33. Fujibayashi Y, Nohara R, Hosokawa R et al (1996) Metabolism and kinetics of iodine-123-BMIPP in canine myocardium. J Nucl Med 37:757–761

34. Galassi AR, Centamore G, Fiscella A et al (1995) Comparison of rest-redistribution thallium-201 imaging and reinjection after stress-redistribution for the as-

sessment of myocardial viability in patients with left ventricular dysfunction secondary to coronary artery disease. Am J Cardiol 75:436–442

35. Germano G, Kiat H, Karvanogh PB et al (1995) Automatic quantification of ejection fraction from gated myocardial perfusion SPECT. J Nucl Med 36:2138–2147

36. Gioia G, Milan E, Giubbini R et al (1996) Prognostic value of tomographic rest-redistribution thallium 201 imaging in medically treated patients with coronary artery disease and left ventricular dysfunction. J Nucl Cardiol 3:150–156

37. Go RT, Marwick TH, MacIntyre WJ et al (1990) A prospective comparison of rubidium-82 PET and thallium-201 SPECT myocardial perfusion imaging utilizing a single dipyridamole stress in the diagnosis of coronary artery disease. J Nucl Med 31:1089–1905

38. Grandin C, Wijns W, Melin JA et al (1995) Delineation of myocardial viability with PET. J Nucl Med 36:1543–1552

39. Gropler RJ, Geltman E, Sampathkumaran K et al (1992) Functional recovery after coronary revascularization for chronic coronary artery disease is dependent on maintenance of oxidative metabolism. J Am Coll Cardiol 20:569–577

40. Gunalp B, Dokumaci B, Uyan C et al (1993) Value of dobutamine technetium-99m-sestamibi SPECT and echocardiography in the detection of coronary artery disease compared with coronary angiography. J Nucl Med 34:889–894

41. Gupta NC, Esterbrooks DJ, Hilleman DE, Mohiuddin SM (1992) Comparison of adenosine and exercise thallium-201 single-photon emission computed tomography (SPECT) myocardial perfusion imaging. The GE SPECT multicenter adinosine study group. J Am Coll Cardiol 19:248–257

42. Hachamovitch R, Berman DS, Kiat H et al (1996) Exercise myocardial perfusion SPECT in patients without known coronary artery disease: incremental prognostic value and use in risk stratification. Circulation 93:905–914

43. Hacot JP, Bojovic M, Delonca J et al (1993) Comparison of planar imaging and single-photon emission computed tomography for the detection and localization of coronary artery disease. Int J Card Imaging 9:113–119

44. Haque T, Furukawa T, Takahashi M, Kinoshita M (1995) Identification of hibernating myocardium by dobutamine stress echocardiography: comparison with thallium-201 reinjection imaging. Am Heart J 130:553–563

45. Hashimoto T, Buxton DB, Krivokapich J et al (1994) Responses of blood flow, oxygen consumption, and contractile function to inotropic stimulation in stunned canine myocardium. Am Heart J 127:1250–1262

46. He Z-X, Darcourt J, Guignier A et al (1993) Nitrates improve detection of ischemic but viable myocardium by thallium-201 reinjection SPECT. J Nucl Med 34:1427–1477

47. Heller GV, Herman SD, Travin MI et al (1995) Independent prognostic value of intravenous dipyridamole with technetium-99m sestamibi tomographic imaging in predicting cardiac events and cardiac-related hospital admissions. J Am Coll Cardiol 26:1202–1208

48. Hendel RC, Leppo JA (1995) The value of perioperative clinical indexes and dipyridamole thallium scintigraphy for the prediction of myocardial infarction and cardiac death in patients undergoing vascular surgery. J Nucl Cardiol 2:18–25

49. Heo J, Kegel J, Iskandrian AS et al (1992) Comparison of same-day protocols using technetium-99m-sestamibi myocardial imaging. J Nucl Med 33:186–191

50. Heo J, Wolmer I, Kegel J, Iskandrian AS (1994) Sequential dual-isotope SPECT imaging with thallium-201 and technetium-99m-sestamibi. J Nucl Med 35:549–553

51. Heyndrickx GR, Wijns W, Vogelaers D et al (1993) Recovery of regional contractile function and oxidative metabolism in stunned myocardium induced by 1-hour circumflex coronary artery stenosis in chronically instrumented dogs. Circ Res 72:901–913

52. Hilton TC, Thompson RC, Williams HJ et al (1994) Technetium-99m sestamibi myocardial perfusion imaging in the emergency room evaluation of chest pain. J Am Coll Cardiol 23:1016–1022

53. Hoffmann R, Lethen H, Kleinhans E et al (1993) Comparative evaluation of bicycle and dobutamine stress echocardiography with perfusion scintigraphy and bicycle electrocardiogram for identification of coronary artery disease. Am J Cardiol 72:555–559

54. Inglese E, Brambilla M, Dondi M et al (1995) Assessment of myocardial viability after thallium-201 reinjection or rest-redistribution imaging: a multicenter study. The Italian group of nuclear cardiology. J Nucl Med 36:555–563

55. Iqbal A, Gibbons R, Zinsmeister A et al (1994) Prognostic value of exercise radionuclide angiography in a population-based cohort of patients with known or suspected coronary artery disease. Am J Cardiol 74:119–124

56. Iskandrian AS (1996) Myocardial viability: Unresolved issues. J Nucl Med 37:794–797

57. Iskandrian AS, Heo J, Kong B et al (1989) Use of technetium-99m isonitrile (RP-30A) in assessing left ventricular perfusion and function at rest and during exercise in coronary artery disease, and comparison with coronary arteriography and exercise thallium-201 SPECT imaging. Am J Cardiol 64:270–275

58. Iskandrian AS, Lamlek J, Ogilby JD et al (1992) Early thallium imaging after percutaneous transluminal coronary angioplasty: tomographic evaluation during adenosine-induced coronary hyperemia. J Nucl Med 33:2086–2089

59. Iskandrian AS, Chae SC, Heo J et al (1993) Independent and incremental prognostic value of exercise single-photon emission computed tomographic (SPECT) thallium imaging in coronary artery disease. J Am Coll Cardiol 22:665–670

60. Johnson LL, Lerrick KS, Coromila J et al (1987) Measurement of infarct size and percentage myocardium infarcted in a dog preparation with single photon emission computed tomography, thallium-201 and indium-111 monoclonal antimyosin Fab. Circulation 76:181–190

61. Kang WJ, Lee DS, J-K Chung et al (1997) Performance of gated Tc-99m-MIBI myocardial SPECT in the diagnosis of coronary artery disease. Korean J Nucl Med 31:50–56

62. Kayden DS, Sigal S, Soufer R et al (1991) Thallium-201 for assessment of myocardial viability: quantitative comparison of 24-hour redistribution imaging with imaging after reinjection at rest. J Am Coll Cardiol 18:1480–1486

63. Kawamoto M, Tamaki N, Yonekura Y et al (1994) Combined study with ^{123}I fatty acid and ^{201}Tl to assess ischemic myocardium: comparison with thallium redistribution and glucose metabolism. Ann Nucl Med 8:47–54

64. Khaw B, Yasuda T, Gold HK et al (1987) Acute myocardial infarct imaging with indium-111-labeled monoclonal Fab. J Nucl Med 28:1671–1678

65. Kiat H, Maddahi J, Roy LT et al (1989) Comparison of technetium-99m methoxy isobutyl isonitrile and thallium-201 for evaluation of coronary artery disease by planar and tomographic methods. Am Heart J 117:1–11

66. Kiat H, Van-Train KF, Maddahi J et al (1990) Development and prospective application of quantiative 2-day stress-rest Tc-99m methoxy isobutyl isonitrile SPECT for the diagnosis of coronary artery disease. Am Heart J 120:1255–1266

67. Kiat H, Van-Train KF, Friedman JD et al (1992) Quantitative stress-redistribution thallium-201 SPECT using prone imaging: methodologic development and validation. J Nucl Med 33:1509–1515

68. Kiat H, Germano G, Friedman J et al (1994) Comparative feasibility of separate or simultaneous rest thallium-201/stress technetium-99m-sestamibi dual-isotope myocardial perfusion SPECT. J Nucl Med 35:542–548

69. Kiat H, Iskandrian AS, Villegas BJ et al (1995) Arbutamine stress thallium-201 single-photon emission computed tomography using a computerized closed-loop delivery system. Multicenter trial for evaluation of safety and diagnostic accuracy. The international arbutamine study group. J Am Coll Cardiol 26:1159–1167

70. Knapp FF Jr, Franken P, Kropp J (1995) Cardiac SPECT with iodine-123-labeled fatty acids: evaluation of myocardial viability with BMIPP. J Nucl Med 36:1022–1030

71. Knuuti MJ, Saraste M, Nuutila P et al (1994) Myocardial viability: fluorine-18-deoxyglucose positron emission tomography in prediction of wall motion recovery after revascularization. Am Heart J 127:785–796

72. Lakkis NM, Mahmarian JJ, Verani MS (1995) Exercise thallium-201 single photon emission computed tomography for evaluation of coronary artery bypass graft patency. Am J Cardiol 76:107–111

73. Lee DS, Yoon SN, Kim KB et al (1997) Predictive values of gated myocardial SPECT for wall motion improvement after bypass surgery. Korean J Nucl Med 31:43–49

74. Lee DS, Yoon SN, Lee WW et al (1997) Transient prolonged stunning by dipyridamole stress proved by post-stress (1 hour) and 24 hour Tc-99m-MIBI gated SPECT. J Nucl Med 38:15P (abstract)

75. Lee KL, Pryor DB, Pieper KS et al (1990) Prognostic value of radionuclide angiography in medically treated patients with coronary artery disease. Circulation 82:1705–1717

76. Le Feuvre C, Banbion N, Aubry N et al (1996) Assessment of reversible dyssynergic segments after acute myocardial infarction: dobutamine echocardiography versus thallium-201 single photon emission computed tomography. Am Heart J 131:668–675

77. Lette J, Tatum JL, Fraser S et al (1995) Safety of dipyridamole testing in 73 806 patients: The multicenter dipyridamole safety study. J Nucl Cardiol 2:3–17

78. Levy W, Cerqueira M, Matsuoka D et al (1992) Four radionuclide methods for left ventricular volume determination: comparison of a manual and automated technique. J Nucl Med 33:763–770

79. Machecourt J, Longere P, Fagret D et al (1994) Prognostic value of thallium-201 single-photon emission computed tomographic myocardial perfusion imaging according to extent of myocardial defect: study in 1 926 patients with follow-up at 33 months. J Am Coll Cardiol 23:1096–1106

80. Mahmarian JJ, Verani MS (1991) Exercise thallium-201 perfusion scintigraphy in the assessment of coronary artery disease. Am J Cardiol 67:2D–11D

81. Mahamrian JJ, Pratt CM, Nishimura S et al (1993) Quantitative adenosine ^{201}Tl single-photon emission computed tomography for the early assessment of patients surviving acute myocardial infarction. Circulation 87:1197–1210

82. Mahmarian JJ, Mahmarian AC, Marks GF et al (1995) Role of adenosine thallium-201 tomography for defining long-term risk in patients after acute myocardial infarction. J Am Coll Cardiol 25:1333–1340

83. Mahmood S, Gunning M, Bomanji JB et al (1995) Combined rest thallium-201/stress technetium-99m-tetrofosmin SPECT: feasibility and diagnostic accuracy of a 90-minute protocol. J Nucl Med 36:932–935

84. Mantysaari M, Kuikka J, Mustonen J et al (1992) Noninvasive detection of cardiac sympathetic nervous dysfunction in diabetic patients using ^{123}I metaiodobenzylguanidine. Diabetes 41:1069–1075

85. Manyari DE, Knudtson M, Kloiber R, Roth D (1988) Sequential thallium-201 myocardial perfusion studies after successful percutaneous transmural coronary artery angioplasty: delayed resolution of exercise-induced scintigraphic abnormalities. Circulation 77:86–95

86. Marie P-Y, Danchin N, Durand JF et al (1995) Long-term prediction of major ischemic events by exercise thallium-201 single-photon emission computed tomography. Incremental prognostic value compared with clinical, exercise testing, catheterization and radionuclide angiographic data. J Am Coll Cardiol 26:879–886

87. Marwick T, Willemart B, D'Hondt AM et al (1993) Selection of the optimal nonexercise stress for the evaluation of ischemic regional myocardial dysfunction and malperfusion, comparison of dobutamine and adenosine using echocardiography and ^{99m}Tc-MIBI single photon emission computed tomography. J Nucl Med 87:345–354

88. Marzullo P, Parodi O, Reisenhofer B et al (1993) Value of rest thallium-201/technetium-99m sestamibi scans and dobutamine echocardiography for detecting myocardial viability. Am J Cardiol 71:166–172

89. Massardo T, Gal R, Grenier R et al (1990) Left ventricular volume calculation using a count-based ratio method applied to multigated radionuclide angiography. J Nucl Med 31:450–456

90. Matsunari I, Fujino S, Taki J et al (1996) Impaired fatty acid uptake in ischemic but viable myocardium identified by thallium-201 reinjection. Am Heart J 131:458–465

91. Matzer L, Kiat H, Wang FP et al (1994) Pharmacologic stress dual-isotope myocardial perfusion single-photon emission computed tomography. Am Heart J 128:1067–1076

92. Maublant JC, Marcaggi X, Lusson J-R et al (1992) Comparison between thallium-201 and technetium-99m methoxyisobutyl isonitrile defect size in single-photon emission computed tomography at rest, exercise and redistribution in coronary artery disease. Am J Cardiol 69:183–187

93. Mazzanti M, Germano G, Kiat H et al (1996) Fast technetium-99m-labeled sestamibi gated SPECT for evaluation of myocardial function. J Nucl Cardiol 3:143–149

94. McFalls EO, Duncker DJ, Krams R et al (1992) Recruitment of myocardial work and metabolism in regionally stunned porcine myocardium. Am J Physiol 32:724–731

95. McFalls EO, Ward H, Fashingbauer P et al (1995) Myocardial blood flow and FDG retention in acutely stunned porcine myocardium. J Nucl Med 36:637–643

96. Merlet P, Valette H, Dubois-Rande J-L et al (1992) Prognostic value of cardiac metaiodobenzylguanidine imaging in patients with heart failure. J Nucl Med 33:477–479

97. Milan E, Zoccarato O, Terzi A et al (1996) Technetium-99m-sestamibi SPECT to detect restenosis after successful percutaneous coronary angioplasty. J Nucl Med 37:1300–1305

98. Miller DD, Stratmann HG, Shaw L et al (1994) Dipyridamole technetium 99m sestamibi myocardial tomography as an independent predictor of cardiac event-free survival after acute ischemic events. J Nucl Cardiol 1:172–182

99. Miller TD, Christian TF, Hopfenspirger MR et al (1995) Infarct size after acute myocardial infarction measured by quantitative tomographic ^{99m}Tc sestamibi imaging predicts subsequent mortality. Circulation 92:334–341

100. Morguet AJ, Munz DL, Klein HH et al (1992) Myocardial distribution of indium-111-antimyosin Fab and technetium-99m-sestamibi in experimental nontransmural infarction. J Nucl Med 33:223–228

101. Mori T, Minamiji K, Kurongane H et al (1991) Rest-injected thallium-201 imaging for assessing viability of severely asynergic regions. J Nucl Med 23:1718–1724

102. Nguyen T, Heo J, Ogilby JD, Iskandrian AS (1990) Single photon emission computed tomography with thallium-201 during adenosine-induced coronary hyperemia; correlation with coronary arteriography, exercise thallium imaging and two-dimensional echocardiography. J Am Coll Cardiol 16 (6):1375–1383

103. Nishimura S, Mahmarian JJ, Boyce TM, Verani MS (1991) Quantitative thallium-201 single-photon emission computed tomography during maximal pharmacologic coronary vasodilation with adenosine for assessing coronary artery disease. J Am Coll Cardiol 18:736–745

104. Obrador D, Ballester M, Carrio I et al (1994) Presence, evolving changes, and prognostic implications of myocardial damage detected in idiopathic and alcoholic dilated cardiomyopathy by In-111 monoclonal antimyosin antibodies. Circulation 89:2054–2061

105. Ohtani H, Tamaki N, Yonekura Y et al (1990) Value of thallium-201 reinjection after delayed SPECT imaging for predicting reversible ischemia after coronary artery bypass grafting. Am J Cardiol 66:394–399

106. Palmas W, Bingham S, Diamond GA et al (1995) Incremental prognostic value of exercise thallium-201 myocardial single-photon emission computed tomography late after coronary artery bypass surgery. J Am Coll Cardiol 25:403–409

107. Panza JA, Dilsizian V, Laurienzo JM et al (1995) Relation between thallium uptake and contracile response to dobutamine: implication regarding myocardial viability is patients with chronic coronary artery disease and left ventricular dysfunction. Circulation 91:990–998

108. Port SC (1994) The role of radionuclide ventriculography in the assessment of prognosis in patients with CAD. J Nucl Med 35:721–725

109. Potts JM, Borges-Neto S, Smith LR et al (1991) Comparison of bicycle and treadmill radionuclide angiocardiography. J Nucl Med 32:1918–1922

110. Pozzoli MM, Fioretti PM, Salustri A et al (1991) Exercise echocardiography and technetium-99m MIBI single-photon emission computed tomography in the detection of coronary artery disease. Am J Cardiol 67:350–355

111. Quinones MA, Verani MS, Haichin RM et al (1992) Exercise echocardiography versus ^{201}Tl single-photon emission computed tomography in evaluation of coronary artery disease. Analysis of 292 patients. Circulation 85:1026–1031

112. Ragosta M, Beller GA, Watson DD et al (1993) Quantitative planar rest-redistribution Tl-201 imaging in detection of myocardial viability and prediction of improvement in left ventricular function after coronary artery bypass surgery in patients with severely depressed left ventricular function. Circulation 86:1630–1641

113. Ritchie JL, Bateman TM, Bonow RO et al (1995) Guidelines for clinical use of cardiac radionuclide imaging: a report of the American Heart Association/American College of Cardiology task force on assessment of diagnostic and therapeutic cardiovascular procedures, committee on radionuclide imaging, developed in collaboration with the American Society of Nuclear Cardiology. Circulation 91:1278–1303

114. Sawada SG, Allman KC, Muzik O et al (1994) Positron emission tomography detects evidence of viability in rest technetium-99m sestamibi defects. J Am Coll Cardiol 23:92–98

115. Schafers M, Matheja P, Hasfeld M et al (1996) The clinical impact of thallium-201 reinjection for the detection of myocardial hibernation. Eur J Nucl Med 23:407–413

116. Segall GM, Atwood JE, Botvinick EH et al (1995) Variability of normal coronary anatomy: implications for the interpretation of thallium-SPECT myocardial perfusion images in single-vessel disease. J Nucl Med 36:944–951

117. Senior R, Bhattacharya S, Manspeaker P et al (1993) ^{99m}Tc-antimyosin antibody imaging for the detection of acute myocardial infarction in human beings. Am Heart J 126:536–542

118. Senior R, Glenville B, Basu S et al (1995) Dobutamine echocardiography and thallium-201 imaging predict functional improvement after revascularization in severe ischemic left ventricular dysfunction. Br Heart J 74:358–364

119. Sinusas AJ, Trautman KA, Bergun JD et al (1990) Quantification of area at risk during coronary occlusion and degree of myocardial salvage after reperfusion with technetium-99m-hexakis-2-methoxyisobutyl isonitrile. Circulation 82:1573–1581

120. Soufer R, Dey HM, Ng CK, Zaret BL (1995) Comparison of sestamibi single-photon emission computed tomography with positron emission tomography for estimating left ventricular myocardial viability. Am J Cardiol 75:1214–1219

121. Stanton MS, Tuli MM, Radtke NL (1989) Regional sympathetic denervation after myocardial infarction in humans detected noninvasively using I-123-metaiodobenzylguanidine. J Am Coll Cardiol 14:1519–1526

122. Stewart RE, Schwaiger M, Molina E et al (1991) Comparison of rubidium-82 positron emission tomography and thallium-201 SPECT imaging for detection of coronary artery disease. Am J Cardiol 67:1303–1310

123. Stratmann HG, Younis LT, Wittry MD et al (1995) Dipyridamole technetium-99m sestamibi myocardial tomography in patients evaluated for elective vascular surgery: Prognostic value for perioperative and late cardiac events. Am Heart J 131:923–929

124. Taki J, Nakajima K, Bunko H et al (1994) Twenty-four-hour quantitative thallium imaging for predicting beneficial revascularization. Eur J Nucl Med 21:1212–1217

125. Taki J, Nakajima K, Matsunari I et al (1995) Impairment of regional fatty acid uptake in relation to wall motion and thallium-201 uptake in ischaemic but

viable myocardium: assessment with iodine-123-labelled beta-methyl-branched fatty acid. Eur J Nucl Med 22:1385–1392

126. Tamaki N, Ohtani H, Yamashita K et al (1991) Metabolic activity in the areas of new fill-in after thallium-201 reinjection: comparison with positron emission tomography using fluorine-18-deoxyglucose. J Nucl Med 32:673–678

127. Tamaki N, Kawamoto M, Takahashi N et al (1993) Prognostic value of an increase in fluorine-18 deoxyglucose uptake in patients with myocardial infarction: comparison with stress thallium imaging. J Am Coll Cardiol 22:1621–1627

128. Uren NG, Camici PG, Melin JA et al (1995) Effect of aging on myocardial perfusion reserve. J Nucl Med 36:2032–2036

129. Vanoverschelde J-L J, Melin JA, Bol A et al (1992). Regional oxidative metabolism in patients after recovery from reperfused anterior myocardial infarction: relation to regional blood flow and glucose uptake. Circulation 85:9–21

130. Vanoverschelde J-L J, Gerber BL, D'Hondt A-M et al (1995) Preoperative selection of patients with severely impaired left ventricular function for coronary revascularization. Role of low-dose dobutamine echocardiography and exercise-redistribution-reinjection thallium SPECT. Circulation 92 [Suppl II]:II37–II44

131. Van-Train KF, Garcia EV, Maddahi J et al (1994) Multicenter trial validation for quantitative analysis of same-day rest-stress technetium-99m-sestamibi myocardial tomograms. J Nucl Med 35:609–618

132. Wallis J, Supine P, Borer J et al (1993) Prognostic value of left ventricular ejection fraction response to exercise during long-term follow-up after coronary artery bypass graft surgery. Circulation 88 (II):99–109

133. Whalley DR, Murphy JJ, Frier M et al (1991) A comparison of same day and separate day injection protocols for myocardial perfusion SPECT using ^{99m}Tc-MIBI. Nucl Med Com 12:99–104

134. Wichter T, Hindricks G, Lerch H et al (1994) Regional myocardial sympathetic dysinnervation in arrhythmogenic right ventricular cardiomyopathy. An analysis using ^{123}I-meta-iodobenzylguanidine scintigraphy. Circulation 89:667–683

135. Yamada T, Tamaki N, Morishima S et al (1992) Time course of myocardial infarction evaluated by indium-111-antimyosin monoclonal antibody scintigraphy: clinical implications and prognostic value. J Nucl Med 33:1501–1508

136. Yamanichi Y, Kusuoka H, Morishita K et al (1995) Metabolism of iodine-123-BMIPP in perfused rat hearts. J Nud Med 36:1043–1050

137. Yamakado K, Takeda K, Kitano K et al (1992) Serial change of iodine-123 metaiodobenzylguanidine (MIBG) myocardial concentration in patients with dialted cardiomyopathy. Eur J Nucl Med 19:265–270

138. Yeo JS, Lee DS, Kang KW et al (1996) Diagnostic accuracy of rest Tl-201/stress Tc-99m-MIBI myocardial SPECT in the diagnosis of coronary artery disease. Korean J Nucl Med 30:112–117

139. Yoon SN, Lee DS, Kim KB et al (1996) Viability assessment with Tl-201 rest-24 hour delay redistribution SPECT before coronary artery bypass graft in coronary artery disease. Korean J Nucl Med 30:493–501

140. Zimmermann R, Mall G, Rauch B et al (1995) Residual Tl-201 activity in irreversible defects as a marker of myocardial viability. Clinicopathological study. Circulation 91:1016–1021

12 Collateral Circulation in the Superior Vena Cava Syndrome

A. M. Mahmud, T. Isawa, and T. Teshima

The superior vena cava syndrome (SVCS), first described in 1757 by William Hunter [1], bears considerable importance for both the physician and the patient. It is a known complication of thoracic neoplasms, with lung cancer accounting for 67%–82% of cases [2].

Impeded venous return through the superior vena cava or its major tributaries due to their partial or complete stenosis gives rise to the constellation of clinical and radiographic findings that constitute the syndrome [3]. Dyspnea and swelling of the face and upper extremities are the cardinal features [4–8]. Persistence of obstruction or compression of the central veins causes retrograde blood flow which eventually culminates in the diversion of blood through certain collateral pathways. The opening of collateral circulatory channels provides symptomatic relief to the patient, but this is enigmatic because:

- It indicates persistent compression of the central veins.
- Obstruction may be missed clinically when gradual development of partial obstruction, allowing establishment of sufficient collateral circulation, prevents appearance of the typical features [9].
- During clinical assessment, relief of edema by collaterals may provide a false sense of relief.
- There is increased risk of hemorrhage during surgery in cases with collaterals.

In contrast, however, collateral circulation which adequately decompresses the upper compartment veins obviates the need for bypass surgery [2] and allows high-dose radiation therapy. In the case of poor collaterals radiation-induced edema may aggravate the situation [10].

In view of the above facts, precise understanding of the collateral pathways is extremely important in the successful management of this syndrome.

Initially reported in 1966 by Rosenthall [11], radionuclide venography (RNV) using ^{99m}Tc is a convenient, safe, and noninvasive imaging procedure [2, 12] which has substantially improved our understanding of the collateral circulation in SVCS [13, 14]. Its safety has been very well documented in Ahmann's review of 96 studies, in which not even a single untoward incident occurred [15]. RNV has the following advantages:

- Provides accurate and detailed information about collateral circulatory pathways in SVCS patients.

- Can detect presence of thrombus. In such patients, anti-cancer therapy needs to be supplemented by thrombolytics.
- Allows preoperative visualization of critical collateral pathways which if disrupted during surgery may lead to postoperative deterioration.
- May be used to confirm patency of bypass grafts.
- In addition to imaging, it can be utilized for studying hemodynamic changes in SVCS patients and their post-therapy assessment [16].

Major collateral pathways are tabulated and illustrated in Table 12.1 and Fig. 12.1. Factors that influence the extent of collateral formation and determine which pathway develops include site, extent, and duration of occlusion rather than the size of the lesion [17]. Uncommon pathways of collateral circulation include systemic-pulmonary venous shunting [18], direct shunting between right subclavian vein and left ventricle [19, 20], the portal vein via paraumbilical veins [21, 22], external jugular vein [16], and cerebral sinuses [14].

It is evident from Table 12.1 that the azygos venous system serves as the major collateral pathway, a view supported by other authors [2, 3]. This is attributed to its several interconnections which allow shunting of blood through veins that either bypass the SVC obstruction or drain into the inferior vena cava (IVC). Accordingly, in patients who have occlusion below the azygos orifice or involving it, clinical features are more prominent and distressing. The importance of the azygos system has been documented in an animal model for SVCS by Carlson [23].

It should be noted that collateral pathways are not always clinically discernible since it is the deep veins that are involved. In some cases, however, superficial tributaries of these veins are visible clinically. RNV gives an elaborate picture of the collateral circulatory pathways by being able to visualize the deep venous systems.

According to Sy and Lao, certain useful identifying points of various collateral veins are:

Table 12.1. Major collateral pathways seen in SVCS (modified from [3])

Shunt	Intermediary	System
Obstruction above the azygos vein		
Jugular venous arch	Contralateral brachiocephalic	SVC
Lateral thoracic	Superior intercostal, azygos	SVC
Cervical venous network	Vertebral venous plexus, azygos	SVC
Internal thoracic	Anterior and posterior intercostal azygos	SVC
Obstruction below the azygos vein or involving its orifice		
Lateral thoracic	Thoraco epigastric, superficial epigastric	IVC
Internal thoracic	Superior epigastric, inferior epigastric	IVC
Lateral thoracic	Posterior intercostal, azygos	IVC
Cervical venous network	Vertebral venous plexus, azygos	IVC

Cervical venous network as defined by Muramatsu et al. [14]

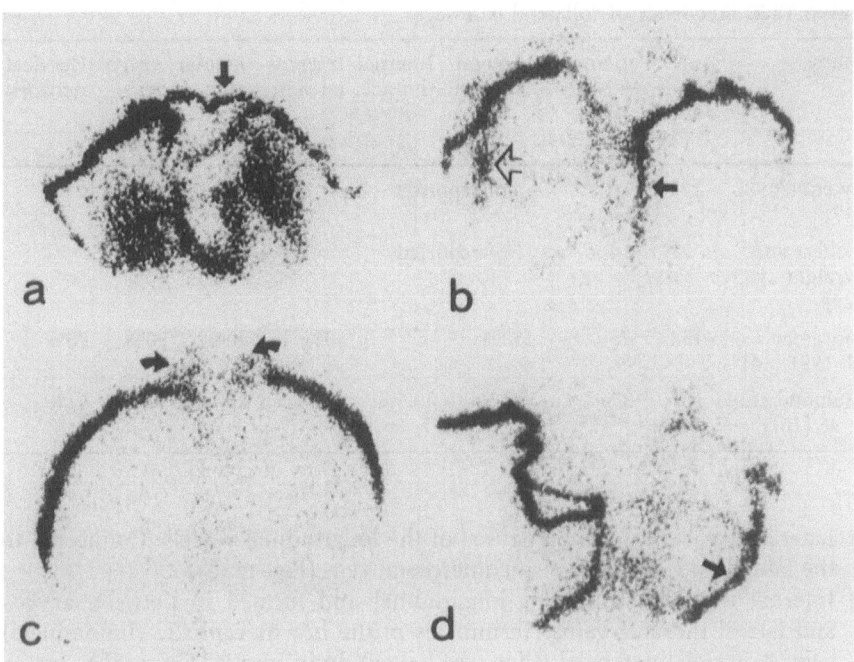

Fig. 12.1 a–d. Major collateral pathways. **a** Jugular venous arch (*arrow*). **b** Lateral thoracic vein (*open arrowhead*) and internal thoracic vein (arrow). **c** Cervical venous network (*arrows*). **d** Lateral thoracic vein draining into thoracoepigastric vein (*arrow*)

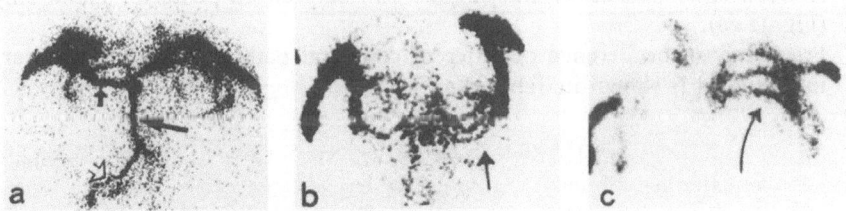

Fig. 12.2 a–c. Identifying points of certain collateral veins. **a** Azygos vein (*long arrow*) is connected to the medial end of the superior intercostal vein (*short arrow*) and the lower tributaries give a "crab leg" appearance (*open arrowhead*). **b** Anterior intercostal veins: note superior *concavity* (*arrow*). **c** Posterior intercostal veins seen on posterior view; note superior *convexity* (*arrow*). (**b,c** By permission of the publisher from [17])

■ Azygos vein: most medial of the longitudinal vessels. This may be confused with the SVC, but the differentiating points are: (a) azygos appears longer than SVC and does not merge into the cardiac silhouette, (b) is connected to the medial end of the superior intercostal vein, (c) posterior intercostal veins drain into it (see below), and (d) it has musculophrenic tributaries at its lower end which give a "crab leg" appearance (Fig. 12.2a).

Table 12.2. Frequency of collateral pathways

Study	Patients		Lateral thoracic	Internal thoracic	Intercostal vein	Jugular arch	Azygos vein	Cervical network
	Total	With collaterals						
Sy et al. 1982 [17]	123	26	Not reported					
Coltart and Wraight 1985 [24]	27	14	Not reported					
Muramatsu et al. 1991 [14]	133	73	50%	–	50%	40%	50%	25%
Mahmud et al. 1996 [16]	107	37	40.5%	40.5%	40.5%	27%	16%	21%

- Lateral thoracic vein: most lateral of the longitudinal vessels. Connected to the lateral end of the superior intercostal vein (Fig. 12.1b).
- Internal thoracic vein: it is longitudinal and located in between azygos and lateral thoracic veins. Terminates in the brachiocephalic (innominate) vein. Anterior intercostal veins (see below) drain into it (Fig. 12.1b).
- Anterior intercostal veins: horizontally situated multiple vessels, parallel to each other, with superior *concavity*. Drain into internal thoracic vein (Fig. 12.2b).
- Posterior intercostal veins: similar to anterior intercostals but have a superior *convexity* and drain into azygos. Can be seen on posterior views only (Fig. 12.2c).
  Frequency of occurrence of different collateral pathways as found in various studies is shown in Table 12.2.

Acknowledgement. The authors are grateful to Ms. Yuko Ogata for providing technical assistance during the study.

References

1. Hunter W (1757) The history of an aneurysm of the aorta with some remarks on aneurysm in general. Med Observ Inq 1:323–357
2. Nieto AF, Doty DB (1986) Superior vena cava obstruction, clinical syndrome, etiology and treatment. Curr Prob Surg 10:442–484
3. Mehta MP, Kinsella TJ (1995) Superior vena cava syndrome. In: Roth JA, Ruckdeschsl JC, Weisenburger TH (eds) Thoracic oncology. Saunders, Philadelphia, pp 239–257
4. Schraufnagel DE, Hill R, Leech JA et al (1981) Superior vena caval obstruction: is it a medical emergency? Am J Med 70:1169–1174
5. Parish JM, Marschke RF, Dines DE et al (1981) Etiological considerations in superior vena cava syndrome. Mayo Clin Proc 36:407–413

6. Armstrong BA, Perez CA, Simpson JR et al (1987) Role of irradiation in the management of superior vena cava syndrome. Int J Radiat Biol Phys 13:531–539

7. Chen JC, Bongard F, Klein SR (1990) A contemporary perspective on superior vena cava syndrome. Am J Surg 160:207–211

8. Yellin A, Rosen A, Riechert N, Lieberman Y (1990) Superior vena cava syndrome. The myth – the facts. Am Rev Respir Dis 141:1114–1118

9. Yedlicka JW, Schultz K, Moncada R et al (1989) CT findings in superior vena cava obstruction. Semin Roentgen 24:84–90

10. Son JH, Wetzel RA, Wilson WJ (1968) ^{99m}Tc pertechnetate scinti photography as diagnostic and follow-up aids in major vascular obstruction due to malignant neoplasm. Radiology 91:349–357

11. Rosenthall L (1966) Applications of gamma-ray scintillation camera to dynamic studies in man. Radiology 86:634–639

12. Van Houtte P, Fruhling J (1981) Radionuclide venography in the evaluation of superior vena cava syndrome. Clin Nucl Med 6:177–183

13. Maxfield WS, Meckstroth GR (1969) Tc-99m superior vena cavography. Radiology 92:913–918

14. Muramatsu T, Miyamae T, Doi Y (1991) Collateral pathways observed by radionuclide superior cavography in 70 patients with superior vena caval obstruction. Clin Nucl Med 16:332–336

15. Ahman FR (1984) A reassessment of the clinical implications of the superior vena cava syndrome. J Clin Oncol 2:961–969

16. Mahmud AM, Isawa T, Teshima T et al (1996) Radionuclide venography and its functional analysis in the superior vena cava syndrome. J Nucl Med 37:1460–1464

17. Sy WM, Lao RS (1982) Collateral pathways in superior vena caval obstruction as seen on gamma images. Br J Radiol 55:294–300

18. Gale B, Chen C, Chun KJ et al (1990) Systemic to pulmonary venous shunting in superior vena cava obstruction: unusual myocardial and thyroid visualization. Clin Nucl Med 15:246–250

19. Muramatsu T, Mashimo M, Miyamae T et al (1987) Rare collateral pathway in superior vena cava obstruction: the development of venous shunts between systemic veins and the left heart. Clin Nucl Med 12:241

20. Taki J, Bunko H, Tonami N et al (1990) Shunt between right subclavian vein and the left heart in superior vena cava obstruction due to lung cancer. Clin Nucl Med 15:251–253

21. Desai AG, Park CH (1983) Cavo-portal shunting in superior and inferior vena caval obstruction. Clin Nucl Med 8:365–368

22. Suneja SK, Teal JS (1989) Discrepant sulfur colloid and radioparticle liver uptake in superior vena cava obstruction: case report. J Nucl Med 30:113–116

23. Carlson HA (1934) Obstruction of the superior vena cava: an experimental study. Arch Surg 29:669–677

24. Coltart RS, Wraight EP (1985) The value of radionuclide venography in superior vena cava obstruction. Clin Radiol 36:415–418

13 Mediastinum

E. E. KIM

Introduction

The mediastinum constitutes a compartmented septum or partition which divides the thorax vertically. It is traditionally divided into two major compartments, the superior and the inferior, the latter being divided into anterior, middle, and posterior compartments. The superior possesses little practical importance as a separate division, defined as that area bounded superiorly by the thoracic inlet and inferiorly by a line drawn from the manubriosternal angle to the intervertebral disc between the fourth and fifth thoracic vertebrae.

The anatomic boundaries of the mediastinum are as follows: lateral, the parietal pleural reflections along the medial aspects of both lungs; superior, the thoracic inlet; inferior, the diaphragm; anterior, the sternum; and posterior, the anterior surfaces of the thoracic vertebral bodies. The anterior compartment contains the thymus gland and the anterior mediastinal lymph nodes. The middle compartment contains the heart, aortic arch, vena cava, brachiocephalic vessels, phrenic and vagus nerves, trachea and main bronchi and their contiguous lymph nodes, and the pulmonary vessels. The posterior compartment contains the esophagus, descending aorta, thoracic duct, azygos and hemiazygos veins, sympathetic and vagus nerves, and posterior mediastinal lymph nodes.

Recently the American Thoracic Society offered a new classification of mediastinal lymph nodes using the aortic and azygos arches as reference points. At the present time computed tomography (CT) is the gold standard for the noninvasive evaluation of mediastinal masses. It depicts subtle difference in absorption or attenuation of X-rays, making it possible to differentiate air, fat, fluid, contrast agent, and calcium with great specificity. However, it has a limitation in differentiating active tumors from posttreatment changes.

Lymphoma

The term lymphoma has been used to describe a large number of diverse lymphoproliferative disorders. Approximately 8% of all cancers diagnosed in the United States are either leukemia or lymphoma. Hodgkin's disease is a re-

latively uncommon tumor responsible for less than 1% of all newly diagnosed cancer in the United States each year, and non-Hodgkin's lymphoma
accounts for 4%. Approximately 30 000 new cases of lymphocytic lymphoma
occur each year in the United States. The incidence increases monotonically
with age [12]. Every year approximately 13 000 persons die from this disease.
Four distinct histological subtypes of Hodgkin's disease have been described:
lymphocytic predominate (10%–15%), nodular sclerosing (30%–70%), mixed
cellularity (20%–40%), and lymphocytic depletion (5%–15%).

Rappaport [17] classified lymphomas on the basis of their pattern of
growth (nodular or diffuse) and the degree of differentiation of the predominant malignant cell (well-differentiated lymphocytic, poorly differentiated
lymphocytic, histiocytic, and mixed). In general patients with diffuse well-
differentiated lymphocytic, nodular poorly differentiated lymphocytic, and
nodular mixed lymphocytic/histiocytic lymphomas follow a more or less in-
dolent course, and those with nodular histiocytic, diffuse mixed, and diffuse
histiocytic lymphomas tend to have an aggressive course. In contrast to
Hodgkin's disease, where relatively little is known about the lineage of the

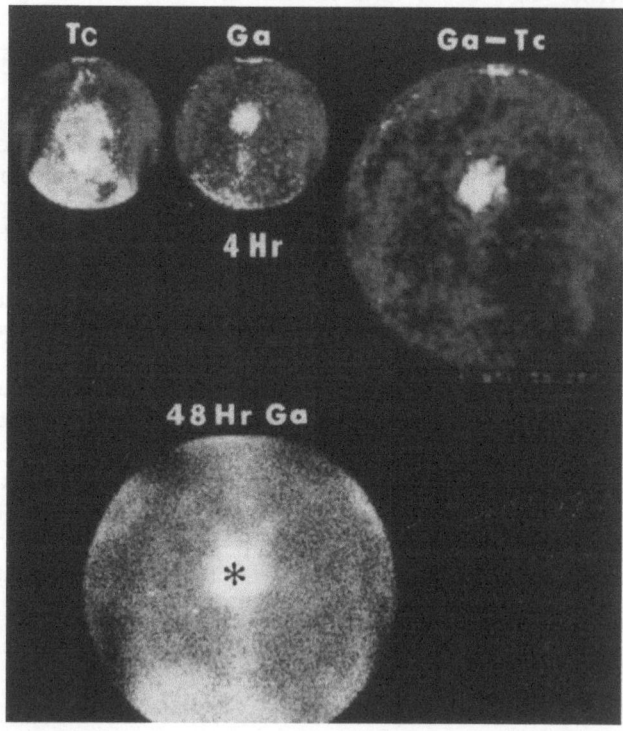

Fig. 13.1. Hodgkin's disease. Anterior static image of the chest 48 h following the injection of ^{67}Ga-citrate shows a focal area of markedly increased activity (*) in the
upper mediastinum. Note the tumor identified at 4 h by the subtraction (^{67}Ga-citrate
– ^{99m}Tc-human serum albumin) technique

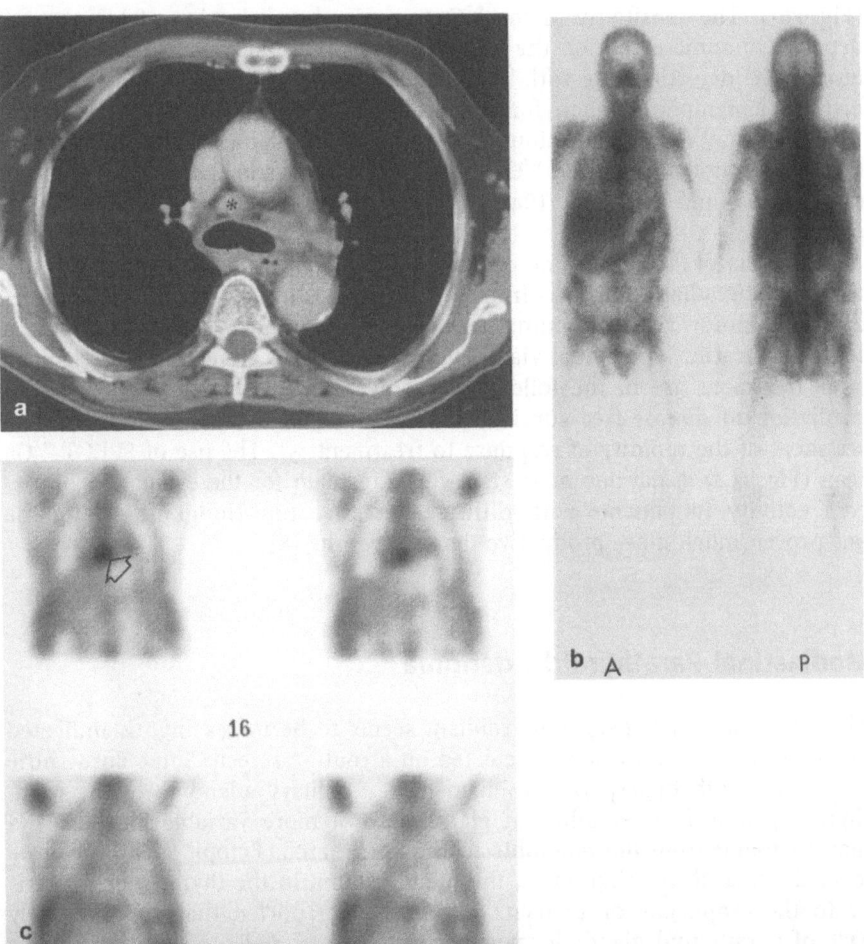

Fig. 13.2a. Axial image of the chest CT shows a nodular subcarinal lesion (*) in a lymphoma patient. **b** Anterior and posterior whole body images of ⁶⁷Ga scan show minimally increased activities in hilar areas, representing reactive hyperplasia of hilar nodes. There is no focal increased activity in the lymphatic chain. **c** SPECT of the chest shows a focal area of markedly increased uptake (*arrow*) of ⁶⁷Ga in the subcarinal lymphatic chain

Reed Sternberg cell, non-Hodgkin's lymphomas are derived from B and T cells. Clinical stage is the extent of disease as defined by the history, physical examination, X-ray, and nuclear imaging studies. Following clinical staging, biopsy evaluation of specific tissues using invasive techniques provides information on the pathological stage [13]. Hodgkin's disease can be cured in nearly 75% of patients whereas non-Hodgkin's lymphomas are cured in fewer than 25%.

⁶⁷Ga scan has been used during the entire process of evaluating lymphoma patients including initial staging and evaluation of therapeutic response

(Fig. 13.1). The sensitivity of the ^{67}Ga scan in the evaluation of lymphomas depends to some extent on the cell type and on the size and location of the lesion. The detection rate with ^{67}Ga scan is greater for Hodgkin's disease and histiocytic lymphoma than for lymphocytic or mixed lymphoma [6]. The ^{67}Ga scan may not detect lesions less than 1 cm in diameter, and the necrotic tissue does not concentrate ^{67}Ga-citrate. ^{67}Ga scan shows a high sensitivity (78%–100%) and specificity (84%–94%) in the detection of mediastinal lymphoma.

By means of ^{67}Ga scan one can distinguish mediastinal widening secondary to postirradiation fibrosis from that due to recurrent lymphoma. The mediastinal tumor site continuing to demonstrate uptake after therapy is a strong indication of residual viable lymphoma. The current uses of ^{67}Ga scan after treatment are in the following: (a) evaluation of a residual mass, (b) prediction of disease-free survival, (c) diagnosis of recurrence, and (d) assessment of the rapidity of response to treatment [5]. The use of SPECT ^{67}Ga scan (Fig. 13.2) at day 100 after stem-cell transplant for the evaluation of disease activity in patients with diffuse aggressive non-Hodgkin's lymphoma has proven much more productive than CT results [8].

Mediastinal Parathyroid Adenoma

The prevalence of hyperparathyroidism seems to be increasing, as indicated by an elevated serum calcium detected on a routine screen. Some 80%–90% of patients with hyperparathyroidism have a solitary adenoma of the parathyroid glands [19]. Parathyroid glands have a more variable location and may be found from the mandible to the aortic arch. Ectopic glands may be located lateral to the thyroid, in the mediastinum, in the thymus, or posterior to the esophagus or pharynx. It has been reported that approximately 62% of parathyroid glands located below the lower poles of the thyroid are within 0.5 cm of the lower pole of the thyroid gland; an additional 13% are within 1 cm and a further 7% within 2 cm. Glands located further caudally and into the superior mediastinum are much less common.

CT can provide high-resolution anatomic detail of the mediastinum, but it does not usually demonstrate a parathyroid adenoma in the posterior mediastinum. The sensitivity of CT for parathyroid adenomas is approximately 70% for initial or recurrent hyperparathyroidism but only 43% for ectopic parathyroid adenomas [4]. Experience with magnetic resonance imaging shows similar sensitivity and specificity to those of CT. Mediastinal glands cannot be evaluated by ultrasound.

In the case of patients who have already had an operative procedure for hyperparathyroidism demonstrated hypercalcemia and elevated parathyroid hormone, ^{201}Tl/^{99m}Tc subtraction scintigraphy [21] can help define ectopic parathyroid tissue in the mediastinum, thymus, or other locations within the neck. First, 1 mCi ^{201}Tl is injected, thereby eliminating the need for the downscatter image of 1 mCi ^{99m}Tc-pertechnetate. An anterior ^{201}Tl view of

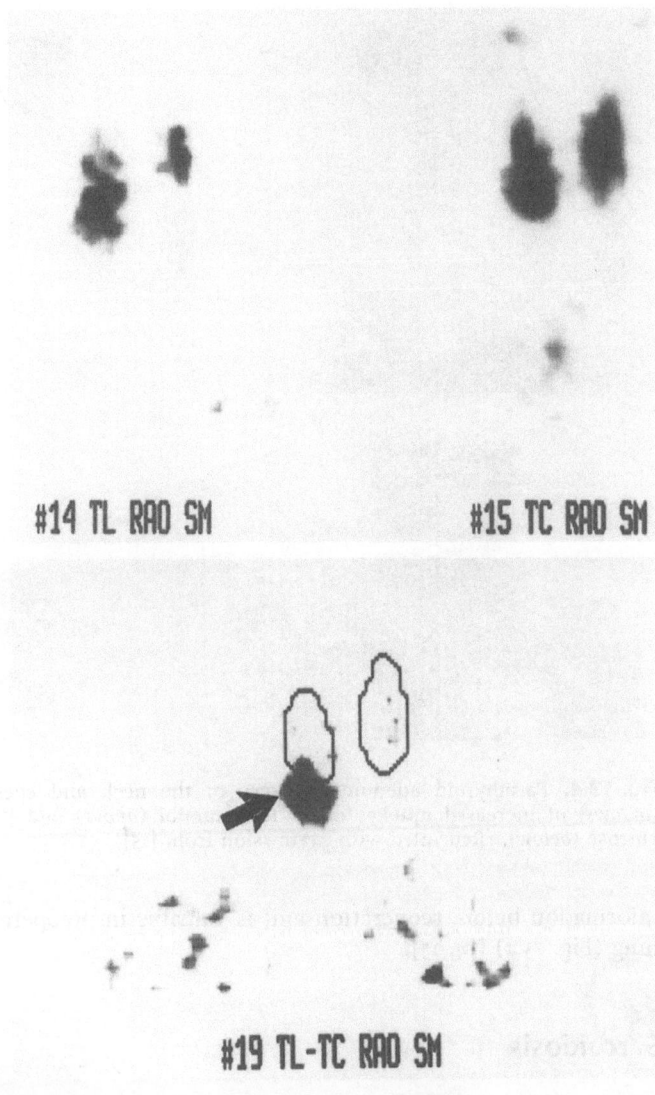

Fig. 13.3. Subtraction (^{201}Tl – ^{99m}Tc-pertechnetate) image (*below*) shows a parathyroid adenoma (*arrow*) in the inferior pole of right thyroid lobe

the chest is acquired with a parallel-hole collimator to localize ectopic thyroid glands (Fig. 13.3). In recent studies ^{99m}Tc-sestamibi has proven the most useful tracer for detecting parathyroid adenomas [3]. Increased perfusion, mitochondria-rich cells, abundant mitochondria, functional activity, and cellularity are possible explanations for the tumor uptake of sestamibi [16]. Fluoro-2-deoxy-D-glucose positron-emission tomography provides accurate

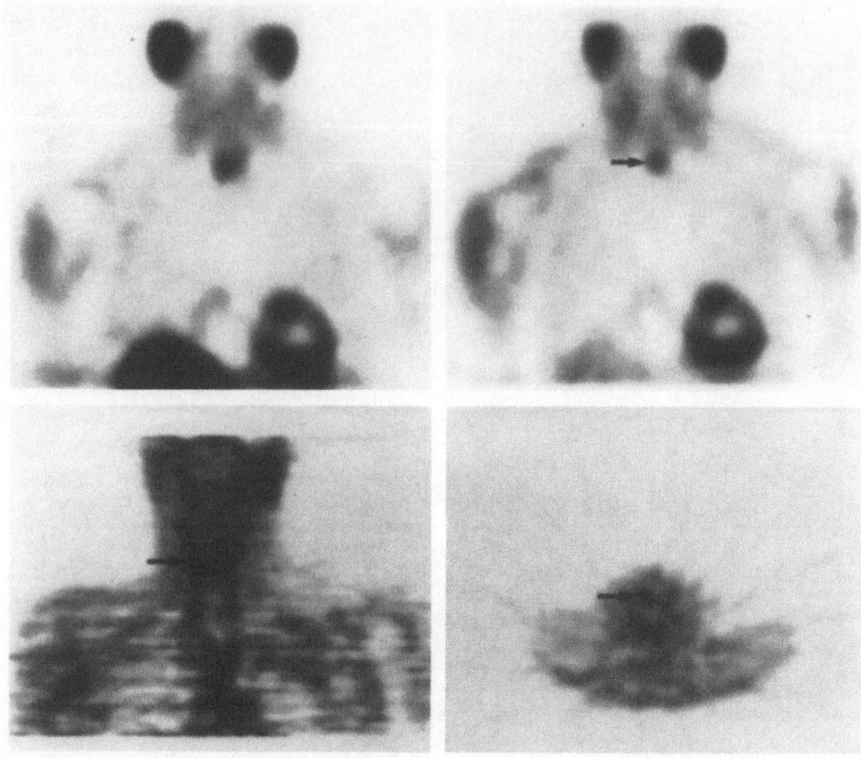

Fig. 13.4. Parathyroid adenoma. Images of the neck and chest show focal areas (*arrows*) of increased uptakes of ^{99m}Tc-sestamibi (*above*) and [^{18}F]fluoro-2-deoxy-D-glucose (*below*). (Reprinted with permission from [15])

information before reoperation and is valuable in preoperative surgical planning (Fig. 13.4) [14, 15].

Sarcoidosis

Sarcoidosis is a systemic granulomatous disease most commonly affecting young to middle-aged adults. Its etiology may be infectious or immunological. Approximately 50% of patients with sarcoidosis are asymptomatic, and symptoms consist of dyspnea and dry cough when symptoms are present at diagnosis, which is usually suggested from a routine chest radiograph. Hilar and peripheral lymph nodes are involved in 80% of sarcoid patients [20]. Gallium scintigraphy is used to evaluate the activity of alveolitis and lymphadenopathy in patients with sarcoidosis. Approximately 50% of patients with biopsy-confirmed sarcoidosis have evidence of extrathoracic involvement by ^{67}Ga imaging. ^{67}Ga scan is also used to guide the course of treatment with steroids [1].

Achalasia, Scleroderma, and Barrett's Esophagus

Esophageal motility disorders include achalasia, diffuse esophageal spasm, nutcracker esophagus, and nonspecific motor disorders. In addition, systemic diseases such as systemic sclerosis and diabetes mellitus have esophageal manifestations. These disorders cause dysphagia, odynophagia, and chest pain. Esophageal transit scintigraphy is useful clinically under the following conditions [10]: (a) when esophageal manometry is unavailable or not tolerated, (b) when manometry is equivocal or negative, but a reasonable suspicion of disease remains, and (c) when clinical management is aided by monitoring for serial change or response to therapy.

Achalasia is a disease of unknown etiology that is characterized by lack of esophageal peristalsis and failure of the lower esophageal sphincter to relax normally after swallowing [2]. The absence of the ganglion cells within the myenteric plexus, vagal nerve degeneration, and changes in the dorsal motor nuclei of the vagus have been found. The barium swallow characteristically reveals a widened esophagus, often with smooth tapering distally into bird beak appearance. In the early stage of the disease the esophageal widening may be minimal, and the diagnosis can be made from manometric findings, which are aperistalsis in the esophageal body and incomplete relaxation in the lower esophageal sphincter. Virtually all patients have solid food dysphagia; weight loss and respiratory symptoms are also common. Approximately one-half the patients experience substernal chest pain. Their symptoms may be difficult to evaluate objectively, especially following dilation. Radionuclide esophageal emptying studies [7] provide an objective way of monitoring a patient's course, evaluating the severity of the disorder, deciding when redilation is required, and comparing various therapeutic results. Achalasia causes a marked delay in esophageal clearance and transit time with the liquid bolus technique (Fig. 13.5). The typical esophageal segmental pattern is relatively flat in all segments, with little evidence of bolus propagation. The scintigraphic findings are not pathognomonic of achalasia and could occur in other conditions, such as scleroderma or mechanical esophageal obstruction. Gastroesophageal reflux is not a prominent feature in achalasia.

Scleroderma is a generalized connective tissue disorder, and the atrophy of muscularis mucosa and its replacement with collagen result in esophageal dysfunction. Most patients show prolonged (greater than 50 s) transit time and abnormal percentage clearance by radionuclide transit techniques [11]. Barrett's esophagus [9] is defined as replacement of the normal squamous mucosa in the distal esophagus with columnar epithelium resembling that found in the stomach. Gastroesophageal reflux (Fig. 13.6) can be demonstrated in a high percentage of patients. It has been hypothesized that following mucosal destruction from repeated reflux, multipotential cells reepithelialize the involved area with cells typical of those found in the stomach. Barrett's esophagus is considered a premalignant condition, and the estimated risk is 30–40 times greater than that in the general population.

Radiographic features include evidence of gastroesophageal reflux, benign stricture, deep esophageal ulcer, and findings of esophagitis. Mamometric examination reveals a decreased lower esophageal sphincter pressure, and pH probe confirms the presence of reflux. Radionuclide studies have shown mild delay in the esophageal clearance of liquid swallows. Barrett's epithelium has been demonstrated in fewer than one-half of patients following the injection of ^{99m}Tc-pertechnetate, and false-positive results may be due to swallowed activity in saliva.

The syndrome with noncardiac chest pain or dysphagia associated with an elevation in the mean amplitude of distal esophageal peristalsis has been

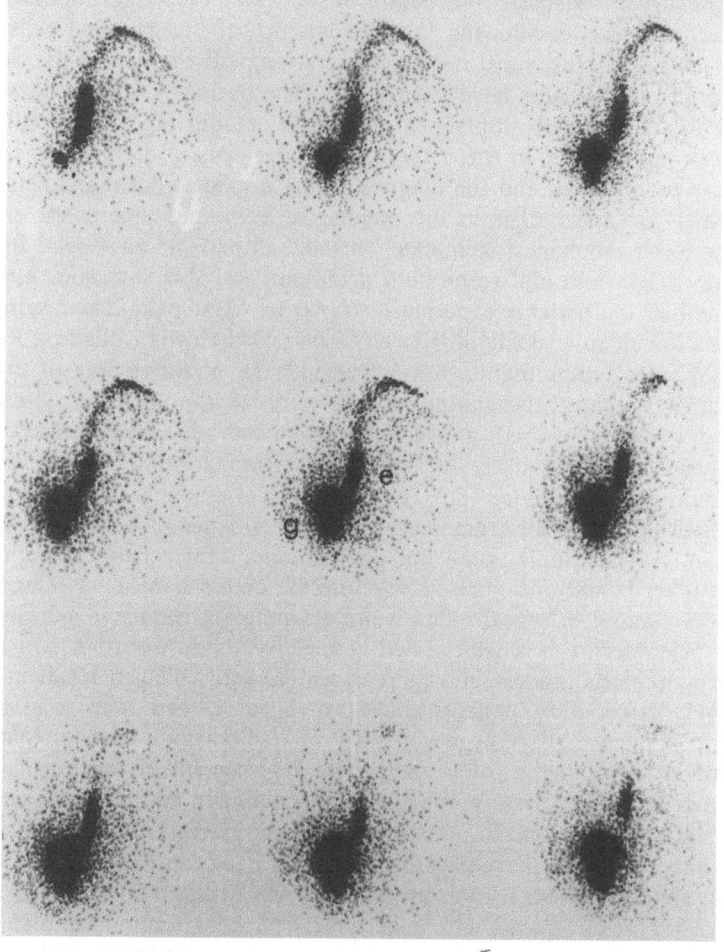

Fig. 13.5. Achalasia. Serial images of the anterior chest following the ingestion of 15 ml water containing 300 μCi ^{99m}Tc-labeled sulfur colloid show a marked delay of the activity (e) in esophageal clearance and transit time

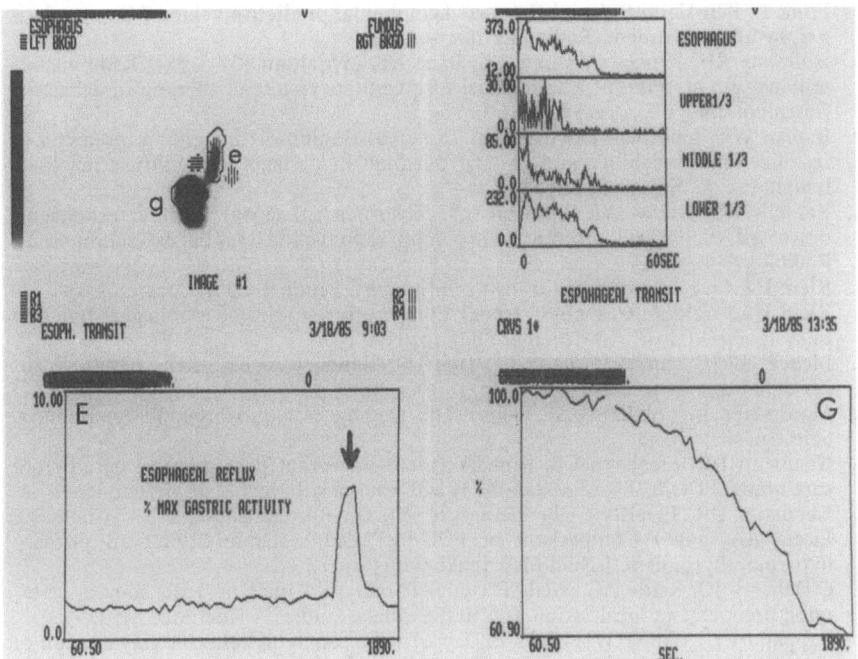

Fig. 13.6. Gastroesophageal reflux. Computer-assisted esophageal time-activity curve (*E*) shows a development of peak activity (*arrow*) indicating a reflux. Gastric emptying (*G*) appears normal

termed "nutcracker esophagus" [17]. Esophageal mamometry shows progression of the peristaltic wave and relaxation of the lower esophageal sphincter. Liquid bolus transit studies suggest that the transit time is delayed only when associated simultaneous contractions are superimposed on the regular peristaltic wave.

References

1. Beckerman C, Szidon JP, Pinsky S (1985) The role of gallium-67 in the clinical evaluation of sarcoidosis. Semin Nucl Roentgenol 20:400–409
2. Bonavina L, Nosadini A, Bardini R (1992) Primary treatment of esophageal achalasia. Long-term results of myotomy and Dor fundoplication. Arch Surg 127:222–226
3. Casara D, Rubello D, Saladini G (1991) Clinical role of Tc-99m MIBI scintigraphy in parathyroid imaging, a comparative study with Tl-201 scintigraphy, echography and CT. Eur J Nucl Med 18:531–535
4. Erdman WA, Breslau NA, Weinreb JC (1989) Noninvasive localization of parathyroid adenomas: a comparison of X-ray computerized tomography, ultrasound, scintigraphy and MRI. Magn Reson Imaging 7:187–194
5. Front D, Israel O (1995) The role of Ga-67 scintigraphy in evaluating the results of therapy of lymphoma patients. Semin Nucl Med 15:60–71

6. Front D, Ben-Haim S, Israel O (1992) Lymphoma: predictive value of Ga-67 scintigraphy after treatment. Radiology 182:359–363

7. Holloway RH, Krosin G, Lange RC, Baue AE, McCallum RW (1983) Radionuclide esophageal emptying of a solid meal to quantitate results of therapy in achalasia. Gastroenterology 84:771–776

8. Kaplan WD, Jochelson MS, Herman TS (1990) Gallium-67 imaging: a predictor of residual tumor viability and clinical outcome in patients with diffuse large-cell lymphoma. J Clin Oncol 8:1966–1970

9. Karvelis KC, Drane WE, Johnson DA, Silverman ED (1987) Barrett's esophagus: decreased esophageal clearance shown by radonuclide esophageal scintigraphy. Radiology 162:97–99

10. Klein HA (1995) Esophageal transit scintigraphy. Semin Nucl Med 25:306–317

11. Klein HA, Wald A, Graham T (1992) Comparative studies of esophageal function in systemic sclerosis. Gastroenterology 102:1551–1556

12. Menck HR, Garfinkel L, Dodd GD (1991) Preliminary report of the national cancer data base. Cancer 41:7–11

13. Moormeier JA, Williams SF (1990) The staging of non-Hodgkin's lymphomas. Sem Oncol 17:43–48

14. Neumann DR, Esselstyn CB, Kim EY (1996) Recurrent postoperative parathyroid carcinoma: FDG-PET and sestamibi-SPECT findings. J Nucl Med 37:2000–2001

15. Neumann DR, Esselstyn CB, MacIntyre WJ, Go RT, Obuchowski NA, Chen EQ, Licata AA (1996) Comparison of FDG-PET and sestamibi-SPECT in primary hyperparathyroidism. J Nucl Med 37:1809–1815

16. O'Doherty JO, Kettle AG, Wells P (1992) Parathyroid imaging with Tc-99m sestamibi: preoperative localization and tissue uptake studies. J Nucl Med 33:313–318

17. Rappaport H, Winter WJ, Hicks EB (1956) Follicular lymphoma. A reevaluation of its position in the scheme of malignant lymphoma, based on a survey of 253 cases. Cancer 9:792–821

18. Richter JE, Blackwell JN, Wu WC, Johns DN, Cowan RJ, Castell DO (1987) Relationship of radionuclide liquid bolus transit and esophageal manometry. J Lab Clin Med 109:217–224

19. Taillefer R, Boucher Y, Potvin C, Lambert R (1992) Detection and localization of parathyroid adenomas in patients with hyperparathyroidism using a single radionuclide imaging procedure with Tc-99m sestamibi (double-phase study). J Nucl Med 33:1801–1807

20. Sharma OP (1983) Diagnosis of sarcoidosis. Arch Intern Med 143:1418–1419

21. Winzelberg GG, Hydovitz JD, O'Hara KR (1985) Parathyroid adenomas evaluated by Tl-201/Tc-99m pertechnetate subtraction scintigraphy and high-resolution ultrasonography. Radiology 155:231–235

14 Bony Thoracic Cage

Y.-W. Bahk

Introduction

The bony thoracic cage consists of the ribs, sternum, and thoracic spine, in addition to the humerus, clavicle, and scapula of the shoulder girdle. Also there are many small and one large (discovertebral) articulations in the thorax. These are the sternoclavicular, manubriosternal, and costosternal joints around the sternal manubrium; the acromioclavicular, glenohumeral, and coracoclavicular joints in the shoulder, and the discovertebral, apophyseal, and costovertebral joints in the spine. The thoracic cage may be affected with various disorders, including inflammation, infection, trauma, sports injury, tumors, tumorous conditions, arthritides, and a number of specific entities such as Tiezte's disease, Freiberg's disease, condensing osteitis of the clavicle, sterenocostoclavicular hyperostosis, and Paget's disease.

Radiography usually suffices for the diagnosis of these conditions. More often than not, however, the radiographic diagnosis is inconclusive because of the smallness and irregularity of the thoracic bones and joints and their overlap with the mediastinal structures. This is true particularly when subjects have marked porosis or obesity that reduce bone density. In such situations bone scintigraphy is indispensable and in fact plays a decisive role.

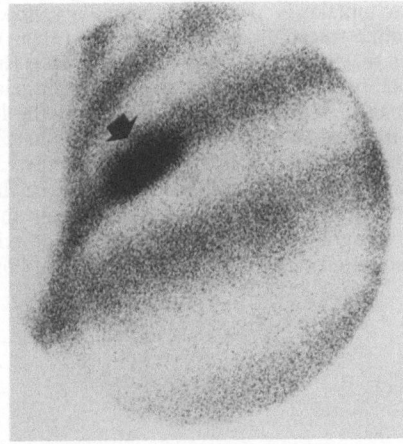

Fig. 14.1. The classic coaxial or longitudinal distribution of tracer uptake in rib metastasis. Posterior pinhole bone scan of the left sixth rib shows intense segmental tracer uptake in the posterior axillary line (*arrow*). The uptake is homogeneous and coaxially aligned

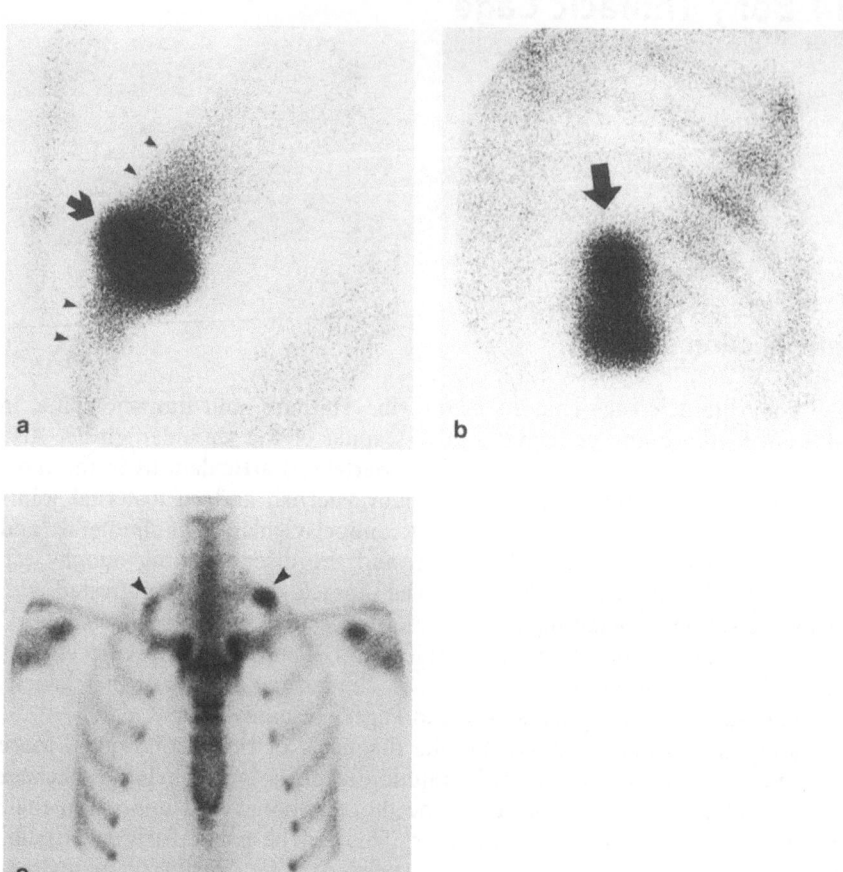

Fig. 14.2 a–c. Scintigraphic manifestations of various rib fractures. **a** Posterior pinhole scintigram of the left tenth rib with a fresh fracture shows a transaxial intense tracer uptake in the posterior axillary line. The fracture is indicated by an intense bandlike tracer uptake in the center (*arrow*) that is flanked on both sides by less intense reactive tracer uptake (*arrowheads*). Note the basic difference between the alignments of "hot" areas in the rib, transaxial in fracture and coaxial in metastasis (Fig. 14.1). **b** Anterior pinhole scan of the left fourth rib in another patient with an old fracture shows the fracture to be sharply defined without low uptake zones (*arrow*). **c** Anterior planar scan of the chest with fatigue fractures in both first ribs shows spotty increased tracer uptake in the fractures. Both were clinically painful (*arrowheads*). The left-sided fracture with more intense tracer uptake was clearly seen on radiography, but the right-sided one with less intense uptake could not be detected, attesting to a greater sensitivity of bone scan

Rib Cage

The ribs are frequent seats of malignant metastasis and fracture. Radiographic diagnosis of established metastasis is not difficult. Frequently, however, small osteolytic or osteoblastic lesions are concealed, especially when the ribs are severely porotic. It is well known that radiography cannot detect all painful metastases in the ribs. Bone scan is sensitive, revealing such lesions weeks ahead of radiographic manifestation. On scintigraphy the great majority of metastases present as "hot" lesions and some as "cold" lesions. The appearances are spotty, segmental, or rarely diffuse, typically having a longitudinal or coaxial alignment in the ribs (Fig. 14.1). Osteomyelitis, osteitis, and tuberculosis may produce similar "hot" areas, but they are usually solitary in occurrence. Among tumors, multiple myelomas are well known for presenting as diffuse photopenic lesions unless complicated with pathological fracture.

The rib fracture strongly resembles metastasis, manifesting a patchy "hot" area. Pinhole scintigraphy, however, can distinguish the transaxial "hot" area of fracture from the coaxial "hot" area of metastasis. The "hot" area of a fresh rib fracture is usually flanked by a zone of less intense uptake on both sides (Fig. 14.2 a). With time the less intense zones gradually disappear, and the "hot" area of fracture in the center becomes sharply defined (Fig. 14.2 b). Bone scan is highly sensitive in detecting occult fractures in the ribs (Fig. 14.2 c). During open thoracic surgery the ribs are likely to be traumatized by rib spreaders, resulting in fracture and periosteal stripping or tear. The costovertebral joints may also be severed, subluxated, and fractured. Such injuries often defy radiographic detection, especially when they are in porotic bones and joints. Bone scintigraphy is an excellent alternative, portraying the signs of the injured periosteum, fractured rib, and severed joint (Fig. 14.3).

Tietze's disease, benign mesenchymoma, fibro-osseous lesion, and focal hematopoietic hyperplasia are unique to the ribs [1]. The ribs may be af-

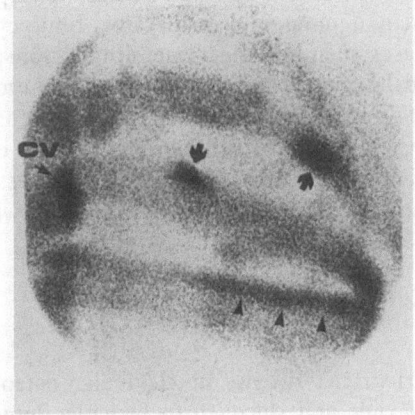

Fig. 14.3. Various rib injuries caused by the use of rib spreaders. Posterior pinhole bone scan of the right mid-chest shows spotty tracer uptake in occult fractures (*arrows*), linear uptake in the stripped periosteum (*arrowheads*), and cigar-shaped uptake in the severed costovertebral joint (*cv*)

Fig. 14.4. Multicameral defects in aneurysmal bone cyst. Anterior pinhole bone scan of the left seventh rib portrays three septated cystic defects (*open arrows*). The lesion is expansile and well demarcated medially by the costochondral junction (*arrow*)

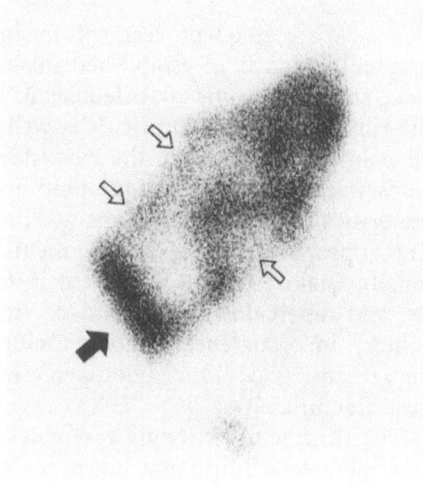

Fig. 14.5. "C" and "inverted C" signs of Tietze's disease. Anterior pinhole bone scan of the first costochondral junctions shows C-shaped and inverted C-shaped tracer uptake in the right and left costochondral junction, respectively (*arrows*)

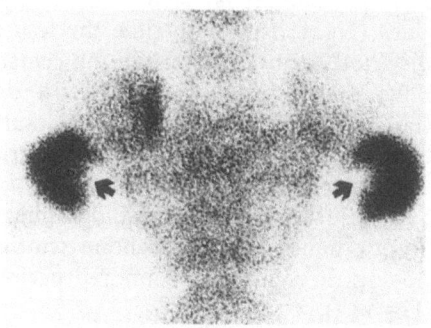

fected with tumors and tumorous conditions such as eosinophilic granuloma, fibrous dysplasia, Paget's disease of bone, osteochondroma, chondrosarcoma, osteosarcoma, all lymphomas, Ewing's sarcoma and rarely enchondroma, hemangioma, and aneurysmal bone cyst [1]. On scintigraphy all of these diseases manifest the same simple nonspecific "hot" areas except for aneurysmal bone cyst which produces a photopenic lesion that is often multicameral (Fig. 14.4). Interestingly, Tietze's disease manifests the typical "C" or inverted "C" sign in costochondral junctions of the first few ribs (Fig. 14.5) [2]. The sign reflects the inflammatory process that is localized in the costochondral junction, the lateral bony margin of which is medially concave.

Clavicle and Sternum

Friedrich's disease or clavicular osteochondrosis, condensing osteitis of the clavicle and sternocostoclavicular hyperostosis are all unique to the clavicle,

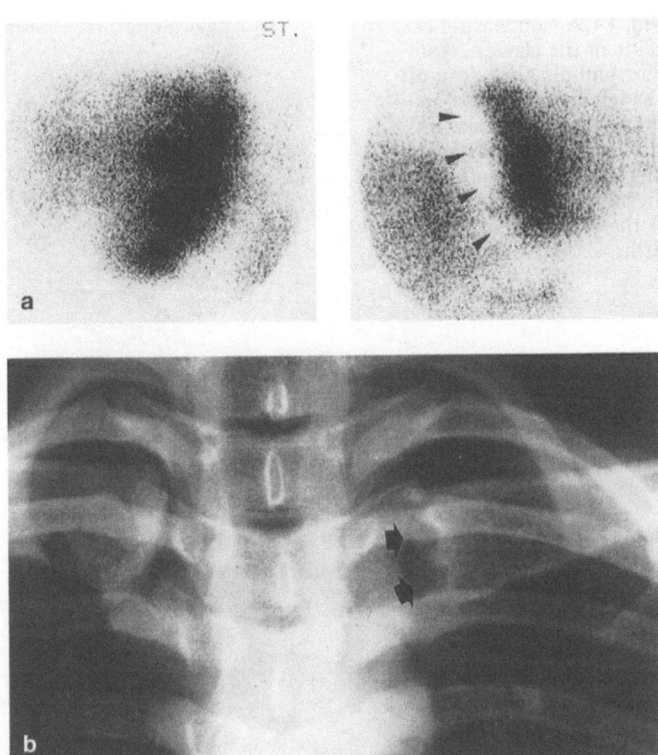

Fig. 14.6 a, b. Osteochondrosis of the clavicle (Friedrich's disease). **a** Anterior pinhole bone scans of the both medial clavicles (two separate acquisitions) show scalloped photon defect in the sternal end of the left clavicle with widened sternoclavicular joint (*arrowheads*). Note that the affected bone accumulates tracer less intensely than the mate, denoting relative avascularity. Unequal size is due to different magnification factors. **b** Anteroposterior radiogram of the clavicles shows sclerotic scalloped sternal end of the left clavicle with widened sternoclavicular joint (*arrows*)

each manifesting a characteristic scintigraphic sign. Friedrich's disease is the clavicular version of avascular necrosis, analogous to the well-known Legg-Perthes disease [3]. Radiographic findings include lucent defect with a scalloped sclerotic margin in the sternal end of the clavicle. The adjacent sternoclavicular joint is widened. On scintigraphy a scalloped defect appears in the sternal end with widening of the adjacent sternoclavicular joint (Fig. 14.6) [4]. The tracer uptake in the diseased bone appears somewhat lower than in normal, suggesting ischemia.

Condensing osteitis of the clavicle is another rare nonspecific inflammatory disease of the clavicle that was first described by Brower et al. [5]. Although the clinical symptoms and radiographic findings strongly resemble those in Friedrich's disease, etiologically it is related to mechanical stress and not to avascular necrosis [5, 6]. Typical alterations are seen in the lower aspect of the sternal end, frequently in association with a narrowed sterno-

Fig. 14.7. Condensing osteitis of the clavicle. Anterior pinhole bone scan of the left clavicle shows increased tracer uptake in the lower aspect of the sternal end (*arrows*) and sternoclavicular joint that is the seat of secondary arthrosis (*arrowheads*)

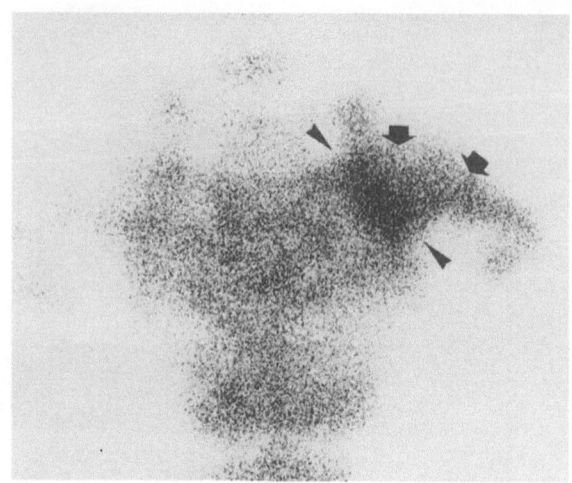

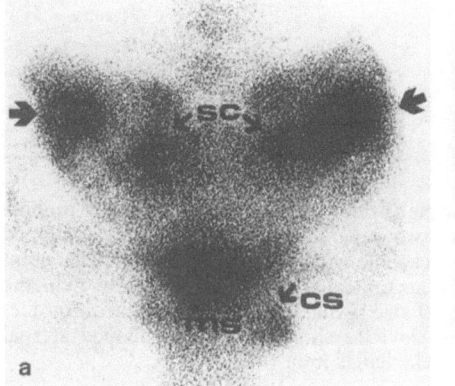

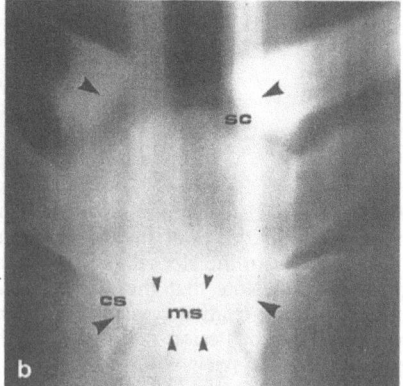

Fig. 14.8 a, b. Sternocostoclavicular hyperostosis. **a** Anterior pinhole scan of the sternum portrays intense tracer uptake specifically in the sternoclavicular (*sc*), manubriosternal (*ms*) and costosternal (*cs*) joints. Findings resemble pansy flower. **b** Anteroposterior conventional X-ray tomography of the sternum shows hyperostosis in the three joints in **a** and between the clavicle and first ribs

clavicular joint which may have cystic change [6]. The scintigraphic finding of this disease has been described by Teates et al. [7], who noted increased activity in the lesion. These authors correctly observe that planar scan finding is not specific. Pinhole scintigraphy, however, can localize the increased radioactivity specifically to the lower aspect of the sternal end of the clavicle with the obliteration of the sternoclavicular joint (Fig. 14.7). We noted that the tracer uptake in condensing osteitis of the clavicle is typically diffuse whereas that of Friedrich's disease is discrete and less intense.

Fig. 14.9. Sternal body fracture. Anterior pinhole bone scan of the sternum shows extremely intense double-line tracer uptake with an intervening photopenic zone in the proximal aspect of the sternal body (*arrow*). Note mild tracer uptake in normal manubriosternal junction (*msj*). Distinction between fracture and normal joint was impossible on the ordinary planar scan

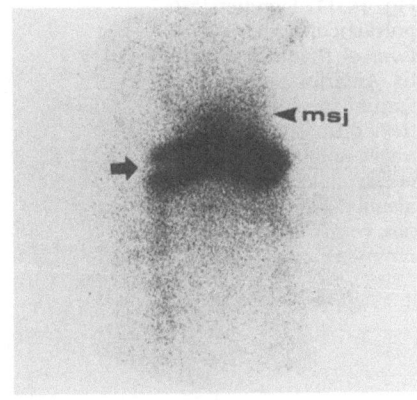

Fig. 14.10. Asymmetric monarticular manifestation of osteoarthritis. Anterior pinhole bone scan of the right sternoclavicular joint shows irregularly increased tracer uptake in the sternum (*lower arrow*) and sternal clavicular end with articular narrowing (*upper arrow*). Note that the most intense tracer uptake occurs in the immediate periarticular bones. *CL,* Clavicle; *MS,* manubrium sterni

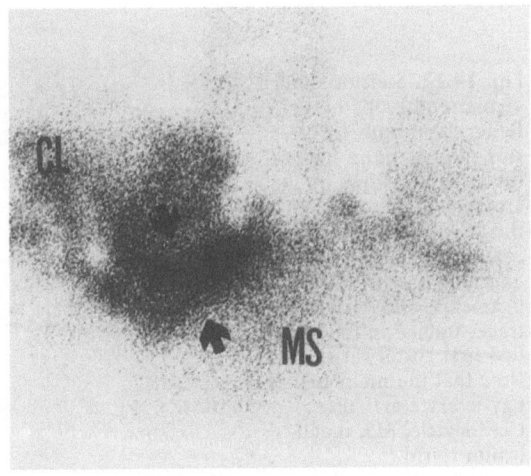

Sternocostoclavicular hyperostosis is a relatively new and rare disease. The pathology shows a chronic nonsuppurative inflammatory process with diffuse hyperostotic reaction involving the sternum, upper ribs, clavicles, and regional soft tissue [8]. Radiography may reveal bone formation that diffusely obliterates the three bones and their interspaces. The ordinary bone scan manifestation of the disease has been reported by Sartoris et al. [9], who observed an increased tracer uptake in the lesional area. Interestingly, pinhole scintigraphy portrays the tracer uptake specifically in and among the clavicles, sternum, and first ribs, giving rise to a "pansy flower" appearance which is pathognomonic (Fig. 14.8) [10].

Fractures are rather common in the clavicles and sternum. Radiography may suffice for their diagnosis, so that a bone scan is not needed. Frequently, however, the fracture in the sternum that is thin and flat does require a bone scan, especially when it is porotic. As with any other fractures,

Fig. 14.11. Symmetrical polyarticular manifestations of rheumatoid arthritis. Anterior pinhole bone scan of the sternum portrays diffusely increased tracer uptake in the sternoclavicular (*arrows*) and manubriosternal articulation (*msa*). Note perfect symmetry of pathology

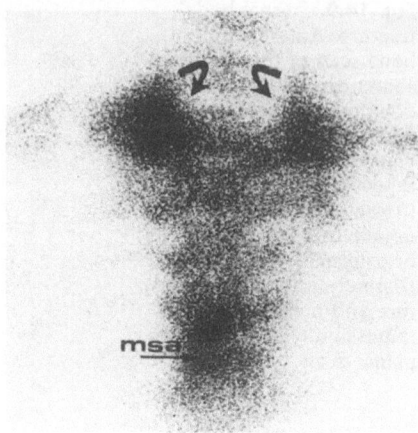

Fig. 14.12. Sternocostoclavicular enthesopathy in Reiter's syndrome. Anterior pinhole bone scan of the sternum shows increased tracer uptake in the sternoclavicular and costoclavicular (*medial and lateral arrowhead*) ligaments, and very intense tracer uptake in the ossified first costal cartilage. Note that the main pathology is extra-articular. *CL*, Clavicle; *MS*, manubrium sterni

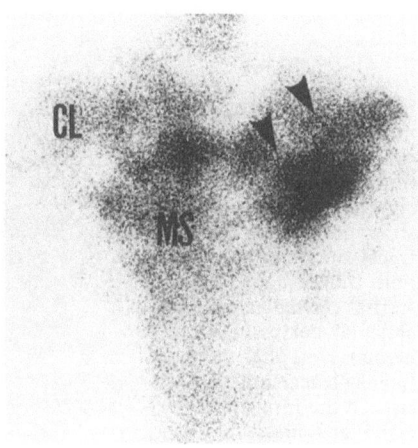

the sternal fracture is easy to detect by bone scintigraphy. An important exception is a fracture that is close to the manubriosternal junction which normally the accumulates tracer intensely. Fortunately, pinhole scintigraphy readily distinguishes such a fracture from the normal manubriosternal junction (Fig. 14.9). The infection and radiation osteitis of the sternum and clavicle may also cause a segmental or patchy increased tracer uptake.

The sternoclavicular, acromioclavicular, and manubriosternal joints are frequently affected with osteoarthritis and rheumatoid arthritis. Osteoarthritis is typically mono- or pauciarticular and eccentric. As the radiographic alterations differ between the two diseases, so too are their scan alterations. The radiographic alterations of osteoarthritis are eccentric articular eburnation, spur formation, small subcortical cysts, and joint space narrowing. On bone scan such radiographic alterations are represented by small areas of mottled, spotty, or patchy increased tracer uptake that are usually discrete

Fig. 14.13. Photopenic myeloma with eggshell-type rupture of the sternal body. Anterior pinhole bone scan of the sternum shows expansile photopenic change involving the first two segments of the sternal body. The lesions (*outlined*) are recognized as such by broken eggshell-like tracer uptake in fractured cortical bone (*arrows*). *MS*, manubrium sterni

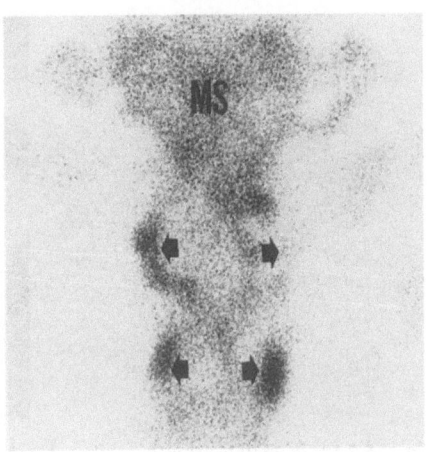

and confined to the periarticular bones with narrowed joint (Fig. 14.10) [11]. In contrast, rheumatoid arthritis typically involves synovial joints in the extremities. In general it is polyarticular, bilateral, and symmetrical. The articular changes are concentric within a joint. Involvement of the clavicular and sternal joints is also not rare [12]. The scintigraphic findings mirror the radiographic alterations, manifesting diffuse and concentric tracer uptake in polyarticular and symmetrical fashion (Fig. 14.11).

Reiter's syndrome is another interesting disease characterized by nonspecific inflammation in the tendon and capsule insertion about a joint, typically in the lower limb [13, 14]. Clinically the syndrome consists of a triad of arthritis, usually mono- or pauciarticular, urethritis, and conjunctivitis [13, 14]. The manubriosternal joint may be involved [15]. We have seen three cases of Reiter's syndrome that involved the sternoclavicular joint (Fig. 14.12).

As with the ribs, the clavicles and sternum are often affected with metastasis, myeloma, aneurysmal bone cyst, Ewing's sarcoma, histiocytosis X, and Paget's disease. Bone scintigraphy shows intense tracer uptake that is segmental or patchy in appearance. As is well known, myelomas and aneurysmal bone cyst are photopenic unless complicated with pathological fracture (Fig. 14.13). Another entity of scintigraphic interest is Paget's disease, which involves the clavicle in 11% [16]. An extremely intense tracer uptake has been described in Paget's disease [17]. Recent pinhole scan study has shown that in Paget's disease intense tracer uptake occurs typically in the cortex and periphery of bone (see below) [18].

Shoulder Girdle

The shoulder girdle is comprised of the humerus, scapula, and clavicle as well as the glenohumeral, acromioclavicular, and coracoclavicular joints. As with any other bones and joints of the thorax, those of the shoulder girdle

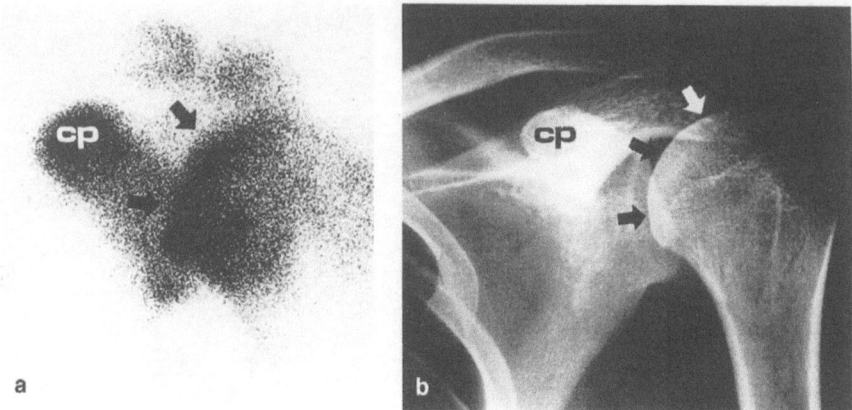

Fig. 14.14 a, b. Osteoarthritis in the glenohumeral joint. **a** Anterior pinhole bone scan of the left shoulder shows increased tracer uptake in the centromedial aspect of the humeral head (*arrows*). Minimal flattening is seen. The increased tracer uptake in the coracoid process is physiological (*cp*). **b** Anteroposterior radiogram shows minimal cortical thickening in the centromedial aspect of the humeral head (*arrows*). *cp*, Coracoid process

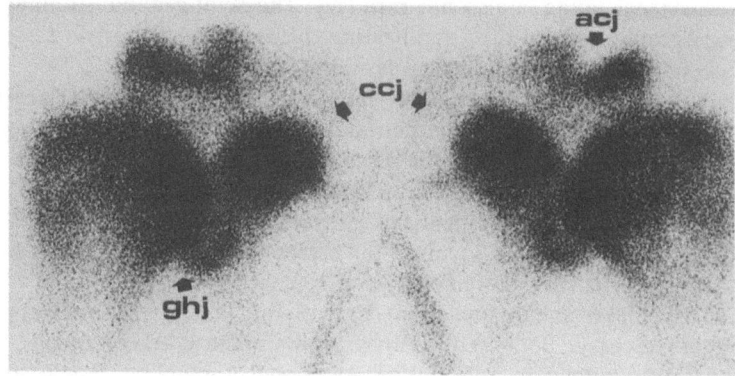

Fig. 14.15. Symmetric polyarticular lesions of rheumatoid arthritis. Anterior pinhole bone scans of both shoulders (two acquisitions) reveal perfect symmetrical tracer uptake in the acromioclavicular joints (*acj*), glenohumeral (*ghj*), and coracoclavicular joints (*ccj*)

are frequently affected with various infections, inflammation, traumatic injuries, tumors and tumorous conditions. Among others, fractures, osteoarthritis and rheumatoid arthritis, and calcium hydroxyapatite crystal deposition disease are of scintigraphic interest. Bone scan is very helpful in the diagnosis of some of these diseases, particularly arthritides and occult fractures.

As discussed in reference to the sternum and clavicle, osteoarthritis is usually mono- or pauciarticular, and on scintigraphy it manifests areas of spotty or patchy increased tracer uptake in the articular bones (Fig. 14.14).

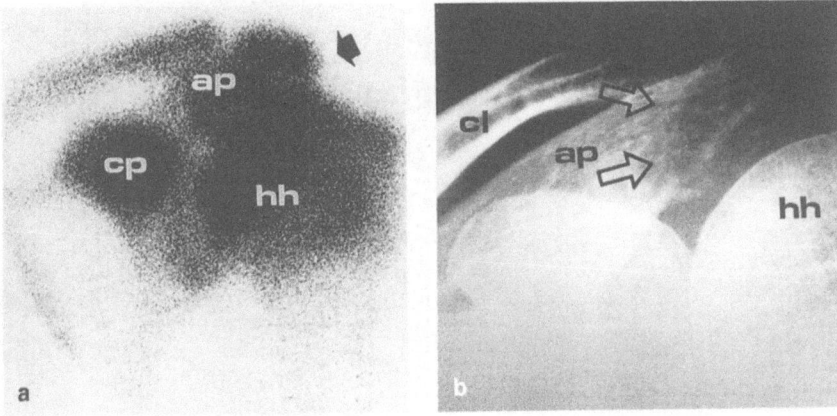

Fig. 14.16a, b. Subacromial bursitis with a bone erosion. **a** Anterior pinhole bone scan of the left shoulder shows intense tracer uptake in the eroded acromion process (*ap*) with the most prominent uptake occurring in the under surface (*arrow*). Tracer uptake appears to be intensified also in the humeral head (*hh*) and coracoid process (*cp*) in response to inflammation. **b** Anteroposterior radiogram shows marked erosion in the undersurface of the acromion process (*ap, arrows*). *cl*, Clavicle

Fig. 14.17. Cortical and peripheral tracer uptake in Paget's disease. Posterior pinhole scintigram of the left scapula portrays intense tracer uptake typically in the lateral margin (*arrows*), the glenoid process and spine (*single arrow*) and the acromion process (*ap*). The finding is pathognomonic of Paget's disease

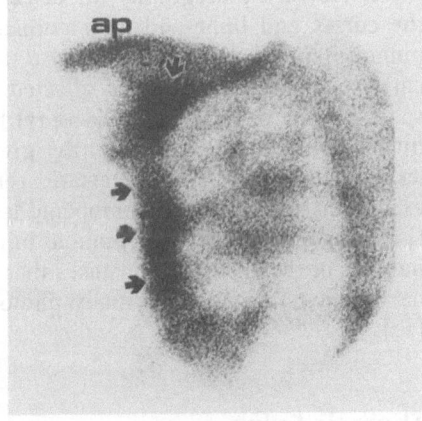

The increased tracer uptake is not diffuse but discrete and eccentric within the confinement of a joint that is often narrowed. Rheumatoid arthritis is polyarticular, bilateral, and symmetrical, manifesting diffuse and concentric increased tracer uptake in the synovia and subchondral bones of joints (Fig. 14.15). Articular space may be widened first in the acute phase but eventually become narrowed. Calcific tendinitis and bursitis or calcium hydroxyapatite crystal deposition disease may show minimal to moderate increase in tracer accumulation in the calcified tendon or bursa and in the eroded regional bone (Fig. 14.16).

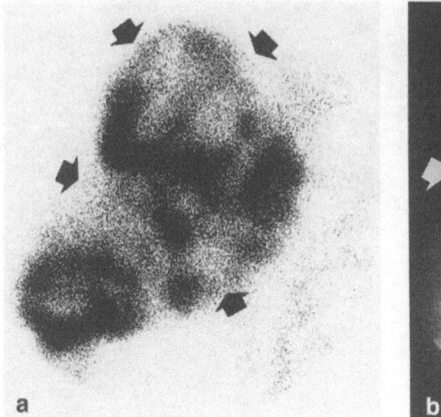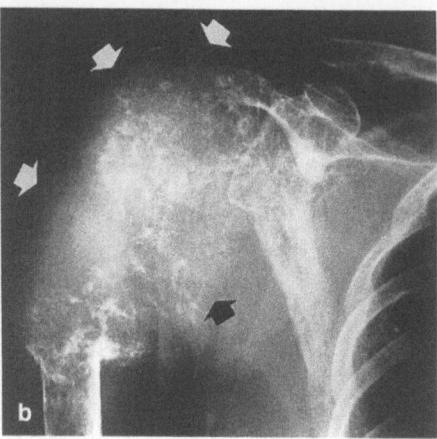

Fig. 14.18a,b. Photopenic lesion of metastatic renal cell carcinoma. **a** Anterior pinhole bone scan of the right proximal humerus shows a large expansile lesion with multiple photopenic areas intermingled with mottled "hot" areas (*arrows*). **b** Anteroposterior radiogram reveals a large irregular expansile osteolytic lesion with melting bone (*arrows*)

Paget's disease of bone frequently involves the humerus (31%) and scapula (24%) [16]. On radiography the disease manifests thickening of trabeculae in the cortex and bone-end with pumice bone change. As mentioned already, pinhole scintigraphy reveals intense tracer uptake to occur specifically in the cortex and the periphery of affected bones with the narrowing of marrow space in long or flat bone (Fig. 14.17) [18]. Malignant metastases are common in the bones of the shoulder, the great majority of which present as "hot" lesions. Myelomas and metastatic renal cell carcinoma are two notorious exceptions that produce photopenic lesions on bone scintigraphy (Fig. 14.18) [19]. Our experience with pinhole bone scan has indicated that not a small number of the skeletal metastases that appear to be simply "hot" on the ordinary planar images are actually photopenic in nature or at least partially so [20].

Thoracic Spine

The thoracic spine consists of one large and many small irregular anatomical parts and the discovertebral, apophyseal, and costovertebral articulations. Radiography shows the spine overlapped by the mediastinal organs, ribs, sternum, and clavicles, often interfering with accurate observation. This is true particularly when the subject is obese, osteoporotic, or crooked. Bone scintigraphy has been shown to be extremely helpful in such situations (see Fig. 3.6).

The thoracic spine is a common seat of metastasis, infection, and fracture. Radiography is essential, but its value is often considerably limited by the

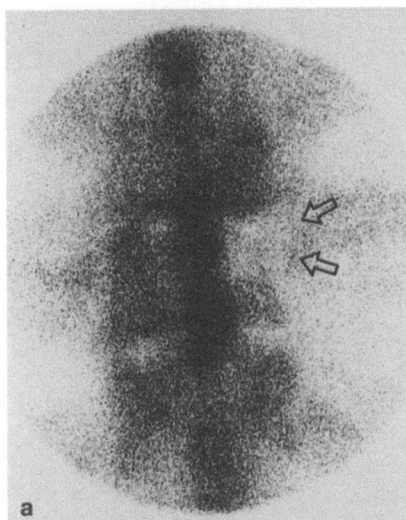

Fig. 14.19 a–c. Characteristic pinhole bone scan signs of metastasis, infection, and compression fracture of the spine. **a** Posterior pinhole bone scan of T10 shows a patchy "cold" area in the right half of the vertebral body (*arrows*) representing metastatic breast cancer. **b** Posterior pinhole bone scan of T10 and T11 shows the classic "sandwich" sign of infective spondylitis. Note that disc space is narrowed (*arrow*). **c** Posterior pinhole bone scan of the thoracolumbar junction shows intense tracer uptake localized to the endplates of T11, T12, and L1, denoting compression fractures (*arrows*). Note that, unlike in infective spondylitis, disc spaces are well preserved, an important differential point

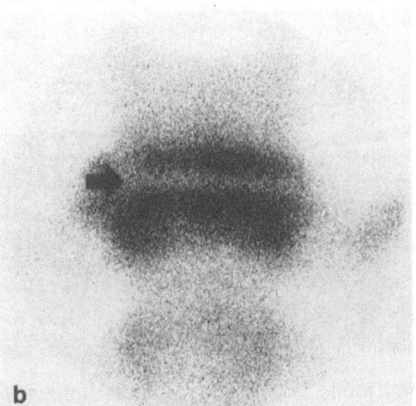

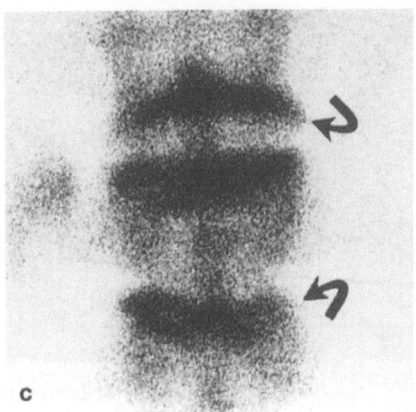

anatomical characteristics of the spine. Bone scan plays an important role in portraying specific signs in many of these diseases [21]. Metastasis may present as either patchy or segmental "hot" or "cold" area in the vertebra (Fig. 14.19 a). Their location and appearances are characteristic. The intervertebral disc space is not affected in metastasis. Infective spondylitis, both bacterial and tuberculous, produces the "sandwich" sign which is comprised of intense tracer uptake in two apposing endplates with narrowed disc space between (Fig. 14.19 b). The sign reflects diskitis with the spread of infection to the endplates above and below. On the other hand, the compression fracture of the spine may cause intense tracer uptake that is localized in the endplate. Fractured endplates are either depressed or arcuated (Fig. 14.19 c).

As with the ribs, the costovertebral joints may also be severed or fractured by the use of rib spreaders during an open thoracic surgery. Radiographic

Fig. 14.20. Typical costovertebral articular sever-
ance caused by the rib
spreaders. Posterior pin-
hole bone scan of the midthoracic spine in a patient
with severed costocorpor-
eal joints during a recent
lower left lobectomy sur-
gery reveals cigar-shaped
intense tracer uptake in
the costocorporeal joints of
T6 and T7 (*arrows*). Small
roundish increased tracer
uptake in the costotrans-
verse joints indicate sub-
luxation (*arrowheads*)

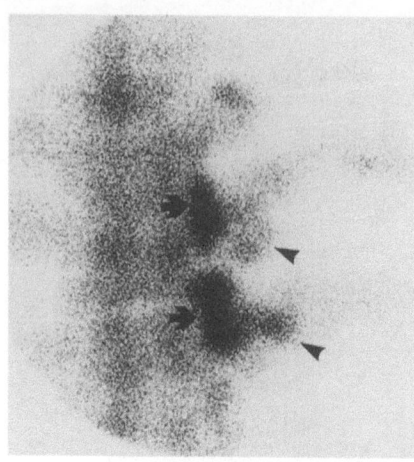

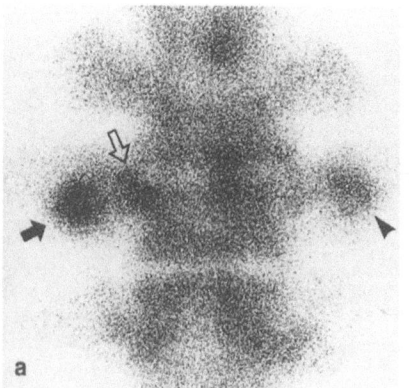
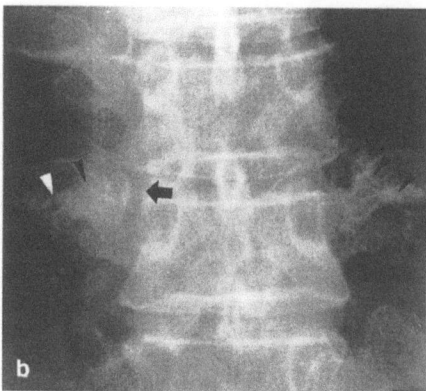

Fig. 14.21 a, b. Osteoarthritis of costovertebral joints. **a** Posterior pinhole bone scan
of T9 vertebra shows increased tracer uptake in the right costotransverse (*solid arrow*)
and costocorporeal joints (*open arrow*) and left costocorporeal joint (*arrowheads*).
Side is reversed on print to match with radiography. **b** Anteroposterior radiogram
reveals typical osteoarthritic changes including joint space narrowing and periarticular sclerosis in the costovertebral joints (*arrow, arrowheads*)

detection of such lesions may not always be easy because of the small dimension and overlapping of the joints. On scintigraphy, however, such injuries
can be clearly indicated by cigar-shaped, spotty, or mottled increased tracer
uptake in the paravertebral regions (Fig. 14.20). The location and appearance
of the tracer uptake are so unique that their recognition may not be difficult.

The osteoarthritis of the costocorporeal and costotransverse joints of the
thoracic spine is a frequent cause of back pain, but their radiographic diagnosis is not convincing in all cases. Bone scan is sensitive, revealing the
characteristic spotty increased tracer uptake in the juxtavertebral location.

Fig. 14.22. The "centipede" sign of ankylosing spondylitis of the thoracic spine. Composite posterior pinhole bone scan of the thoracic spine portrays diffuse obliteration of intervertebral, interspinous, apophyseal and costovertebral joints (*arrows*).
CCJ, Costocorporeal joint;
CTJ, costotransverse joint

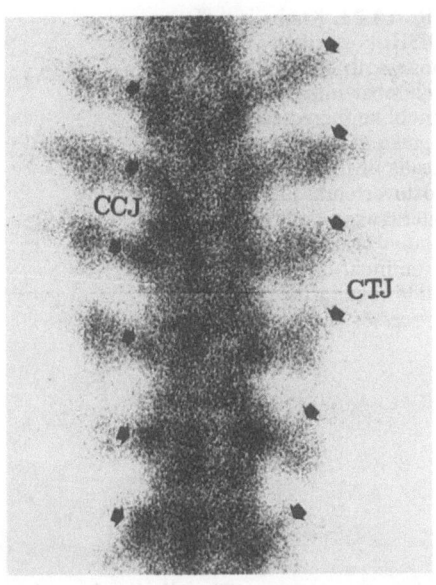

Pinhole scintigraphy is still more sensitive and specific, efficiently detecting and identifying minor osteoarthritic changes in the costotransverse and costocorporeal joint (Fig. 14.21). Ankylosing spondylitis is a nonspecific inflammatory disease of the sacroiliac joints and the spine. It differs from rheumatoid arthritis in that the main pathological changes occur in entheses and not in the synovial joint [22]. Radiographically, it is characterized by the diffuse fibrosis, calcification, or ossification of the discovertebral and other small accessory vertebral joints and longitudinal ligaments. Bone scan may portray diffusely increased tracer uptake in the longitudinal, interspinous, and supraspinous ligaments as well as in the apophyseal and costovertebral joints, creating the peculiar "centipede" sign in the thoracic spine (Fig. 14.22). The sign is considered to be the scintigraphic representation of the "bamboo" spine alteration seen on radiography.

Diffuse idiopathic skeletal hyperostosis (DISH) is a common disease of the thoracic spine in the elderly. The radiographic alterations include diffuse flowing calcification or ossification in the anterolateral aspects of more than four contiguous vertebrae [23]. Typically, the disc spaces are not involved. In some patients the heads of the ribs at the costovertebral articulations [24] and the spinous processes are also involved [25]. Bone scan demonstrates diffusely increased tracer uptake along the thoracic or thoracolumbar spine. At a glance, the findings strongly mimic ankylosing spondylitis. However, closer observation reveals that DISH spares the discovertebral and apophyseal joints. When the costal heads are involved, there may be seen small ovoid increased tracer uptake in the lateral aspects of the intervertebral spaces in the midthoracic spine and in the lateral parts of the vertebral bodies in the lower thoracic spine (Fig. 14.23). Increased tracer uptake may also be seen in the

Fig. 14.23. Knob sign of DISH. Posterior pinhole bone scan of the thoracolumbar junction shows knoblike increased tracer uptake in the hypertrophic heads of the ribs near the costovertebral joints at the lateral aspects of vertebral bodies (*black arrows*). Prominent uptake in the midline is in the spinous processes (*white arrows*)

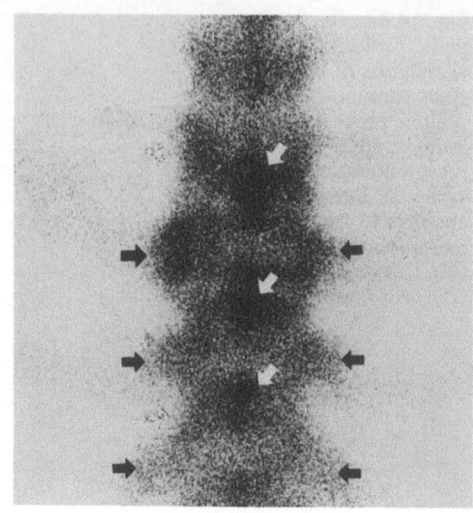

spinous processes. The distinction of tracer uptake in the specific sites of the vertebra is imperative for differential diagnosis of DISH and ankylosing spondylitis.

References

1. Mirra JM (1989) Unique tumors of the ribs. In: Mirra JM (ed) Bone tumors. Lea and Febiger, Philadelphia, pp 1519–1548
2. Yang WJ, Bahk YW, Chung SK et al (1994) Pinhole skeletal scintigraphic manifestations of Tietze's disease. Eur J Nucl Med 21:947–952
3. Friedrich H (1924) Über ein noch nicht beschriebenes, der Perthesschen Erkrankung analoges, Krankheitsbild des sternalen Clavikelendes. Dtsch Z Chir 187:385–398
4. Bahk YW (1994) Friedrich's disease. In: Bahk YW (ed) Combined scintigraphic and radiographic diagnosis of bone and joint diseases. Springer, Berlin Heidelberg New York, p 143
5. Brower AC, Sweet DE, Keats TE (1974) Condensing osteitis of the clavicle: a new entity. Am J Roentgenol 12:17–21
6. Bahk YW (1994) Condensing osteitis of the clavicle. In: Bahk YW (ed) Combined scintigraphic and radiographic diagnosis of bone and joint diseases. Springer, Berlin Heidelberg New York, p 56
7. Teates CD, Brower AC, Williamson BRJ et al (1978) Bone scans in condensing osteitis of the clavicle. South Med J 71:736–738
8. Sonozaki H, Azuma A, Okai K et al (1979) Clinical features of 22 cases with "inter-sterno-costo-clavicular ossification": a new rheumatic syndrome. Arch Orthop Unfallchir 95:13–22
9. Sartoris DJ, Schreiman JS, Kerr R et al (1986) Sternocostoclavicular hyperostosis: a review and report of 11 cases. Radiology 158:125–128
10. Bahk YW, Chung SK, Kim SH (1992) Pinhole scintigraphic manifestations of sternocostoclavicular hyperostosis. Korean J Nucl Med 26:155–159
11. Bahk YW (1994) Degenerative joint diseases. In: Bahk YW (ed) Combined scintigraphic and radiographic diagnosis of bone and joint diseases. Springer, Berlin Heidelberg New York, pp 73–97

12. Resnick D, Niwayama G (1988) Rheumatoid arthritis. In: Resnick D, Niwayama G (eds) Diagnosis of bone and joint disorders, 2nd edn. Saunders, Philadelphia, pp 955-1067

13. Reiter H (1916) Über eine bisher unerkannte Spirochaeteninfektion. Dtsch Med Wochenschr 42:1535-1536

14. Willkens RF, Arnett FC, Bitter T et al (1981) Reiter's syndrome: evaluation of preliminary criteria for definite disease. Arthritis Rheum 24:844-849

15. Candardjis G, Saudan Y, De Bosset P (1978) Etude radiologique de l'articulation manubrio-sternale dans la pelvispondylite rhumatismale et le syndrome de Reiter. J Radiol Electrol Med Nucl 59:93-97

16. Meunier PJ, Salson C, Mathieu L et al (1987) Skeletal distribution and biochemical parameters of Paget's disease. Clin Orthop 217:37-44

17. Serafini AN (1976) Paget's disease of the bone. Semin Nucl Med 6:47-58

18. Bahk YW, Park YH, Chung SK, Chi JG (1995) Bone pathologic correlation of multimodality imaging in Paget's disease. J Nucl Med 36:1421-1426

19. Kim EE, Bledin AG, Gutierrez C (1983) Comparison of radionuclide images and radiographs for skeletal metastases from renal cell carcinoma. Oncology 40:284-286

20. Bahk YW (1994) Tumors and tumorous conditions of bone. In: Bahk YW (ed) Combined scintigraphic and radiographic diagnosis of bone and joint diseases. Springer, Berlin Heidelberg New York, pp 183-217

21. Bahk YW, Kim OH, Chung SK (1987) Pinhole collimator scintigraphy in the differential diagnosis of metastasis, fracture, and infections of the spine. J Nucl Med 28:447-451

22. Resnick D, Niwayama G (1988) Ankylosing spondylitis. In: Resnick D, Niwayama G (eds) Diagnosis of bone and joint disorders, 2nd edn. Saunders, Philadelphia, pp 1103-1170

23. Resnick D, Shaul SR, Robins JM (1975) Diffuse idiopathic skeletal hyperostosis (DISH): Forestier's disease with extraspinal manifestations. Radiology 115:513-524

24. Mironov A, Ziegler F (1983) Unterschiedliche Stadien von Hyperostose der Rippenköpfchen bei Spondylosis Hyperostotica. Fortschr Röntgenstr 139:416-420

25. Resnick D, Niwayama G (1988) Diffuse idiopathic skeletal hyperostosis (DISH): ankylosing hyperostosis of Forestier and Rotes-Querol. In: Resnick D, Niwayama G (eds) Diagnosis of bone and joint disorders, 2nd edn. Saunders, Philadelphia, p 1571

15 Breast Cancer

E. E. KIM

Breast cancer is the most common malignancy of women in North America and is the leading cause of death in women between the ages of 40 and 55. In 1995 approximately 182000 women in the United States will have been diagnosed with breast cancer, and 46000 women will die of this disease [20].

Women routinely undergo physical examination and mammography to screen for breast cancer; however, both have diagnostic limitations. Symptoms and signs of breast cancer are not always distinctive and sometimes are not evident during physical examination. Some breast abnormalities are not detected because they are not palpable, and in some cases cystic lesions cannot be distinguished easily from solid lesions by means of palpation. Mammography is the only imaging method recommended for cancer screening; however, the role of mammography is still in question, with 20% false negative rate for nonpalpable cancer [4]. Although the positive predictive value of mammography is 15%–30% in the United States, mammographic detection, preoperative localization, stereotaxic core biopsy, fine-needle aspiration, and excisional biopsy of suspected or occult abnormalities are the standard diagnostic workup [12]. Mammography cannot be used alone reliably to differentiate between benign and malignant lesions. The most important role of ultrasound is the differentiation between cystic and solid masses. While ultrasound is 96%–100% accurate in identifying a cyst, it is less reliable in differentiating between benign and malignant solid masses [10]. Ultrasound appears to be more accurate than mammography for determining actual tumor size and guides fine-needle aspiration or core biopsy [5]. In recent years contrast-enhanced magnetic resonance imaging has been added to the list of imaging techniques for breast lesions [7].

Accurate determination of the extent of a given tumor and possible multifocality is essential when a breast-conserving surgical approach is considered. Since axillary lymph node involvement is an important prognostic factor, almost every patient with invasive breast cancer undergoes an axillary dissection. This surgical procedure also has a nonnegligible morbidity. There is certainly a need for reliable noninvasive diagnostic technique that can detect axillary lymph node metastasis in clinically negative nodes and confirm clinically positive nodes. Such techniques would be useful a complement to existing diagnostic procedures and could help eliminate many unnecessary biopsies and axillary dissections.

Detection of breast cancer and axillary metastasis have been evaluated using several radionuclide imaging techniques with various radiopharmaceuticals such as: ^{99m}Tc-labeled methylene disphosphonate (MDP), ^{99m}Tc-labeled sestamibi, ^{201}Tl-labeled chloride, ^{67}Ga-labeled citrate, [^{18}F]fluoro-2-deoxyglucose (FDG), [^{11}C]methionine, ^{18}F-labeled estradiol, ^{18}F-labeled tamoxifen, and ^{111}In-labeled octreotide.

Scintimammography with ^{201}Tl-labeled chloride, which is a myocardial perfusion agent but taken by active tumor cells through the sodium-potassium pump system, showed a sensitivity of 98% in a series of 44 palpable breast tumors, thus allowing correct diagnosis of carcinomas larger than 10 mm. Among benign lesions only 3 of 13 adenomas were positive whereas fibrocystic and/or fat necrotic lesions were negative [19]. ^{201}Tl is not a proper tracer for tumor detection because of suboptimal physical characteristics for imaging, washout, and redistribution in tumors. Because of more favorable emission characteristics of ^{99m}Tc, sestamibi is a good alternative to ^{201}Tl for the detection of various tumors. It is likely that many factors are simultaneously involved in sestamibi tumor uptake, including cationic charge, lipophilicity, blood flow, transcapillary exchange, interstitial transport, and the negative intracellular charge of both mitochondria and cell membranes. It is known that ^{99m}Tc-sestamibi is taken up by the mitochondria using some form of active transport, but that it is passively transferred across the cell membrane.

Recent publications have reported positive results of ^{99m}Tc-sestamibi uptake in various tumors including gliomas, bone tumors, thyroid, parathyroid tumors, and breast tumors [2] (Fig. 15.1). ^{99m}Tc-sestamibi scintimammography showed a high sensitivity (91%–92%) and specificity (89%–94%) for detecting primary breast cancer, with positive and negative predictive values of 81%–97% and 81%–95%, respectively (Fig. 15.1). False-positive cases with fi-

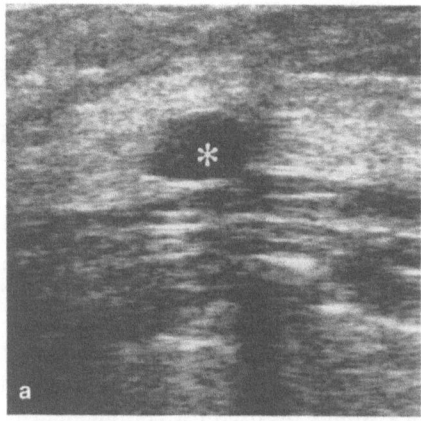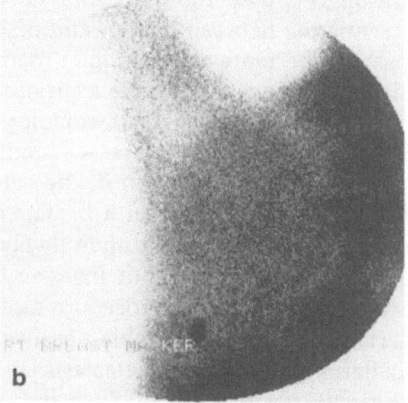

Fig. 15.1 a. Ultrasound of right breast shows a nodular hypoechoic lesion (*). **b** Anterior-oblique image of right breast using ^{99m}Tc-sestamibi shows no focal area of increased activity. Biopsy confirmed a fibroadenoma

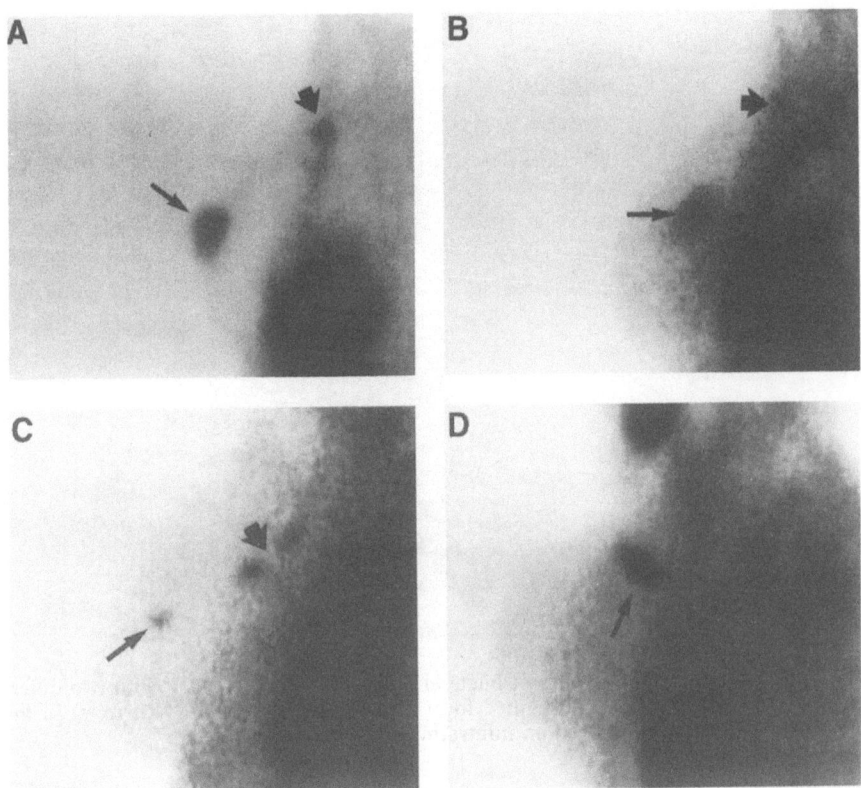

Fig. 15.2 A–D. ^{99m}Tc-sestamibi scintimammography from four different patients. **A–C** Primary breast cancers (*thin arrows*) and metastatic axillary lymph nodes (*thick arrows*). **D** Malignant follicular lymphoma in. (Reprinted with permission from [16])

broadenoma and fibrocystic disease and false-negative cases [13] with small or diffuse cancer or cancer in the medial aspect of the large breast have been reported [11]. The sensitivity of scintimammography using ^{99m}Tc-sestamibi to detect metastatic lymph nodes was 84% and the specificity was 90% (Fig. 15.2) [13, 15].

Extraskeletal accumulation of ^{99m}Tc-MDP has often been reported in some malignant tumors including breast cancer [21]. For images collected at 10–20 min, possibly related to increased vascularity, the sensitivity of ^{99m}Tc-MDP scintimammography (Fig. 15.3) was 92% in patients with histologically confirmed breast cancer (158/172) and 4.7% in patients with confirmed benign lesions (3/63). The specificity was 95% while the positive predictive value and negative predictive value were 98% and 81%, respectively [15]. Metastatic axillary lymph nodes larger than 3 cm avidly concentrate ^{99m}Tc-MDP and are most recognizable on the early images. Tracer uptake is not correlated with tumor histotype or grading. The use of oblique lateral views improves imaging of smaller lesions and lesions located in the inner quadrants.

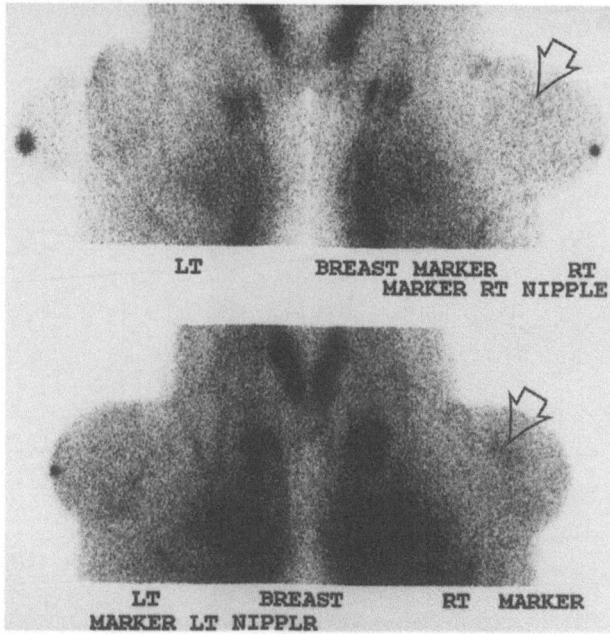

Fig. 15.3. Oblique-lateral images of bilateral breasts using ^{99m}Tc-MDP with two different intensity sets shows an ill-defined focal area of increased activity (*arrows*) in the right breast. Surgery confirmed an infiltrating adenocarcinoma

The mammographic patterns are usually classified as definitely positive, highly suspicious, indeterminate, and definitely negative.

Positron emission tomography (PET) has been used to study a pathophysiology of various cancers. Because most tumors have high glycolytic rates, FDG is a suitable PET agent both for detecting cancer and for monitoring responses to treatment [8]. Sensitivity for detection of pathologically confirmed primary breast cancer was 100%, 62%, and 87% with FDG PET, mammography, and ultrasound, respectively; and sensitivity for detection of initial nodal involvement was 77%, 70% and 87%, respectively [3]. FDG PET is also valuable in monitoring the effect of preoperative chemotherapy in patients with locally advanced breast cancer, with better sensitivity for primary breast cancer and better specificity for nodal metastasis than ultrasound [1]. Estrogen-receptor (ER) positive breast cancers not only have a more favorable prognosis than do ER-negative cancers, but also ER status determines the likelihood of response to hormonal therapy. There may be a relationship between the ER status of breast cancer and their FDG uptake, for example, ER-negative tumors would be expected to have lower tumor FDG uptake than more aggressive ER-negative tumors [18]. It has been confirmed that PET using 16α-[^{18}F]fluoro-17β-estradiol (FES) is a reliable in vivo technique for evaluating the ER status of primary or metastatic breast cancer. The overall rate of agreement between the results of in vitro ER assays and the results

Fig. 15.4 A, B. Mammary lymphoscintigraphy in two different patients showing sentinel axillary lymph nodes (*arrowheads*) by ^{99m}Tc-labeled antimony sulfide colloids drained from injection sites (*IS*) around breast cancers. (Reprinted with permission from [17])

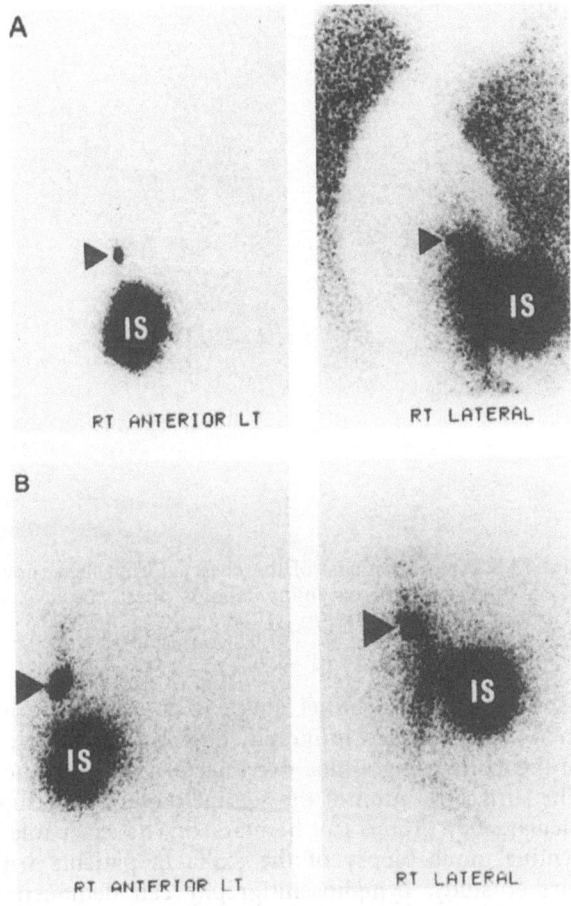

of FES PET was 88% [6]. Tamoxifen is a nonsteroidal antiestrogenic drug that is widely used for breast cancer. PET using [^{18}F]fluorotamoxifen has been shown to be useful in predicting the effect of tamoxifen therapy in patients with ER-positive breast cancer [9].

There have been many studies reporting the use of lymphoscintigraphy in patients with breast cancer. These have included axillary, internal mammary, and intramammary lymphoscintigraphy. Axillary lymphoscintigraphy has been used in the preoperative search for nodal metastases or to assess the completeness of axillary dissection postoperatively or intraoperatively [14]. Internal mammary lymphoscintigraphy has been used in attempts to diagnose nodal metastases and to locate the internal mammary nodes for radiation treatment planning [17]. Studies of intramammary lymphoscintigraphy comprise a variety of techniques to diagnose nodal metastases. The lymphatic drainage pattern using ^{99m}Tc-labeled antimony sulfide colloid varies from patient to patient depending on the tumor site and does not always follow

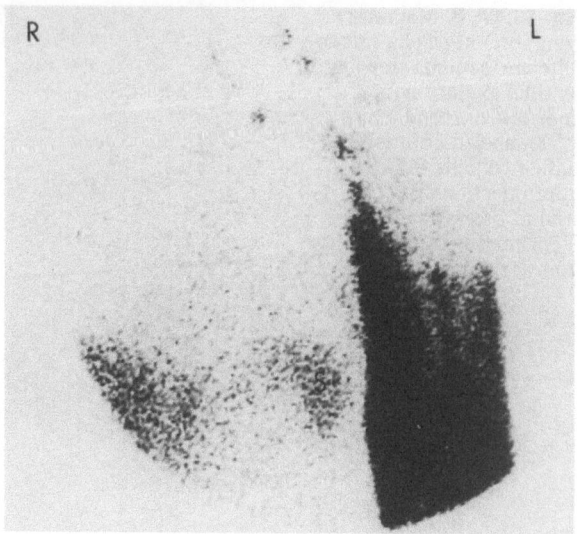

Fig. 15.5. Anterior image of the chest and left arm show a marked dermal retention of ^{99m}Tc-labeled filtered sulfur colloids up to the level of middle upper arm. Some activities in liver and spleen (*s*)

expected routes. Sentinel nodes in the axilla are located, which emphasizes the role of lymphoscintigraphy during surgical detection of the sentinel node in the axilla using a blue dye injection and also the gamma-probe (Fig. 15.4). The surface location of the sentinel node in the supraclavicular and infraclavicular node groups can be marked. The exact role of lymphoscintigraphy in sentinel node biopsy of the axilla in patients with breast cancer requires further study. Lymphoscintigraphy can demonstrate the exact obstruction site of lymphatic drainage in patients with lymphedema following the mastectomies (Fig. 15.5).

References

1. Adler LP, Crowe JP, Al-Kaisi NK, Sunshine JL (1993) Evaluation of breast masses and axillary lymph nodes with F-18 2-deoxy-2-fluoro-D-glucose PET. Radiology 187:743–750
2. Balon HR, Fink-Bennett D, Stoffer SS (1992) Tc-99m sestamibi uptake by recurrent Hunthle cell carcinoma of the thyroid. J Nucl Med 33:1393–1395
3. Bassa P, Kim EE, Inoue T, Wiong FCL, Korkmaz M, Yang DJ, Wong W-H, Hicks KW, Buzdar AU, Podoloff DA (1996) Evaluation of preoperative chemotherapy using PET with F-18 fluorodeoxyglucose in breast cancer. J Nucl Med 37:931–938
4. Bird R, Wallace T, Yankaskas B (1992) Analysis of cancers missed at screening mammography. Radiology 184:613–617
5. Boetes C, Mus RDM, Holland R, Barentsz JO, Strijk SP, Wobbes T, Hendriks JHCL, Ruys SHJ (1995) Breast tumors: comparative accuracy of MR imaging relative to mammography and US for demonstrating extent. Radiology 197:743–747

6. Dehdashti F, Mortimer JE, Siegel BA, Griffieth LK, Bonasera TJ, Fusselman MJ, Detert DD, Cutler D, Katzenellenbogan JA, Welch MJ (1995) Positron tomographic assessment of estrogen receptors in breast cancer: comparison with FDG-PET and in vitro receptor assays. J Nucl Med 36:1766–1774

7. Harms SE, Flaming DP, Hesley KL (1993) MR imaging of the breast with rotating delivery of excitation off resonance: clinical experience with pathologic correlation. Radiology 187:493–501

8. Hawkins RA, Hoh C, Dahlbom M (1991) PET cancer evaluation with FDG. J Nucl Med 32:1555–1558

9. Inoue T, Kim EE, Wallace S, Yang DJ, Wong FCL, Bassa P, Cherif A, Delpassand E, Buzdar A, Podoloff DA (1996) PET using F-18 fluorotamoxifen to evaluate therapeutic responses in patients with breast cancer. Cancer Biotherapy Radiopharm 11:235–245

10. Jackson V (1990) The role of US in breast imaging. Radiology 177:305–311

11. Khalkhali I, Cutrone JA, Mena IG, Diggles IE, Venegas RJ, Vargas HI, Jackson BL, Khalkhali S, Moss JF, Klein SR (1995) Scintimammography: the complementary role of Tc-99m sestamibi prone breast imaging for the diagnosis of breast carcinoma. Radiology 196:421–426

12. Kopans DB (1992) The positive predictive value of mammography. AJR 158:521–526

13. Maublant J, de Latour M, Mestas D, Clemenson A, Charrier S, Feillel V (1996) Tc-99m sestamibi uptake in breast tumor and associated lymph nodes. J Nucl Med 37:922–925

14. McLean RG, Ege GN (1986) Prognostic value of axillary lymphoscintigraphy in breast cancer patients. J Nucl Med 27:1116–1124

15. Piccolo S, Lastoria S, Mainolfi C, Muto P, Bazzicalupo L, Salvatore M (1995) Tc-99m methylene diphosphonate scintimammography to image primary breast cancer. J Nucl Med 36:718–724

16. Taillefer R, Robidoux A, Lambert R, Turpin S, Laperriere J (1995) Tc-99m sestamibi prone scintimammography to detect primary breast cancer and axillary lymph node involvement. J Nucl Med 36:1758–1765

17. Uren RF Howman-Giles RB, Thompson JF, Malouf D, Ramsey-Stewart G, Niesche FW, Renwick SB (1995) Mammary lymphoscintigraphy in breast cancer. J Nucl Med 36:1775–1780

18. Wahl RL, Cody R, Fisher S (1991) FDG uptake before and after estrogen receptor stimulation: feasibility studies for functional receptor imaging. J Nucl Med 32:1011–1015

19. Waxman AD, Ramanna L, Memsic LD (1993) Thallium scintigraphy in the evaluation of mass abnormalities of the breast. J Nucl Med 34:18–23

20. Wingo PA, Tong T, Bolden S (1995) Cancer statistics. Cancer 5:8–30

21. Worsley DF, Lentle BC (1993) Uptake ofi Tc-99m MDP in primary amyloidosis with a review of the mechanisms of soft-tissue localization of bone-seeking radiopharmaceuticals. J Nucl Med 34:1612–1615

Subject Index